Key Clinical Topics in

Trauma

JP

Preface

There has been a significant transformation in the organisation of trauma services and the clinical management of patients in the last decade. Trauma care has a higher profile than ever before, and more patients are surviving than would have been expected only a few years ago. Trauma networks have been developed, with effective transport platforms connecting trauma units and major trauma centres. Organisational change has occurred in parallel with clinical advances, and classic questions regarding fluids, imaging and operative intervention have been answered at least in part.

A significant number of these advances arose from the provision of medical care by the Defence Medical Services in Iraq and Afghanistan and from the efforts of those in the UK responsible for the further management of these challenging injuries. We make no apologies, therefore, for the over representation of such individuals amongst the authors of topics in *Key Clinical Topics in Trauma*. Having said this, our contributors represent a wide range of centres of excellence in trauma management both in the UK and abroad.

We hope that this book provides readers with access to the most up-to-date thinking and practice in clinical traumatology. We have tried to ensure that all the important areas of trauma care are covered, and we have also included an admittedly personal selection of more unusual topics which are either establishing themselves in clinical practice or are likely to do so in the future (for example REBOA and lyophilised plasma).

We would like to thank all those who have helped us identify topic contributors, and most importantly the contributors themselves for devoting their time and effort to *Key Clinical Topics in Trauma*.

The editors' royalties from the sales of this book are donated in their entirety to the organisation Trauma Care UK (www.traumacare.org.uk), an organisation dedicated to promoting excellence in trauma management. We urge you to consider joining it.

Keith Porter
Ian Greaves
Derek Burke
March 2016

Contents

Contributors

Neil Abeysinghe MBBS BSc(Hons) MRCP UK
FRCA DIMC RCS Ed FFICM PGCert Med Ed
Topic 23
Consultant in Critical Care, University
Hospitals Birmingham NHS Foundation Trust,
Birmingham, UK

David Alexander MA(Hons) CPsychol PhD
FBPS FRSM(Hon) FRCPsych
Topic 68
Emeritus Professor, Robert Gordon University,
Aberdeen, UK; Principal Adviser, Police
Scotland, UK

Seyed Ali MBBS MSOrth MChOrth
FRCS(Tr&Orth)
Topics 27, 28
Consultant Foot and Ankle Surgeon, University
Hospitals Birmingham NHS Trust, Birmingham,
UK

Steve Amerasekera MB BChir MA (Cantab)
MRCP FRCR
Topic 39
Consultant Radiologist in Musculoskeletal
and Trauma Imaging, University Hospitals
Birmingham NHS Foundation Trust,
Birmingham, UK

Amit Anand MB ChB
Topic 77
Trainee in Orthopaedic Surgery, West Midlands
Rotation, UK

Alex K Ball MBChB MSc MD FRCP
Topic 70
Consultant in Rehabilitation Medicine, North
Staffordshire Rehabilitation Centre, Haywood
Hospital, Stoke-on-Trent, UK

Khalid G Baloch MBChB FRCS FRCS(Tr&Orth)
Topic 77
Consultant Trauma and Orthopaedic Surgeon,
University Hospitals Birmingham NHS Trust,
Birmingham, UK

Tom Barker BSc(MedSci) MBChB DMCC MRCS
RAMC
Topic 56
Research Fellow, Academic Department of
Military Surgery and Trauma, Royal Centre for
Defence Medicine, Birmingham, UK

Edward G B Barnard FCEM RN
Topics 13, 18
Consultant in Emergency Medicine, Defence
Medical Services, Lichfield, UK

Antonio Belli MD FRCS FRCS(SN)
Topics 53, 54
Professor of Trauma Neurosurgery, School
of Clinical and Experimental Medicine,
College of Medical and Dental Sciences,
Institute of Biomedical Research, University of
Birmingham, Birmingham, UK

Steven Bland FCEM RN
Topic 20
Consultant in Emergency Medicine and
Defence Speciality Advisor in CBRN Medicine,
Defence CBRN Centre, Lichfield, Salisbury, UK

Charlotte Booth FCEM RAMC
Topic 74
Consultant in Emergency Medicine, Defence
Medical Services, Lichfield, UK

Deepa Bose MBBS FRCS(Tr&Orth)
Topic 48
Consultant in Trauma and Limb Reconstruction,
University Hospitals Birmingham NHS Trust,
Birmingham, UK

Richard J Bowman MB ChB MCEM LLM
Topic 78
Trainee in Emergency Medicine, University
Hospital Coventry and Warwickshire NHS Trust,
Coventry, UK

John Breeze PhD MRCS MFDS
Topic 64
Specialty Registrar in Maxillofacial Surgery,
Royal Centre for Defence Medicine,
Birmingham Research Park, Birmingham, UK

Robert Briard MRCS FRCR RAMC
Topics 37, 38, 40
Consultant in Interventional Radiology,
Defence Medical Services, Lichfield, UK

Ilana Delroy Buelles FRCA
Topics 5, 6, 51, 82
Specialty Registrar in Anaesthesia,
Royal Bournemouth Hospital,
Bournemouth, UK

Derek Burke FRCSEd FCEM FRCPCH
Topic 61
Medical Director and Consultant in Paediatric
Emergency Medicine, Sheffield Children's NHS
Foundation Trust, Sheffield, UK

Samuel K L Chan MBChB MRCS FRCS(Tr&Orth)
Topic 77
Specialty Trainee in Trauma and Orthopaedics,
Robert Jones and Agnes Hunt Orthopaedic
Hospital NHS Foundation Trust, Oswestry, UK

Darren Chester FRCS(Plast)
Topic 33
Consultant in Hand and Plastic Surgery,
Worcester Royal Infirmary, Worcester, UK

Julian Cooper BSc(Hons) MB ChB(Hons)
FRCS(Tr&Orth)
Topics 22, 63
Consultant in Orthopaedic Trauma,
University Hospitals Birmingham NHS Trust,
Birmingham, UK

Mike Craigen MBBS FRCS(Orth) FRCS(Ed) Dip
Hand Surg(Euro)
Topic 93
Consultant in Orthopaedics and Hand Surgery,
Royal Orthopaedic Hospital, Birmingham, UK

Claire Dawkins MA MB BChir MRCS RAF
Topic 91
Medical Officer, Royal Air Force Medical Branch,
Birmingham, UK

Christopher Day BSc(Hons) MB BCh MRCS
FRCR
Topics 37, 39, 40
Consultant in Vascular and Interventional
Radiology University Hospitals of North
Midlands NHS Trust, UK

Catherine Doran MD FRCS
Topic 47
Consultant Military General Surgeon, University
Hospitals Birmingham NHS Foundation Trust,
Birmingham, UK

Heidi Doughty MB BChir FRCPath
Topic 49
Consultant in Transfusion Medicine, NHS Blood
and Transplant, Birmingham, UK

Linda Dykes FCEM
Topic 58
Consultant in Emergency Medicine, Ysbyty
Gwynedd, Gwynedd, UK

Ismail Fathallah FRCS
Topic 28
Senior Clinical Fellow, University Hospitals
Birmingham NHS Trust, Birmingham, UK

Paul Fenton MB ChB FRCS (Tr&Orth)
Topic 30
Consultant in Orthopaedic Surgery,
University Hospitals Birmingham NHS
Foundation Trust, Birmingham, UK

Navin Furtado BSc MBBS MSc(Eng) FRCS(Neuro
Surg)
Topic 42
Consultant in Neurosurgery and Spinal Surgery,
University Hospitals Birmingham NHS
Foundation Trust, Birmingham, UK

Yunus Gokdogan MB BS FCEM
Topic 55
Consultant in Emergency Medicine, West
Middlesex University Hospital, London, UK

Paul Hunt MD FCEM
Topic 89
Consultant in Emergency Medicine, Defence
Medical Services, Lichfield, UK

Jan O Jansen FRCS FFICM
Topic 73
Consultant in General Surgery and Intensive
Care Medicine, Aberdeen Royal Infirmary,
Aberdeen, UK

Andrew Johnston DMCC FRCP RAMC
Topic 12
Consultant in Intensive Care Medicine,
Defence Medical Services, Lichfield, UK

Socrates Kalogrianitis MBChB FRCS
Topic 76
Consultant in Orthopaedic Surgery,
University Hospitals Birmingham NHS Trust,
Birmingham, UK

Ravichandran Karthikeyan FRCS(Tr&Orth)
PGCE FHEA
Topic 35
Consultant in Trauma and Orthopaedic Surgery,
University Hospitals Birmingham NHS Trust,
Birmingham, UK

Alan Kay L/RAMC
Topic 17
Consultant in Plastic Surgery, Defence Medical
Services, Lichfield, UK

Daniel Kennedy MB BCh BAO FRCA FFICM
Topic 16
Consultant in Critical Care and Anaesthesia, The
Royal London Hospital, London, UK

Mansoor Khan MBBS(Lond) FRCS(GenSurg) AKC
Topic 1
Consultant in Trauma Surgery, St Mary's
Hospital, Imperial College Healthcare NHS Trust,
London, UK

Emrys Kirkman PhD
Topics 44, 45, 46
Principal Scientist, Defence Science and
Technology Laboratory Porton Down,
Salisbury, UK

Kathryn L Kneale MRCS
Topic 24
Trainee in Orthopaedic Surgery, West Midlands
Rotation, UK

Nadeeja Koralage
Topic 74
St Mary's Hospital, London, UK

Dhushy Surendra Kumar MB ChB FCA RSCI
FRCA FICM
Topics 5, 6, 51, 82
Consultant in Critical Care Medicine, Prehospital
Care and Anaesthesia, University Hospitals
Coventry and Warwickshire NHS Trust,
Coventry, UK

Sumitra Lahiri FRCA
Topic 26
Consultant in Anaesthesia and Senior Lecturer
in Anaesthetics, Barts and the London NHS
Foundation Trust, London, UK

Simon Le Clerc FCEM
Topic 89
Consultant in Emergency Medicine, Defence
Medical Services, Lichfield, UK

Caroline Leech MBChB FRCEM FIMC RCSEd
Topics 36, 66, 79
Consultant in Emergency Medicine and
Prehospital Medicine, University Hospital
Coventry and Warwickshire NHS Trust,
Coventry, UK

Ari K Leppaniemi MD PhD DMCC
Topic 25
Chief of Emergency Surgery, Meilahti Hospital
Abdominal Center, Helsinki, Finland

Will Lester MBChB BSc FRCP FRCPath PhD
Topic 9
Consultant in Haematology, University
Hospitals Birmingham NHS Foundation Trust,
Birmingham, UK

Philippa Lewis MBChB DMCC RAMC
Topic 43
Assistant Regimental Surgeon,
Household Cavalry Regiment, Windsor, UK

Simon B Maclean FRCS(Tr&Orth)
Topics 24, 76
Consultant in Orthopaedic Surgery, University
Hospital Birmingham NHS Foundation Trust,
Birmingham, UK

Rob MacSweeney PhD
Topic 3
Consultant in Intensive Care Medicine,
Royal Victoria Hospital, Belfast, UK

Gerlinde Mandersloot
Topic 16
Consultant in Critical Care Medicine and
Anaesthesia, Barts and the London NHS
Foundation Trust, London, UK

Karanjit S Mangat FRCS(Tr&Orth)
Topics 24, 76
Trainee in Trauma and Orthopaedic Surgery,
Sandwell and West Birmingham Hospitals NHS
Trust, Birmingham, UK

Samir N Massoud MBChB FRCSI FRCS(Orth)
Topic 24
Consultant in Orthopaedic Surgery,
The Royal Orthopaedic Hospital and University
Hospital Birmingham NHS Foundation Trust,
Birmingham, UK

Danny McAuley FRCP MD FFICM
Topic 3
Professor of Intensive Care Medicine, Centre
for Infection and Immunity, Queen's University
of Belfast and Consultant in Intensive Care
Medicine, Royal Victoria Hospital, Belfast, UK

Mark Midwinter CBA MD RN
Topics 47, 71, 75, 92
Consultant in General and Trauma Surgery,
Royal Centre for Defence Medicine,
Birmingham, UK

Jonathan James Morrison MB ChB MRCS PhD
Topic 75
Academic Department of Military Surgery and
Trauma, Royal Centre for Defence Medicine,
Birmingham, UK

Rob Moss FRCA
Topic 19
Consultant in Anaesthesia, University Hospitals
Birmingham NHS Foundation Trust, Birmingham,
UK

Alistair Mountain MBChB FRCS(Tr&Orth) RAMC
Topic 7
Consultant in Trauma and Orthopaedic Surgery,
Defence Medical Services, Lichfield, UK

Christopher Murray MB BCh BAO DipFRCA
Topic 3
Specialty Trainee in Anaesthesia,
Antrim Hospital, Antrim, UK

Rajpal Nandra MBBS BSc(Hons) MRCS
Topics 2, 21, 29
Trainee in Trauma and Orthopaedics, Queen
Elizabeth Hospital Birmingham, UK

James O'Connor MD FACS
Topics 14, 83
Chief, Thoracic and Vascular Trauma Care,
R Adams Cowley Shock Trauma Center,
Baltimore, MD, USA

Breda O'Neill FRCA
Topic 26
Consultant in Anaesthesia, Barts and the
London NHS Foundation Trust, London, UK

Beryl Oppenheim MB BCh FRCPath
Topic 8
Consultant Microbiologist, University
Hospitals, Birmingham NHS Foundation Trust,
Birmingham, UK

Piers Page MBBS MRCSEd
Topics 11, 58, 62, 81, 86, 87, 90
Specialty Registrar in Orthopaedics and
Honorary Clinical Lecturer in Trauma Surgery,
Brighton and Sussex University Hospitals NHS
Trust, Brighton, UK

Paul Parker FIMC FRCSEd(Orth) L/RAMC
Topic 88
Consultant in Orthopaedic Surgery, Defence
Medical Services, Lichfield, UK

Claire Park MBE FRCA
Topic 67
Consultant in Anaesthesia, Defence Medical
Services, Lichfield, UK

Craig Pearce BDS MFDS MBChB FRCSEd(OMFS)
Topic 50
Consultant in Oral and Maxillofacial Surgery,
University Hospital of North Midlands,
Stoke-on-Trent, UK

Jowan G Penn-Barwell MB CHC MSc MRCS RN
Topics 12, 32
Trainee in Trauma and Orthopaedics,
Defence Medical Services, Lichfield, UK

Francis Peart FRCS
Topic 34
Consultant in Plastic Surgery, The Royal
Orthopaedic Hospital, Birmingham, UK

Henrietta Poon MBChB MRCS DMCC
Topic 46
Specialty Registrar in General Surgery,
Academic Department of Military Surgery and
Trauma, Birmingham, UK

Dominic Power MA MB BChir FRCS(Tr&Orth)
Topic 15
Consultant in Hand and Peripheral Nerve
Surgery, University Hospitals Birmingham NHS
Foundation Trust, Birmingham, UK

James Ralph FRCA L/RAMC
Topic 10
Consultant in Anaesthesia, Defence Medical
Services, Lichfield, UK

Jonathan Ritson MRCEM RN
Topic 72
Trainee in Emergency Medicine, St Mary's
Hospital, London, UK

James Dean Ross PhD
Topic 75
Director, Trauma and Clinical Care Research,
59th Medical Wing, Joint Base San Antonio–
Lackland, Texas, USA

Sasha Rossaye MBBCh BSc FRACP
Topic 57
Paediatric Emergency Medicine Specialist,
Children's Emergency Department, Starship
Children's Hospital, Auckland, New Zealand

Robert AH Scott MBBS FRCOphth FRCS(Ed)
DipMedEd DM
Topic 60
Professor of Ophthalmology, Royal College
of Ophthalmologists, London; Consultant
Ophthalmologist, Royal Centre for Defence
Medicine, Birmingham, UK

Davendra M Sharma MB BCh BAO MRCS
MSc(Urol) FRCS(Urol)
Topic 31
Consultant in Urology, St George's Hospital,
London, UK

Danny Sharpe MBBS BSc DipIMC MRCEM
RAMC
Topic 84
Specialty Trainee in Emergency Medicine and
Prehospital Emergency Medicine, St Mary's
Hospital, London, UK

Peter Shirley FRCA FIMC RCSEd FFICM EDIC
Topic 80
Consultant in Intensive Care Medicine and
Anaesthesia, Royal London Hospital, London,
UK

Adikarige Haritha Dulanka Silva BA(Hons)
MA(Hons) MBBChir MPhil(Cantab) MRCS(Eng)
Topics 53, 54
Trainee in Neurosurgery, West Midlands
Rotation, UK

Andy Smith BSc(Hons) MB ChB MRCS(Eng)
FCEM FFSEM(UK) MSc FIMC RCSED
Topic 41
Consultant in Emergency Medicine, Mid
Yorkshire Hospitals NHS Trust, UK

Iain Smith MA MB BChir MSc MRCSEd
Topic 49
Clinical Research Fellow and Specialty Registrar
in General Surgery, Royal Centre for Defence
Medicine and NIHR Surgical Reconstruction and
Microbiology Research Centre, Birmingham, UK

Jason E Smith MD MRCP(UK) FRCEM RN
Topics 13, 18
Consultant in Emergency Medicine, Defence
Medical Services, Lichfield, UK

Adam Stannard BSc MBChB FRCS RN
Topic 91
Consultant in Vascular Surgery, Defence
Medical Services, Lichfield, UK

Arunan Sujenthiran MRCS MBBS BSc(Hons)
Topic 31
Academic Clinical Fellow in Urology & Specialty
Registrar in Urology, London Rotation, UK

Simon Tan MBBS MRCS FRCS(Tr&Orth)
Topic 65
Consultant in Hand and Peripheral Nerve
Surgery, University Hospitals Birmingham NHS
Foundation Trust, Birmingham, UK

Rhys Thomas MBBS FRCA DipIMC RCSEd
Topic 45
Co-Director, Emergency Medical Retrieval and
Transfer Service (EMRTS), Swansea, UK

Sarah Watts PhD
Topics 44, 45, 46
Principal Scientist, Defence Science and
Technology Laboratory Porton Down,
Salisbury, UK

Gemma Winzor MBChB MPH
Topic 52
Specialty Trainee in Medical Microbiology, West
Midlands Rotation, UK

Thomas Woolley MD FRCA
Topic 69
Consultant in Anaesthesia,
Derriford Hospital, Plymouth, UK

Matthew Wordsworth MA(Cantab) MRCS
DMCC RAMC
Topics 17, 85
Trainee in Plastic Surgery, London
Rotation, UK

Chris Wright MB ChB DIMC FCEM RAMC
Topics 4, 72, 74
Consultant in Emergency Medicine, Defence
Consultant Advisor in Prehospital Emergency
Care, St Mary's Hospital, Imperial College
Healthcare NHS Trust, London, UK

Parjam Zolfaghari MBBS PhD FRCA DICM
FFICM
Topic 59
Consultant in Intensive Care Medicine and
Anaesthesia, Royal London Hospital, London, UK

Abdominal trauma

Key points

- Evaluation remains a diagnostic challenge
- Selective nonoperative management is being increasingly adopted following contrast-enhanced CT scan in haemodynamically stable patients with serial clinical assessment by an experienced clinician
- Damage control laparotomy (DCL) is a key component of damage control resuscitation

Introduction

Injuries to the abdomen present a complex diagnostic challenge and continue to cause significant morbidity and mortality whether blunt or penetrating in nature. Regardless of injury type, the initial assessment and management are the same.

Motor vehicle collisions remain one of the commonest causes of blunt abdominal injury and there has been a comparative rise in the incidence of seatbelt-induced abdominal injuries, even though the incidence of head and thoracic injuries has decreased.

Penetrating abdominal trauma is commonly classified into stab wound or ballistic injuries. Both can present with an apparently minor abdominal injury, yet be associated with major intra-abdominal trauma. Ballistic injuries can be further subdivided into low-kinetic energy or high-kinetic energy wounds.

Pathophysiology

Solid organ injury

The commonest organs to be injured in blunt abdominal trauma are the spleen, liver, kidney and pancreas, in that order. In penetrating trauma, the order differs, with the liver being the most commonly affected organ, followed closely by the spleen, kidney and pancreas. Blunt trauma results in injury through two main forces: compression and shearing. Shearing forces result in disruption of the attachment points of an organ and lacerations of the organ and parenchyma. In severe road traffic collisions, this may also result in disruption of the vascular structures supplying the organ. Penetrating injuries are less frequent, but can result in considerable trauma to solid organs, especially as result of gunshot wounds.

Hollow viscus injury

The hollow organs located in the abdominal cavity can be divided into gastrointestinal and urinary viscera. The gastrointestinal viscera consist of the stomach, duodenum, jejunum, ileum, colon and rectum; the urinary viscera are the ureters and urinary bladder (the kidneys are retroperitoneal).

Blunt injury is estimated to cause bowel injury in approximately 1% of patients, with bowel or mesenteric injury resulting from compression against hard structures, from a sudden compressive rise in intraluminal pressure or from shearing forces generated by acceleration and deceleration particularly at fixed points such as the ligament of Treitz (the suspensory muscle of duodenum).

These shearing forces are exerted on the origins of small vessels resulting in avulsion, rupture and intimal injury. The consequence of this may be catastrophic haemorrhage or thrombotic occlusion of the vessel and distal necrosis.

Injuries to the diaphragm

Diaphragmatic injuries are notoriously difficult to diagnose, but should be suspected in casualties who have suffered thoracoabdominal penetrating trauma or blunt injury to the abdomen.

Clinical features

The clinical features of abdominal trauma are largely dependent on the injury pattern and the organs affected. Abdominal examination follows the basic principles of inspection, palpation, percussion and auscultation. Unfortunately, the initial assessment of patients with blunt abdominal trauma is often difficult and is notably inaccurate. Associated injuries, pain and anxiety often cause tenderness and spasm in the abdominal wall and make diagnosis difficult. The most reliable signs and symptoms in alert patients are pain, tenderness, haematemesis, per rectal blood loss, hypovolaemia and evidence of peritonitis. However, large amounts of blood can accumulate in the peritoneal and pelvic cavities without any significant or early changes in the physical examination findings.

A detailed knowledge of the underlying anatomy of the intra-abdominal organs is the key to successfully managing a polytrauma casualty. Bruising or the stigmata of trauma over a particular region of the abdomen may highlight which organs have suffered traumatic insult. The abdominal examination must be thorough and systematic.

Pelvic injury and instability should be assessed radiologically since examination may cause clot dislodgement and consequent haemorrhage.

The presence of a pelvic fracture indicates a raised probability of lower urinary tract injury as well as pelvic and retroperitoneal haematoma. If there is the presence or suspected presence of a urethral injury, a retrograde urethrogram will be needed. In practice, this may be difficult in an acute setting, and a suprapubic catheter may be required.

A sensory examination of the chest and abdomen must be undertaken to evaluate the potential for spinal cord injury.

If present, a spinal cord injury may interfere with the accurate assessment of the abdomen by causing decreased or absent pain perception.

A rectal and vaginal examination should be performed to search for evidence of bone fragment penetration resulting from a pelvic fracture and the stool should be evaluated for gross or occult blood. Rectal tone should be assessed to identify spinal injury and the prostate palpated to identify potential urethral injury.

Evaluation and diagnosis

A number of imaging modalities are available to assist in identifying injuries and monitoring changes in condition:

- Focus abdominal sonography for trauma (FAST) scan
- Plain radiographs
- CT scan of the abdomen
- Interventional angiography

The importance of other investigations and monitoring such as electrocardiography, conventional vital signs, oximetry, capnography and blood gas analysis should not be overlooked.

Blunt trauma

The Eastern Association of Surgery of Trauma (EAST) in the USA has systematically reviewed modalities for the evaluation of blunt abdominal trauma. Radiographs, especially of the chest and pelvis, still remain useful in determining the presence of intrathoracic or abdominal injury. If a spinal injury is suspected, then an erect chest radiograph may not be feasible, thereby limiting diagnosis of free intraperitoneal air.

The FAST scan allows the rapid examination of body cavities by appropriately trained personnel. FAST may be considered to be the initial diagnostic modality for exclusion of haemoperitoneum. In a recent prospective study of 2576 patients, FAST had a sensitivity of 87% and a specificity and negative predictive value of 98% for detecting haemoperitoneum. It will not detect or grade severity of visceral injury alone.

CT with intravenous contrast is recommended for the evaluation of patients with equivocal findings on physical examination, associated neurologic injury, or multiple extra-abdominal injuries. Under these circumstances, patients with a negative CT should be admitted for observation. CT is the diagnostic modality of choice for nonoperative management of solid visceral injuries. The advent of multislice CT has fundamentally changed the way trauma patients are managed. CT has a number of advantages including higher speed of data collection, thinner sections and reduced artifactual abnormality. CT scanning is more often undertaken in the stable patient, and has a sensitivity approaching 98% and specificity of 99%. Its advantage over other investigations is that it is the only investigation which allows imaging of retroperitoneal structures as well as grading of the severity of injury.

Penetrating trauma

Patients with penetrating abdominal trauma are at high risk of life-threatening injuries. While many patients will be in need of emergent operative intervention, some patients may be safely managed nonoperatively.

- Haemodynamic instability, shock, evisceration and peritonitis mandate immediate laparotomy following penetrating abdominal trauma
- Thoracoabdominal stab wounds should be further evaluated with chest X-ray, ultrasonography and laparoscopy or thoracoscopy
- Wounds to the back and flank should be imaged by CT scanning
- Anterior abdominal stab wounds without peritoneal signs of evidence of haemoperitoneum on FAST examination may be followed with serial clinical assessments by an experienced clinician but with a low clinical threshold for operative intervention

- The majority of patients with gunshot wounds are best served by laparotomy, although in select patients a nonoperative approach may be adopted after a negative good quality contrast-enhanced CT scan

Management

A spectrum of modalities is available for the management of abdominal trauma, ranging from clinical observation, through selective nonoperative management to damage control procedures. Interventional angiography is playing an increasing role in the management of solid organ injury; however, in the circumstances of physiological compromise, operative intervention remains the 'gold standard'.

Indications for emergency surgical intervention include traumatic cardiac arrest, unexplained, especially progressive shock, a rigid silent abdomen, evisceration, evidence of intraperitoneal gas or diaphragmatic rupture and gunshot injury. The main aim of damage control surgery, which is a

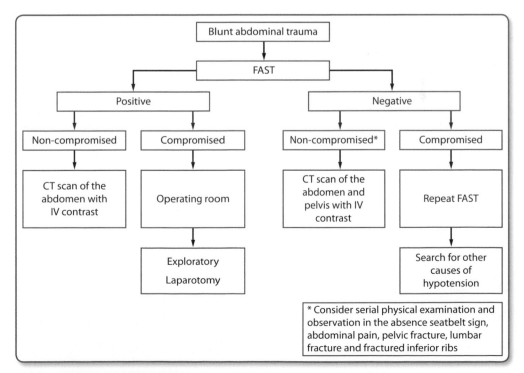

Figure 1 Management of blunt injuries.

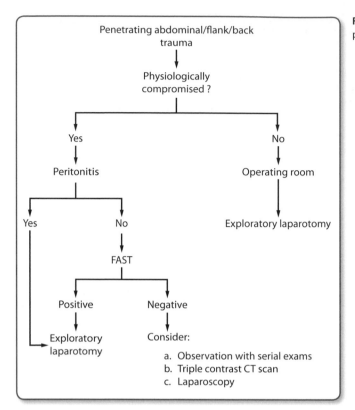

Figure 2 Management of penetrating injuries.

component of damage control resuscitation, is to prevent the lethal triad of hypothermia, coagulopathy and acidosis from occurring, and if it has occurred to enable recovery to take place. **Figures 1** and **2** illustrate potential algorithms for the management of blunt and penetrating injuries.

DCL is a physiological approach to the management of selected critically injured patients where the surgical technique is directed at minimising the metabolic insult, rather than restoring anatomic integrity. The aim is to prevent the development of, or to reverse, an established lethal triad of hypothermia, coagulopathy and acidosis. The priorities in DCL are to control haemorrhage and contamination. Manoeuvres to achieve these objectives include controlling major abdominal vascular structures by medial visceral rotations, supracoeliac aortic compression or clamping, preperitoneal

pelvic packing, perihepatic packing, splenectomy, nephrectomy and bowel resection.

Laparoscopy

In the diagnosis of blunt abdominal injuries, most institutions prefer radiological imaging depending on local resources and experience. The potential benefit of diagnostic laparoscopy is that it can be both diagnostic and therapeutic. There are reported cases in the literature of laparoscopy being utilised with or without the presence of a pneumoperitoneum.

Complications

The complications of abdominal trauma can be divided into local and systemic responses to the insult (**Table 1**), and the time period after the insult at which they occur.

Table 1 Abdominal defects	Local	Systemic
Early	Haemorrhage DVT Organ-specific complications Wound dehiscence	Coagulopathy ARDS Sepsis PE Abdominal compartment syndrome Hypothermia Acidosis Pneumonia
Late	Infection Collection Fistulation	Malnutrition Respiratory failure

DVT, deep vein thrombosis; ARDS, acute respiratory distress syndrome; PE, pulmonary embolism.

Further reading

Biffl WL, Moore EE. Management guidelines for penetrating abdominal trauma. Curr Opin Crit Care 2010; 16:609–617.

Hirshberg A. Chapter 27: Trauma laparotomy. In: Mattox KL, Moore EE, Feliciano DV. Trauma, 7th edn. New York: McGraw-Hill, 2013.

Hoff WS, Holevar M, Nagy KK, et al. Practice management guidelines for the evaluation of blunt abdominal trauma: The EAST practice management guidelines work group. J Trauma 2002; 53:602–615.

Related topics of interest

- Blunt and penetrating cardiac trauma (p. 45)
- Damage control resuscitation and surgery (p. 83)
- Genitourinary trauma (p. 114)
- Selective non-operative management of penetrating abdominal injuries (p. 254)

Abnormal fracture healing

Key points

- Abnormal fracture healing remains a problem in trauma patients despite advances in initial and definitive management
- Both delayed and nonunion of fractures have significant direct and indirect costs to health care providers and the patient
- Promoting smoking cessation, dietary supplementation and early weight bearing will reduce the risk of fracture nonunion

Epidemiology

Despite advances in orthopaedic practice and a greater understanding of fracture biology, the incidence of fracture nonunion remains a concern. Fracture nonunion has direct cost implications for the health services and indirect costs for patients through loss of earnings and additional social care. In the United Kingdom, there are approximately 850,000 new adult fractures each year. In Scotland between 2005 and 2010, the overall incidence of nonunion was 18.4/100,000 per annum, with a peak at 30–40 years of age and a higher incidence in males.

Nonunion in children is considered a rare complication. The immature skeleton has a robust periosteal layer, sufficient vascularity and enhanced healing potential. The risk of nonunion per fracture is low throughout childhood with a risk of approximately 1 in ≤500 per fracture in boys aged under 14 years and in girls of all ages; however, nonunion risk increases to approximately 1 in 200 fractures for older teenage (15–19 years) boys.

Definitions

A fracture is considered to have healed when the patient is pain free during physiological loading of the injured bone; there is no translation at the fracture site on examination and there is adequate consolidation on radiographs. The majority of fractures are expected to unite within 3–4 months of injury in adults. Delayed union is when the fracture heals at a slower rate than expected for a particular bone.

A nonunion exists when repair is not complete within the period expected for a specific fracture, cellular activity at the fracture site ceases and there are no visible progressive signs of healing. According to the United States Food and Drug Administration, a nonunion is established when a minimum of 9 months has elapsed since injury and the fracture show no visible progressive signs of healing for 3 months. It is impractical to apply this to every patient, and the clinician must judge each case individually. Delayed union, nonunion and pseudoarthrosis represent part of the spectrum of bone repair. It is difficult to predict which patient or fracture type will progress to nonunion and an even greater challenge to prevent it.

Diagnosis

- Clinical examination is the cornerstone of diagnosis and will identify tenderness at the fracture site, persistent movement at the fracture site and pain while applying physiological stresses or while weight bearing
- Plain radiographs provide additional information (**Figure 3**). Assessing for fracture consolidation involves evaluating the extent of bridging callous across the

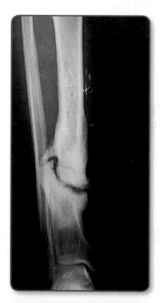

Figure 3
Nonunion of a tibial fracture.

fracture site in two orthogonal views and demonstrating diminishing fracture lines
- High-resolution CT is more sensitive and is used in cases where nonunion is suspected
- Dual-energy X-ray absorptiometry scanning is useful for distinguishing between hypervascular and atrophic nonunion in the early phase
- Diagnostic adjuvants have been developed, such as the orthometer or strain gauge bar, but they are not yet universally used
- Recently, attention has been drawn to biochemical markers. The majority of studies are laboratory based with extensive work carried out on animal models, but encouraging data has been reported on the predictive value of transforming growth factor and alkaline phosphatase

Classification

Weber introduced a classification system based on biological activity at the fracture site. The system is widely used and has stood the test of time. Other classifications exist that are specific to a particular fracture site or injury type.

According to Weber, fracture nonunions are divided into hypervascular (hypertrophic) or avascular (atrophic) types. The hypervascular group has adequate vascularity and biological activity to progress to union but union is limited by bony stability and is evident on radiographs with excessive callus in response to motion at the fracture site. Excessive interfragmentary motion has a detrimental effect on healing. Weber further subdivided this group by radiological appearance (elephant foot, horse hoof and oligotrophic).

Avascular nonunions lack vascularity and biological healing potential and show no evidence of healing. Avascular nonunion can be further subgrouped by the fracture pattern into torsion wedge, comminuted, defect or atrophic fractures. The classification systems are useful in treatment planning. It is important to consider the possibility of infection in all cases, particularly in high-energy open fractures.

Risk factors

Nonunion occurs when there is failure of biology (high-energy injuries with devascularisation), failure of host (nicotine consumption, vascular disease and other comorbidities), failure of mechanics (improper stabilisation) or treatment failure (iatrogenic devascularisation). If the original injury was open, or there has been previous surgery to the limb, there should always be the suspicion of infection as the cause of nonunion. The aetiology is often multifaceted, requiring a host of patient and treatment factors to be managed simultaneously. **Table 2** summarises the common factors associated with nonunion which have been the literature to date.

Bones with a tenuous or precarious blood supply such as the scaphoid or talus are prone to nonunion after fracture, and even conservatively managed patients must be closely followed up. Maintaining vascularity to the fractured bone ends is vital, particularly during surgery. Trauma patients with high-energy mechanisms sustain soft tissue injuries

Table 2 The risk factors for fracture nonunion	
Patient factors	**Fracture-specific factors**
Increasing age	High-energy trauma or injury severity score
Smoking	Soft tissue injury. Larger zone of injury and high Gustilo–Anderson grade
Poorly diabetic control	Large interfragmentary gaps
Osteoporosis	Biomechanical instability
Vitamin D, calcium, or protein deficiency	Infection
Increased alcohol consumption	Prolonged immobilisation
Reduced muscle mass and mechanical stimuli	Perioperative or prolonged nonsteroidal anti-inflammatory drugs use
Postmenopausal females	Complex or comminuted fractures
	Diaphyseal fractures
	Large fracture haematoma

with periosteal stripping. A larger zone of injury is associated with a greater risk of nonunion.

In addition to maintaining vascularity, a favourable local environment at the fracture site is crucial to the proper progression of healing. This is achieved by minimising interfragmentary gaps through accurate reduction and adequate stability through fixation or casting (**Figure 4**). Mechanical stability is required to prevent further insult to callus and to modify osteogenic behaviour to promote healing. Bone cells are sensitive to their environment and mesenchymal cells alter differentiation according to local forces. Hydrostatic forces promote a chondrogenic pathway; however, sheer or tensile forces have a detrimental effect resulting in fibrogenesis. Achieving mechanical stability in osteoporotic bone is challenging; technology such as locking screws where the screw engages into an osteosynthesis device has resulted in increased stiffness of fixation.

Smoking and dietary insufficiency are detrimental to bone healing and potentially modifiable to minimise risk of nonunion. Not only does nicotine cause tissue hypoxia through induced vasoconstriction, it also has inhibitory effects on biological activity and cell maturation required during the early phases of fracture healing.

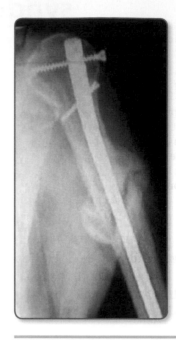

Figure 4 Humeral nonunion treated by nailing.

Conclusion

Nonunion remains a significant problem and socioeconomic burden. Early recognition and appropriate management of patients failing to progress are important; however, there is an increasing focus on modifiable risk factors to minimise risk.

Further reading

Mills LA, Simpson AH. The relative incidence of fracture non-union in the Scottish population (5.17 million): a 5-year epidemiological study. BMJ Open 2013; 3: e002276.

Perren SM. Evolution of the internal fixation of long bone fractures. The scientific basis of biological internal fixation: choosing a new balance between stability and biology. J Bone Joint Surg Br 2007; 84:1093–1110.

Rockwood CA, Green DP, Robert W. Local complications. In: Rockwood CA (ed), Fractures in adults. Philadelphia: Lippincott Williams & Wilkins, 2006:586–592.

Weber BG, Cech O. Pseudarthrosis, pathophysiology, biomechanics, therapy, results. Bern: Hans Huber, 1976.

Related topics of interest

Acute respiratory distress syndrome

Key points

- Acute respiratory distress syndrome (ARDS) is acute hypoxaemic respiratory failure, with bilateral pulmonary infiltrates on either the chest radiograph or CT scan, and at least 5 cmH$_2$O positive end-expiratory pressure (PEEP), and not solely secondary to left heart failure
- Therapeutic strategies for ARDS can be classified as ventilatory or nonventilatory
- The current overall mortality of ARDS is between 30% and 40%

Introduction and epidemiology

Critically ill patients are prone to the development of ARDS, which is characterised by excessive alveolar inflammation and increased permeability pulmonary oedema. This condition is defined by the Berlin criteria, describing the syndrome as acute (<7 days from inciting event) hypoxaemic respiratory failure, with bilateral pulmonary infiltrates on either the chest radiograph (**Figure 5**) or CT scan, in the presence of at least 5 cmH$_2$O PEEP, and not solely secondary to left heart failure. Three mutually exclusive categories are defined, based on the degree of hypoxaemia [partial pressure of oxygen in arterial blood/fraction of inspired oxygen (PaO_2/FiO_2)]:

- Mild (300–200 mmHg)
- Moderate (200–100 mmHg)
- Severe (≤100 mmHg)

ARDS is the clinical manifestation of the underlying alveolar injury termed diffuse alveolar damage, describing the structural damage to the alveolar epithelial–interstitial–endothelial complex, with concomitant impediment to gaseous diffusion, alveolar perfusion, alveolar ventilation and resultant ventilation/perfusion mismatch. Progressive hypoxaemia occurs with increasing extravascular lung water and decreasing lung compliance.

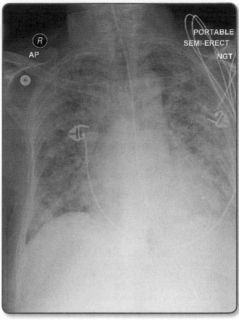

Figure 5 Pulmonary infiltrates in acute respiratory distress syndrome. By courtesy of Lt Col Andy Johnston, Consultant in Respiratory Medicine and Critical Care at Queen Elizabeth Hospital Birmingham.

The incidence of ARDS has been estimated at 79 per 100,000 person-years, with recent randomised controlled, multicentre studies reporting an associated mortality of approximately 30%. Contemporary observational studies, however, fail to report this low mortality, or any decrease over the past decade, and continue to report mortalities of between 30% and 40%. Of the various risk factors, sepsis-related ARDS is associated with a poorer outcome than nonsepsis-related ARDS, and trauma-related ARDS has the lowest incidence and associated mortality of any risk factor.

Pathophysiology

Three sequential pathological phases have been described: an injurious exudative phase, a reparative proliferative phase and a chronic fibrotic phase; although overlap occurs, the fibrotic phase may not develop.

During the exudative phase, lung capillary endothelial cells, alveolar epithelial cells and the associated basement membrane are injured, increasing permeability and allowing the alveolus to be flooded with plasma, plasma proteins, inflammatory cells and other blood constituents.

The proliferative stage is marked by the replication of alveolar type II epithelial cells, with subsequent transdifferentiation into type I epithelial cells, leading to repopulation of the denuded alveolus and return of functional proteins such as surfactant.

The fibrotic stage is characterised by fibrotic tissue deposition, with partial or complete failure of alveolar regeneration. The pathogenesis of trauma-related ARDS differs from other risk factors by having lesser degrees of alveolar endothelial and epithelial injury, combined with greater dysfunction of coagulation/fibrinolysis and increased inflammation.

Risk factors

There are two sets of risk factors for the development of ARDS – pulmonary and nonpulmonary. Pulmonary risk factors include pneumonia, lung contusion, aspiration and inhalational injury; nonpulmonary risk factors include nonpulmonary sepsis, acute pancreatitis, burns and drug overdose. Mechanical ventilation can be harmful if inappropriately administered and may also produce the features of ARDS, even in people without other risk factors [ventilator-induced lung injury (VILI)]. In contrast with elderly medical and surgical patients, trauma patients tend to be younger, with fewer comorbidities, have a different cytokine profile, lower severity of illness scores and suffer less hypotension, which is associated with improved outcome. When mechanically ventilated, this group tends to have intercostal chest drains in situ and higher airway pressures.

Therapy

Therapeutic strategies for ARDS can be classified as ventilatory or nonventilatory.

Ventilatory strategies

Ventilatory strategies are based on the concept of lung protective ventilation, aiming to minimise the potential for ventilatory harm in already injured lungs. Initially noninvasive ventilation may be tried, but it is often unsuccessful. Invasive mechanical ventilation has been extensively studied, with optimal outcomes requiring the adjustment of several ventilator settings to avoid various injurious mechanisms. These include:

- Utilising a physiological tidal volume (6 mL/kg predicted body weight) to prevent excessive lung stretch (volutrauma)
- Minimising high airway pressures (barotrauma)
- Accepting permissive hypercapnia where possible
- Using PEEP to prevent atelectasis and injury from repetitive reopening (atelectrauma)
- Minimising high concentrations of inspired oxygen, and the subsequent generation of inflammatory cytokines (biotrauma)

Whether a higher or lower PEEP in general should be used is uncertain, although meta-analyses suggest that higher PEEP may be more beneficial. Permissive hypercapnia may be dangerous in traumatic brain injury, where hypercapnia worsens intracranial hypertension. If adequate carbon dioxide (CO_2) control is not achievable with conventional mechanical ventilation, extracorporeal CO_2 removal ($ECCO_2R$) may be added, although this approach has not been formally tested. Similarly, targeting an excessive intracranial perfusion pressure may promote the development of ARDS. Two alternative modes of ventilation have been investigated, high-frequency oscillatory ventilation and liquid ventilation, with both being inferior to conventional mechanical ventilation. Should severe ARDS persist despite these measures, two further techniques can be employed to minimise VILI or worsening of ARDS. Early neuromuscular blockade for <48 hours has been associated with improved adjusted mortality in a single randomised controlled trial, while prone positioning has been associated with an enormous 50% relative risk reduction for 28-day mortality (33–16%), again in a single randomised controlled trial.

Nonventilatory strategies

Parallel to ventilator management, once resuscitated, nonshocked patients should receive a restrictive fluid regime, aiming for a cumulative neutral balance over several days. Such an approach is not associated with an increased incidence of circulatory or renal failure. The use of either a pulmonary artery catheter or central venous catheter to guide fluid management is equivalent, which is unsurprising, as cardiac filling pressures bear no relationship to either volaemic status or fluid responsiveness. The optimal feeding regime is unclear, with early trophic enteral feeding possibly being similar to early full-enteral feeding. Antioxidant supplementation to dampen inflammation may be harmful and is not recommended.

Other pharmacotherapies have failed to show a consistent beneficial effect and are not routinely used. Of note, β2-agonists are at best ineffective and at worst harmful if employed solely for ARDS; corticosteroid studies continue to return conflicting results, while adult surfactant trials fail to replicate the success observed in infant respiratory distress syndrome. Routine deep sedation is harmful, and titrated sedoanalgesia to achieve an awake cooperative patient is preferred.

Rescue therapies

Should refractory hypoxaemia persist despite these measures, rescue therapies are initiated. Inhaled nitric oxide, a selective pulmonary vasodilator, has been utilised for its oxygenation effect, although no mortality benefit has been demonstrated. Extracorporeal gas exchange devices are now the primary rescue therapy, although they presently remain unproven. The only contemporary randomised controlled trial, the Conventional ventilation or ECMO for Severe Adult Respiratory failure (CESAR) study, compared management at an extracorporeal membrane oxygenation (ECMO) centre, where the patient may have received either conventional mechanical ventilation or ECMO, with ongoing management at the referring centre, rather than comparing conventional mechanical ventilation with ECMO. $ECCO_2R$ is gaining prominence as a method of reducing mechanical ventilation, and thus minimising VILI, without the need for formal ECMO. It is interesting to reflect on how just 10% of ARDS patients actually die from refractory hypoxaemia; most die from multiorgan failure and sepsis. Post-ARDS, many patients suffer prolonged neuromuscular disability and psychological trauma, with just half returning to work.

Summary

ARDS is a syndrome of increased permeability pulmonary oedema, seen in critically ill mechanically ventilated patients. Therapeutic goals are the avoidance of iatrogenic insults – a positive fluid balance, excessive sedation and harmful ventilation. Few patients die from refractory hypoxaemia, but if it is present, this can be treated with extracorporeal gas exchange when the patient's condition is suitable.

Further reading

Guérin C, Reignier J, Richard J-C, et al. Prone positioning in severe acute respiratory distress syndrome (PROSEVA). New Engl J Med 2013; 368:2159–2168.

The Acute Respiratory Distress Syndrome Network. Ventilation with lower tidal volumes as compared with traditional tidal volumes for acute lung injury and the acute respiratory distress syndrome. N Engl J Med 2000; 342:1301–1308.

The ARDS Definition Task Force. Acute respiratory distress syndrome. The Berlin definition. JAMA 2012; 307:2526–2533.

Related topics of interest

Aeromedical evacuation and retrieval

Key points

- The principle of retrieval medicine is to maintain and enhance the care provided at each stage of the evacuation process, bringing forward a critical care capability to the casualty
- Effective tasking is an essential component of a well-functioning aeromedical service
- Patient packaging and preparation are the keys to an effective retrieval

Introduction

Aeromedical evacuation is a comprehensive term covering the use of air transportation by airplane (fixed wing) or helicopter (rotary), to move patients to and from health care facilities and from accident scenes. Appropriate personnel are able to provide comprehensive prehospital emergency and critical care to all types of patients during evacuation or rescue operations aboard helicopters and fixed wing airframes. Although team composition varies, a doctor is increasingly commonly deployed as a team member alongside paramedics or, less frequently, nurses.

The use of air transport for seriously injured patients dates back to World War I, but its role was expanded dramatically during the Korean and Vietnam conflicts. In civilian practice, helicopters are used to transport patients between hospitals and from trauma scenes; fixed-wing aircraft are used for long-distance transfers. Many recent clinical developments have arisen from the extensive use of aeromedical evacuation in the recent conflicts in Iraq and Afghanistan.

Modern aeromedical retrieval has evolved to become a distinct specialist discipline and, as technology has progressed, so has the level of critical care that can be delivered during transport. The fundamental principle of retrieval medicine is to maintain and enhance the care provided at each stage of the evacuation process.

Advantages

The advantages of medical transport by helicopter include provision of a higher level of care at the scene of trauma and improving access to specialist care in major trauma centres. Helicopter-based emergency medical services (EMS) also provide critical care capabilities during interfacility transport from community hospitals to trauma centres and may be used to facilitate access to casualties in challenging and remote locations.

Indications for air transport

Effective use of helicopter services in trauma depends on the ground responder's ability to determine whether the patient's condition warrants air medical transport. Protocols and training must be developed to ensure that appropriate triage criteria are applied. Excessively stringent criteria may prevent rapid care and transport of trauma victims; relaxed criteria can result in the embarrassing and costly situation of transporting a patient by helicopter only to have the patient discharged in good condition from the emergency department.

Crew and patient safety is the single most important factor to be considered when deciding whether to transport a patient by helicopter. Weather, air traffic patterns and distances (e.g. from the trauma scene to the closest level one trauma centre) must also be considered. Some have questioned the safety of air medical services. While the number of crashes may be increasing, the number of programs and use of services have also increased. Factors associated with fatal crashes of medical transport helicopters include flying at night and during bad weather.

Air ambulances

An air ambulance is a specially fitted and equipped aircraft that transports injured or sick people in a medical emergency or over distances or terrain impractical for a conventional ground ambulance (**Figure 6**). These and related operations are called aeromedical.

Like ground ambulances, air ambulances are equipped with the medical equipment needed for monitoring and treating injured or ill patients (**Figure 7**). Common equipment for air ambulances includes medications, ventilators, electrocardiogram and monitoring units, cardiopulmonary resuscitation equipment and stretchers. A medically staffed and equipped air ambulance provides medical care in flight, while a nonmedically equipped and staffed aircraft simply transports patients without care in flight. Military organisations and North Atlantic Treaty Organisation (NATO) refer to the former as medical evacuation (MEDEVAC) and to the latter as casualty evacuation (CASEVAC).

Organisation

Air ambulance services are provided by a variety of different sources in different parts of the world. There are a number of methods of differentiating types of air ambulance services. These include military and civilian models and services that are government-funded, fee-for-service, donated by a business

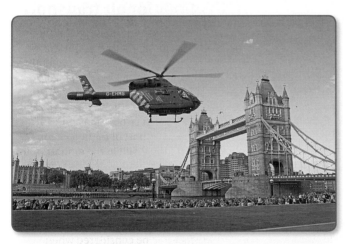

Figure 6 London's air ambulance.

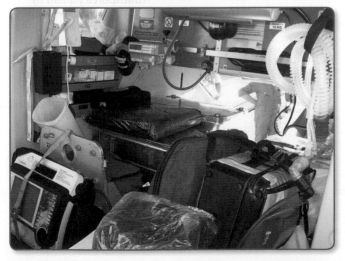

Figure 7 Typical helicopter interior.

enterprise or funded by public donations. Some aircraft are dedicated to the medical role; however, some are multipurpose such as police helicopters used for air ambulance work (e.g. at night when air ambulances cannot fly). Finally, it is reasonable to differentiate by the type of aircraft used, including rotary-wing, fixed-wing or very large aircraft.

Communications

The single most important aspect of conducting successful and safe aeromedical retrieval is communication. Use of a systemic standardised manner of clinical communication is increasingly recommended: an example is SBAR (situation, background, assessment and recommendations).

Medical personnel

The team requires the skills to independently maintain or preferably improve the care of the patient in transit. These will include diagnostic and procedural skills and the ability to apply these in an aeromedical environment. Inexperienced and junior staff should not undertake retrievals without the presence of an experienced team member. Training and continued development are an essential part of the clinical governance of any aeromedical operation. The training should involve the principles and practicalities of retrieval medicine, familiarisation with the equipment and vehicles and the relevant safety and emergency procedures. A diploma in retrieval medicine is now offered by the Faculty of Pre-Hospital Care of the Royal College of Surgeons of Edinburgh.

Patient preparation

Air transport places both physiological and psychological stressors on the acute patient. With smaller airframes, it is necessary to package the patient fully before loading and take-off. With larger airframes (such as the military Chinook – CH47), the treatment and packaging can be done in flight. Once a patient is stabilised for transport, the

same level of care should be maintained throughout the entire retrieval process until the definitive care location is reached.

Standard approach

Adequate preparation for transport must follow the standard <C>ABCDE approach (see p. 63). Air ambulances are increasingly carrying blood products and have the ability to transfuse during flight. It has already been shown that trauma victims have improved outcomes when transfused blood and blood products instead of crystalloid solution. The principles of prehospital transfusion are similar to those which apply in hospital.

An adequate trial of sedation is vital and best conducted before the flight. Acute sedation during flight is risky with little margin for error. The level of consciousness before sedation must be documented. It is increasingly common practice to fully anaesthetise (rapid sequence induction) and intubate patients in order to maintain and ensure a secure unsoiled airway during transfer, as well as to reduce the need for an unexpected emergency induction in flight and to improve the patient experience.

Adequate analgesia, antiemetics (air sickness is common apart from the other causes of nausea following trauma), immobilisation of fractures, thermal control and minimisation of contamination must all be considered.

Equipment

Most aircraft used as air ambulances, with the exception of charter aircraft and some military aircraft, are equipped for advanced life support and have interiors that reflect this. The challenges in most air ambulance operations, particularly those involving helicopters, are the high ambient noise levels and limited amounts of working space, both of which create significant issues for the provision of ongoing care. While equipment tend to be of high-level and conveniently grouped, it may not be possible to perform some assessment procedures, such as chest auscultation, while in flight. In some types of aircraft, the aircraft's design means that some parts of the patient are not physically accessible in flight.

Additional issues occur with respect to pressurisation of the aircraft. Not all aircraft used as air ambulances in all jurisdictions have pressurised cabins, and those that do have typically tend to be pressurised to only 10,000 feet above sea level. These pressure changes require advanced knowledge by flight staff with respect to the specifics of aviation medicine, including changes in physiology and the behaviour of gases. In general, these issues do not apply to helicopter services in the United Kingdom.

Funding

While some air ambulances have other effective methods of funding, in the United Kingdom most air ambulance services remain almost entirely charity funded, as improved cost–benefit ratios are generally achieved with land-based attendance and transfers. Health outcomes, e.g. from London's Helicopter EMS, remain largely the same for both air- and ground-based services. Some countries, such as the UK, use a mix of such systems. In Scotland, the air ambulance service is funded directly, through the Scottish Ambulance Service. In England and Wales, however, the service is funded on a charitable basis via a number of local charities for each region covered, although the service to London receives most of its funding through the National Health Service (NHS).

Great strides were made in the United Kingdom between 2005 and 2008, when independent charities formed the National Association of Air Ambulance Charities (AAAC). This organisation is widely credited for having created the political climate that made the helicopter industry and NHS recognise the enormous contribution charities make to trauma care in the United Kingdom. In 2008, NHS partners joined the association, and it was renamed the Association of Air Ambulances.

Further reading

Milligan JE, Jones CN, Helm DR, Munford BJ. The principles of aeromedical retrieval of the critically ill. Trends in Anaesthesia and Critical Care 2011; 1:22–26.

le Cong M. Aeromedical retrieval. Australian Rural Doctor 2012:12–21.

Isakov AP. Souls on board: helicopter emergency medical services and safety. Ann Emerg Med 2006; 47:357–360.

Marsh AC. A framework for a high performing air ambulance service. UK-Helicopter Emergency Medical Service 2008.

Morrison JJ, Oh J, DuBose JJ, et al. En-route care capability from point of injury impacts mortality after severe wartime injury. Ann Surg 2013; 257:330–334.

Related topics of interest

- Anaesthesia (p. 16)
- Blood product (1:1:1) resuscitation (p. 42)
- Prehospital blood product resuscitation (p. 236)

Anaesthesia

Key points

- Low Glasgow coma score, unprotected/compromised airway, poor ventilation/oxygenation, the need for surgery, control of bleeding, an agitated patient and neuroprotection are the most likely indications for anaesthesia following trauma
- The unconscious patient presents a clinical challenge and standard procedures should account for the risk that hazards have not been identified in advance
- Safe anaesthesia requires careful application of established effective protocols

Potential difficulties

Trauma anaesthesia is potentially extremely challenging, especially in the prehospital environment. The factors which complicate trauma anaesthesia can be divided into patient and environmental factors.

Patient factors

Patient factors which increase the potential difficulty of anaesthesia following trauma include altered or combative behaviour as a result of head injury; hypoxia; drugs or alcohol; maxillofacial or airway trauma resulting in blood/debris in the airway; disrupted anatomy; facial oedema; and where there is a risk of cervical spine injury. Manual in-line stabilisation (MILS) with the collar off should be considered prior to intubation. All trauma patients should be considered to have a full stomach (gastric contents or blood) and so be at risk of aspiration. Haemodynamic instability due to ongoing bleeding (which may be exacerbated by anaesthesia) and rapid desaturation on induction due to difficult preoxygenation, reduced residual capacity and/or chest trauma may occur. High spinal lesions may cause respiratory compromise and neurogenic shock. In the medium term, there is also the risk of rapid development of multiorgan failure (acute respiratory distress syndrome, acute kidney injury, cardiovascular collapse and disseminated intravascular coagulation). The patient may also be suffering from hypothermia, making assessment and intravenous (IV) access more difficult.

Environmental factors

Induction of anaesthesia in the trauma victim is always stressful. Contributing factors which are likely to include an unfamiliar environment often with unfamiliar team members and complex concurrent activity environmental factors are likely to be even more challenging in the prehospital environment.

General anaesthesia

Preparation

Rapid sequence induction of anaesthesia (RSI) with MILS of the neck is most commonly used. A number of components must be present and checked, and use of checklist cards may be useful:

- Equipment must be available for basic and difficult airway management, including suction, a ventilator and infusion pumps as well as surgical airway kit. A bougie should be immediately available and used for all prehospital intubations. The ability to tilt the bed may be needed if the patient regurgitates
- Drugs – these include induction agents, muscle relaxants, vasopressors, fluids, oxygen, drugs to maintain sedation and emergency drugs (see below)
- Personnel – an experienced airway specialist, anaesthetic assistant and an assistant trained person to give drugs and monitor observations must be present and aware of their allocated tasks (as must other members of the team. Tabards may be helpful)
- Monitoring is essential, including pulse oximetry, blood pressure (noninvasive or invasive), three-lead electrocardiograph (ECG), end-tidal carbon dioxide ($EtCO_2$) capnometry or capnography. Whether in or out of hospital, the full range of minimum monitoring as specified in

the Association of Anaesthetists of Great Britain and Ireland (AAGBI) guidelines or local equivalent should be used
- IV and intraosseous access must be established, confirmed to be patent and secure. Ideally at least two lines should be in place. For central access, the subclavian vein is preferred, although neck access may be restricted by the collar. Femoral access is associated with a high risk of infection, but the femoral vein is less likely to collapse in the shocked patient

Investigations including CT scanning will be required for the conformation or elimination of injuries, but these (including plain radiography) and standard bloods, arterial blood gas and ECG must not delay intubation in a patient with airway compromise. Where possible, the patient should be adequately resuscitated prior to induction to mitigate the risk of cardiac arrest on induction – a very significant risk in unidentified and untreated hypovolaemia.

Induction

The patient must be preoxygenated, ideally for 3 minutes. This can be done while equipment is being checked. During this time, the collar is removed and MILS substituted. Consideration should also be given to the position of assistants. One Yankauer suction catheter should be available under the pillow, a second nearby.

Ketamine

Ketamine is increasingly used as it is associated with less hypotension (due to induced sympathetic stimulation) than other agents. Historically, it has been considered contraindicated in head injury patients to a potential risk of increased intracranial pressure (ICP), but review of the original studies has resulted in this being questioned. Ketamine-induced maintenance of mean arterial pressure (MAP) and cerebral perfusion pressure (CPP) along with potential cellular protective mechanisms may indeed lead to an overall neuroprotective effect. Even short periods of hypotension may exacerbate secondary brain injury, thus in certain patients ketamine may be the best current induction drug.

Etomidate

Etomidate has classically been the drug of choice for trauma anaesthesia as its onset is rapid, and associated with relative haemodynamic stability concerns raised regarding prolonged adrenal suppression in sepsis have led to a decline in use as ketamine use has increased Etomidate. It may also cause seizures and platelet inhibition.

Thiopentone

Thiopentone has commonly been used for its rapid onset and effects of reducing ICP, cerebral metabolic rate and seizure termination. However, cardiovascular instability may be exacerbated, and extravasation can cause significant tissue damage.

Propofol

Propofol is a familiar anaesthetic agent with a rapid onset, but causes hypotension especially in haemodynamically unstable patients.

Neuromuscular blockade

Suxamethonium is typically used for muscle relaxation as it has a predictable end point, rapid onset and short duration of action. Its side effects include an increase in ICP and hyperkalaemia. The latter may contraindicate use in major burns (after 48 hours), spinal cord injuries (after 24 hours) and recurrent general anaesthetics in major trauma patients. In addition, the effects of suxamethonium may wear off before the tube is in place and muscle fasciculations may increase the speed of desaturation. A longer acting agent will be needed post-induction.

Rocuronium is increasingly used for RSI (1 mg/kg) due to its rapid onset and consequent good intubating conditions.

Anaphylaxis has been reported, and in the event of a 'can't intubate can't ventilate', reversal can be achieved with Sugammadex.

Cricoid pressure is used to limit aspiration risk; however, caution is required if cervical spine injury is suspected, in which case a two-handed technique (one on front and one on back of the neck) should be used to limit movement. Once intubation has occurred, tube position should be checked by $EtCO_2$

measurement auscultation and chest X-ray and the tube is secured with a tie or tape (bearing in mind the possibility of obstruction of cranial venous outflow in head injury).

Maintenance

Appropriate monitoring must be in place. Propofol by infusion is commonly used for maintenance but caution must be exercised in shocked patients. Opiates reduce anaesthetic requirements and prevent hypertensive surges to stimulation. In theatres, volatile agents are used (noting a reduced mean alveolar concentration requirement in shocked patients). Nitrous oxide may be used, but caution is important in those patients with air-filled cavities (e.g. pneumothorax), undergoing long procedures and with high oxygen requirements.

Ventilation should be with high inspired oxygen and controlled $EtCO_2$ (particularly to help reduce ICP). A simple pneumothorax may tension under positive pressure ventilation and airway pressures must be monitored with a low threshold for chest drain insertion.

A good perfusion pressure is needed in head injury (CPP = MAP − ICP); however, permissive hypotension may be needed to prevent clot disruption in bleeding patients. A conflict therefore may occur in multiply injured patients and treatment priorities will need to be discussed. Cardiac output monitors, urine output and serum lactate may be used to guide fluid replacement. Activation of a major haemorrhage protocol may be required, remembering that bleeding may be occult. Now is the time to establish further venous and arterial access, a urinary catheter, 30° head up tilt to reduce ICP (not if the patient is not hypovolaemic), a nasogastric tube and blood glucose control. Attention must be paid to ensuring that the patient is warmed or remains warm by under-patient heating and warming blankets. When the patient is transferred from the emergency department, standard equipment and a transfer checklist should always be used.

Further reading

Chang LC, Raty SR, Ortiz J, et al. The emerging use of ketamine for anesthesia and sedation in traumatic brain injuries. CNS Neurosci Ther 2013; 19:390–395.

Gwinnutt C, Bethelmy L, Nolan J. Anaesthesia in trauma. Trauma 2003; 5:51–60.

Langeron O, Birenbaum A, Amour J. Airway management in trauma. Minerva Anesthesiol 2009; 75:307–311.

Related topics of interest

- Analgesia (p. 19)
- Damage control resuscitation and surgery (p. 83)
- Penetrating neck injury (p. 227)

Analgesia

Key points

- Pain as a result of trauma carries a significant emotional and psychological burden and exacerbates the physiological stress response
- Ineffective treatment of pain may result when there are concerns about cardiovascular instability, sedation and the risk of respiratory depression
- Early treatment is not only humane but may also assist functional recovery including earlier restoration of movement, reduced chance of debilitating chronic pain and psychological syndromes

Introduction

Pain control can be provided in a number of ways. In many cases, use of a combination of techniques and drugs (a multimodal approach) is most likely to produce pain relief while limiting adverse effects.

Pharmacological methods

After significant trauma, absorption from the gastrointestinal tract is often reduced and the patient may be nil by mouth awaiting surgery, thus intravenous (IV) administration is usually preferred in the acute phase. Small but regular aliquots titrated to effect, while resuscitation is ongoing, are often most effective in the unstable patient. However, in minor trauma, use of standard cheap analgesic agents, sometimes in combination, e.g. paracetamol and a nonsteroidal anti-inflammatory drug (NSAID) or codeine and paracetamol), should not be overlooked. The choice of the most appropriate and effective delivery method [nurse-delivered boluses, patient-controlled anaesthesia (PCA), boluses or infusions] will depend on nursing staff skill levels, the drug used and patient factors. Infusions run the highest risk of respiratory depression.

Simple analgesia

Paracetamol is safe, cheap, effective and reduces opiate requirements when used as part of a multimodal approach. IV paracetamol is very effective and underused, although caution should be exercised in patients with suspected liver disease. NSAIDs provide good analgesia and can be given orally, rectally and intravenously. They should be avoided in the acute stages of severe injury as the risk of acute renal failure, gastric ulcers and bleeding (due to platelet dysfunction) is increased.

Opiates

Opiates provide good pain relief but concerns regarding respiratory depression, impaired gut motility (ileus), nausea, sedation and addiction have perhaps made clinicians over cautious in their use. Burns patients may be particularly sensitive to opiates due to altered plasma protein levels and possibly upregulated opiate receptors. Administration may be oral, transdermal, intramuscular, IV, epidural, intrathecal or intranasal and by bolus or infusion (including PCA). Caution is important in patients with renal dysfunction. There is concern that morphine may exacerbate haemodynamic instability, and impair the immune system's response to infection. Fentanyl has a shorter time of onset than morphine but accumulates when given as an infusion. Remifentanil is effective as an infusion but highly potent with a risk of bradycardia, hypotension and chest wall rigidity (as with high dose fentanyl). Because remifentanil is rapidly metabolised, an additional longer acting agent will often be needed. Hyperalgesia after use has also been described.

Other agents include codeine, although this is not effective in some patients who are unable to metabolise it to morphine. Constipation is common and may be severe, so a stool softener or laxative should be prescribed. Tramadol is as effective as morphine in IV form, but associated with a significant incidence of often severe nausea. There is also a risk of acute severe confusion in the elderly.

Antidepressants, anxiolytics and anticonvulsants

These agents may also play a role, although they are less used in the acute setting. They are of particular value in the treatment of neuropathic pain where their early use may help in preventing progression to chronic pain.

Ketamine

Ketamine has been commonly used in paediatrics for many years and is increasingly used in adults for sedation and analgesia, especially in the prehospital setting. Low doses can be titrated to effect with minimal respiratory depression and maintenance of upper airway reflexes. In the patient in the early stages of shock, haemodynamic status is less affected due to direct sympathetic stimulation. This effect, however, is not maintained as shock progresses. Ketamine induces a dissociated state, with possible distressing hallucinations. Benzodiazepines have been used to counteract the hallucinations; however, the incidence of hallucinations varies, has probably been overstated and symptoms are usually mild with analgesic doses and do not require treatment.

Local anaesthesia

Local anaesthetic infiltration or blocks are an effective but underused method of pain control. At their simplest, local anaesthetic cream may be applied topically. Alternatively, anaesthetic may be infiltrated locally into the tissues or around peripheral or central nerves as a nerve block. Lignocaine or prilocaine is used for speed of onset, though their duration of action is short. Ropivacaine and bupivacaine have a slower onset but longer duration of action. Doses vary according to the weight of the patient and must be calculated carefully to avoid the risk of adverse effects. Practitioners must know the signs of local anaesthetic toxicity and its management.

Concerns regarding local anaesthetic techniques delaying diagnosis of compartment syndromes are long standing and based on case reports rather than substantial clinical evidence. Although dense sensory and motor blocks may lead to delay in diagnosis, with the use of lower dose local anaesthetic mixtures, breakthrough pain will still occur and appropriate levels of suspicion should lead to the diagnosis. Pain can be a variable and alone is a poor indicator of compartment syndrome which should not be relied upon.

Regional pain management will help reduce systemic analgesic requirements and thus their potential complications. Depending on the block, there may be risk of damage to nearby structures as well as potential permanent damage to the nerve itself, although this is rare. Inadvertent block of nearby nerves, e.g. of the phrenic nerve after interscalene block causing hemidiaphragmatic paralysis, may also occur and must be considered preprocedure. Single injections or placement of catheters in order to run continuous infusions are possible. The latter may also be done intraoperatively by the surgeons.

Spinal and epidural anaesthesia

Central neuraxial blocks – spinal and epidural anaesthesia – are very effective. Pain relief without sedation is useful in patients with impaired ventilation due to the pain, e.g. from multiple rib fractures, and may help prevent secondary respiratory failure. Regional techniques may also play a role in beneficially modulating the body's stress response to surgery. This benefit in trauma is unclear since it is impossible to perform the technique before the insult. Contraindications include coagulopathy, local infection, local anaesthetic allergy, patient refusal and trauma involving damage to the spinal cord. Complications include the risk of haematoma (high in the coagulopathic trauma patient), infection, failure of the technique and haemodynamic instability (secondary to sympathetic block). Positioning of the patient to perform the techniques is also likely to be difficult. Local anaesthetic alone or a mixture of local anaesthetic and opiate may be used. The typical opiate side effects are less common than via other routes if the procedure is undertaken correctly.

Nitrous oxide

The most common oxygen/nitrous oxide mixture is Entonox which is a 50% nitrous oxide and 50% oxygen mix and is an effective form of pain relief. Complications include nausea, sedation and acute confusion (although this is rare). Use of Entonox is contraindicated in trauma patients requiring high levels of inspired oxygen to maintain saturations and those with chest trauma or any other gas-filled space and in patients who have been diving.

Nonpharmacological methods

There are a number of effective methods of pain control which are sometimes overlooked. These include immobilisation of fractures (e.g. by splintage, traction splintage or surgical fixation) and reassurance. Distraction by a familiar adult or toy may be at least partially effective in children. Good communication at all times is essential as is an honest assessment of the likely effects of a procedure: inappropriate reassurance will lead to loss of confidence in the clinician, especially by young patients. Other techniques used in the subacute and chronic settings include transcutaneous electronic nerve stimulation machines, hypnosis and psychological support and treatment, e.g. for post-traumatic stress reactions.

Pain management protocols

There is some evidence suggesting that a departmental protocol for pain management in trauma patients reduces time to analgesia administration and leads to more effective control of pain.

Further reading

Davidson EM, Ginosar Y, Avidan A. Pain management and regional anaesthesia in the trauma patient. Curr Opin Anaesthesiol 2005; 18:169–174.

Gage A, Rivara F, Wang J, Jurkovich GJ, Arbabi S. The effect of epidural placement in patients after blunt thoracic trauma. J Trauma Acute Care Surg 2014;76:39–46.

Hedderich R, Ness TJ. Analgesia for trauma and burns. Crit Care Clin 1999;15:167–184.

Related topics of interest

Ankle injuries

Key points

- Fractures around the ankle account for 9% of all fractures
- Ankle fractures are clinically most easily classified according to their site
- Most ankle sprains are lateral ligament complex injuries – anterior talofibular ligament (ATFL) and calcaneofibular ligament (CFL)

Fractures

Fractures around the ankle account for 9% of all fractures and range from simple undisplaced fractures with a stable construct to complex intra-articular injuries associated with disruption of the ankle joint (dislocation). As the stabilising structures around the ankle become disrupted with increasing energy, the more unstable the ankle becomes (**Figure 8**).

Classification

Ankle fractures affect all ages from the skeletal immature through to the elderly population with multiple comorbidities. Fractures of the immature skeleton may be classified using the Salter–Harris classification of physeal injuries. As the skeleton matures, the Tillaux fracture (a Salter–Harris type III fracture through the anterolateral aspect of the distal tibial epiphysis occurring in older adolescents) becomes more common due to the growth plate around the ankle closing (**Figure 9**).

The treatment of immature fractures is to attempt to minimise or prevent any disruption to further growth and thus any effect on the alignment of the ankle. As with any paediatric fracture, it is important to make an early diagnosis in order to minimise the long-term effects.

For the skeletally mature patient, there are two main classification systems for ankle fractures. The Lange–Hansen classification describes the mechanism of injury and the resultant moment causing the fracture. It was originally described in 1948 based on a cadaveric anatomical study of the position of the foot and the rotational force applied. This gives five main mechanisms: supination

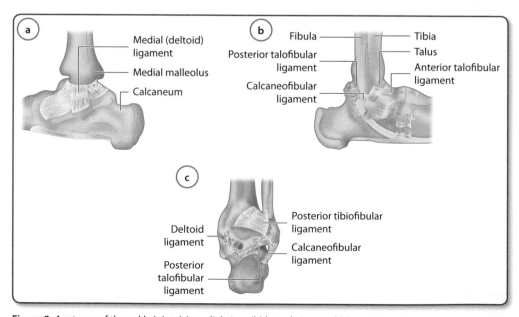

Figure 8 Anatomy of the ankle joint: (a) medial view, (b) lateral view, and (c) posterior view.

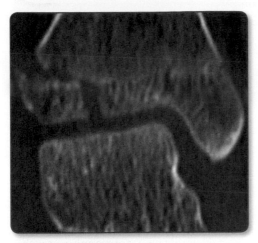

Figure 9 Tillaux fracture.

adduction, supination eversion, pronation eversion, pronation abduction and pronation dorsiflexion. Each of these groups has between two and four subgroups depending on the severity of the injury. A more user-friendly classification for both emergency department staff and orthopaedic surgeons is the Danis–Weber classification (1972) (**Figure 10**). The higher the level of the fracture, the more severe the injury to the syndesmotic ligament and hence the higher the level of instability, the greater the likelihood of subsequent need for surgical management:

- Weber A: Transverse fibular fractures below the level of the ankle joint with intact tibiofibular syndesmosis and deltoid ligament. The medial malleolus may or may not be fractured. These fractures are usually stable.
- Weber B: Fibular fractures at the level of the ankle joint, extending superiorly and laterally up the fibula with possible damage (but not complete rupture) to the tibiofibular syndesmosis and no widening of the distal tibiofibular articulation. The medial malleolus may be fractured or deltoid ligament torn. Stability varies and surgical management may be required.
- Weber C: Fractures of the fibula above the level of the ankle joint with tibiofibular syndesmosis disruption and widened tibiofibular space. The medial malleolus is fractured or the deltoid ligament injured. These fractures require open fixation.

In everyday clinical practice, ankle fractures are most easily classified anatomically into medial malleolar, lateral malleolar, posterior malleolar, bimalleolar or trimalleolar and closed or open and displaced or undisplaced.

Diagnosis

This is usually via X-ray appearance on anteroposterior (AP), true lateral and Mortise views (internal rotation 15°–20°). If there is gross distortion of normal anatomical alignment, CT scanning may be used to delineate the pathology more clearly and aid in surgical planning for reconstruction.

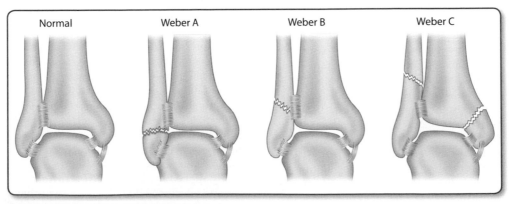

Figure 10 Danis–Weber classification.

Eponymous fractures

There are a number of eponymous fracture types which are sufficiently frequently used to be worth retaining:

- Maisonneuve fracture: a high fibular fracture with talar shift which may be associated with injury to the common peroneal nerve
- Pilon fracture: a complex distal tibial fracture associated with axial loading
- Tillaux fracture (see p. 109)
- Triplane fracture: a fracture involving frontal, lateral and transverse planes
- Bosworth fracture: a low, external rotation fracture of the fibula which becomes entrapped behind the posterior tibia preventing reduction

Assessment

A full history including details of comorbidities and the mechanism of injury is essential. Examination must include documentation of any dislocation or subluxation, neurovascular status and whether the fracture is open or closed. If there is disruption to the vascular supply as a result of dislocation, this usually returns on prompt reduction. An assessment must also be made of the soft tissues and the amount of swelling. Investigation is usually by X-ray sometimes augmented by CT. MRI is rarely of use in the acute phase of an injury.

Treatment

In all cases, the patient should be made comfortable by temporary splintage usually using a below knee backslab with suitable analgesia. Treatment in a functional boot is an effective alternative.

As with any intra-articular fracture, the principles of treatment are anatomical reduction, rigid fixation and early mobilisation. However, the quality of the bone varies significantly with older patients unsurprisingly having worse bone quality. Treatment is based upon the position of the talus underneath the tibial plafond and whether there is talar shift on the AP radiograph. (>1 mm of talar shift can decrease the talar–tibial contact pressures by approximately 42% and may predispose to early degenerative changes).

The actual technical details of surgical management are a matter of some debate and it is more helpful to talk about concepts. In general, nonoperative management with early weight-bearing can be considered for:

- Tip avulsions of lateral or medial malleolar fractures
- Isolated lateral malleolar fractures with <3 mm displacement and no talar shift
- Posterior malleolar fractures with <25% joint involvement or <2 mm step-off

Operative management should be considered when there is:

- Any talar displacement
- A displaced isolated medial malleolar fracture
- A displaced isolated lateral malleolar fracture
- A bimalleolar fracture or bimalleolar-equivalent fracture
- Posterior malleolar fracture with >25% or >2 mm step-off
- Bosworth fracture dislocations
- Ankle instability after manipulation of dislocation

Surgical outcomes

The outcome of surgery should be superior to nonoperative management. Current surgical practice allows for a successful outcome in 90% of cases, but it should be noted that it can take up to 2 years to gain the final result. Adverse outcomes are associated with poor technique, smoking, poor compliance due to educational or mental capacity, excess alcohol, diabetes, increasing age and multiple comorbidities.

A significant advantage of surgical reduction and stabilisation is that it allows the patient to commence early rehabilitation and regain movement more quickly. In an ideal situation, any reconstruction should aid early weight bearing and restore the patient to normality. However, this should be judged on an individual patient basis. Nonoperative management is not without complications relating to prolonged immobilisation and poorly applied casts. The decision to treat nonoperatively should therefore be a positive one.

Ankle sprains

Ankle sprains are common and unfortunately often poorly treated. The mechanism of an ankle sprain is often the same as that which results in a fracture but with less energy. Forty per cent of ankle sprains are associated with sporting activity.

Assessment

A detailed history should be taken, including the individual's usual performance level. Examination should identify the location of ligamentous swelling, bruising (if present) and tenderness. The majority of sprains are of the lateral ligament complex injuries – ATFL two-thirds and CFL one-third. Ligament specific tests are not often useful in the emergency department due to severity of pain. If assessment using the Ottawa rules (see below) is positive, then an X-ray is mandatory to exclude a fracture.

Ottawa rules

If a patient has one or more of the following:
- Bony tenderness around the posterior edge or the tip of the lateral malleolus (distal 6 cm of the fibula)
- Bony tenderness around the posterior edge or the tip of the medial malleolus (distal 6 cm of the tibia)
- An inability to bear weight both immediately and in the emergency department
- An X-ray is indicated

Management

Treatment is with a short period of rest, analgesia, compression and elevation. Early functional bracing in a weight-bearing removable boot is ideal, giving the support of a synthetic cast while allowing early rehabilitation. Early referral to physiotherapy, especially of those who have the most severe swelling and more severe pain, is essential.

Outcomes

Ninety per cent of ankle sprains will heal with no long-term sequelae. Those who have recurrent symptoms or persistent talocrural pain should be referred to a specialist for further assessment. MRI investigation in the acute phase can be useful to help quantify any talar articular injury.

Further reading

Calhoun JH, Laughlin RT. Fractures of the foot and ankle: diagnosis and treatment of injury and disease, 1st edition. Boca Raton: Taylor & Francis, 2005.

Thordarson DB. Orthopaedic surgery essentials: foot and ankle. Philadelphia: Williams & Wilkins, 2004.

Related topics of interest

Antibiotic therapy and infection control

Key points

- Infections continue to be a major cause of morbidity and mortality in patients suffering from traumatic injuries
- Appropriate surgical debridement remains the mainstay of management of infected wounds – antibiotics can be a useful adjunct but courses should be only as long as is necessary and the choice of agent should cover only those bacteria likely to be causing infection
- Trauma patients who have received health care abroad are at risk of carrying multiple resistant organisms which may transmit to other patients – pre-emptive isolation and screening for resistant organisms is required

Background and microbiology

Infections are an important cause of morbidity and mortality in patients who have suffered traumatic injuries. As well as acute infections, they include long-term sequelae such as post-traumatic osteomyelitis which may present many years after the initial trauma. Infections can present at a number of sites, most obviously at a wound site, but also as a result of the management strategies, e.g. ventilator-associated pneumonia and device-associated bloodstream infections.

The micro-organisms causing infections associated with trauma can originate from a number of sources:

Endogenous organisms

The most common source of infection is from the patient's own resident flora which has been disrupted during the traumatic event. These organisms include *Staphylococcus aureus,* β-haemolytic streptococci, and gut organisms such as coliforms and clostridia. Gas gangrene is extremely rarely seen nowadays as a result of improved surgical techniques and the availability of antibiotics.

These endogenous organisms remain the main target of any initial antibiotic treatment or prophylaxis, which is why agents such as flucloxacillin or co-amoxiclav remain the mainstay of treatment.

Environmental organisms

These organisms are acquired from the environment where the injury took place, are often of low pathogenicity and are unlikely to result in infection or other serious consequences. However, there are some notable exceptions:

Clostridium tetani: Tetanus spores are widespread in soil or manure and a high-risk tetanus prone injury is one where there was heavy contamination with material likely to contain tetanus spores with or without extensive devitalised tissue. In such cases, human tetanus immunoglobulin should be given as a precautionary measure for immediate protection, irrespective of the tetanus immunisation history of the patient. Tetanus vaccine given at the time of a tetanus prone injury may not boost immunity early enough to provide protection but provides an opportunity to update that individual's vaccine status.

Aeromonas hydrophila **and other** *Aeromonas* **spp**: These are Gram-negative bacteria which are associated with water-related injuries, especially in freshwater injuries and can cause a range of infections including cellulitis and necrotising fasciitis. They are often resistant to a number of commonly used antibiotics. Treatment involves surgical debridement and appropriate antibiotics – ciprofloxacin is usually considered the drug of choice.

Invasive fungal infections **including** *mucormycosis*: Invasive fungal wound infections are a rare but increasingly commonly reported complication of trauma associated with natural disasters and combat-associated injuries. The common factor appears to be severe wounds which are heavily contaminated with water, soil or debris and the most commonly associated fungi belong to the group causing mucormycosis. A high index of suspicion is required to make the diagnosis which relies on culture of tissue samples on appropriate media as well as histological examination. Aggressive surgical debridement is essential but early antifungal treatment does appear to be an important adjunct and a combination of liposomal amphotericin B and a broad spectrum azole such as posaconazole is recommended.

Pasteurella multocida **associated with cat and dog bites**: These bacteria are commonly found as part of the normal flora of companion animals and can cause serious infections especially following cat bites. The bacteria are relatively resistant to flucloxacillin and always resistant to erythromycin and clindamycin, but susceptible to ciprofloxacin and doxycycline.

Health care-associated organisms

Patients with traumatic injuries can quickly become colonised with, and occasionally infected by, organisms acquired during the first few hours or days of health care. This has become a particular problem with patients who have been injured and treated outside the United Kingdom (UK) and then repatriated as not only can the patient themselves be affected but the organisms can spread rapidly throughout the health care setting. Particular bacteria of concern at the moment include:

Methicillin-resistant *Staphylococcus aureus* **(MRSA):** It is now a routine to screen all admissions to high-risk areas in the UK hospitals. Screening sites should include, as a minimum, a nose swab but axilla and perineum swabs may also be helpful. Panton-Valentine leukocidin MRSA is a particular strain carrying a toxin which can be responsible for severe soft tissue infections and even necrotising pneumonia.

Acinetobacter baumannii: This organism can be multiply antibiotic resistant and also has the ability to survive in the environment for prolonged periods. Multiple samples including any clinical sites, rectal swabs and throat swabs may be helpful in early detection.

Carbapenemase-producing *Enterobacteriaceae*: These include bacteria such as *Escherichia coli* and *Klebsiella* spp. that have acquired genetic material making them resistant to multiple antibiotics including meropenem and imipenem, and therefore very difficult to treat. Any patients transferred from high-risk countries or hospitals must be pre-emptively isolated and rectal swabs taken to detect these organisms.

Diagnosis of trauma-related infections

Diagnosing traumatic wound infections can be extremely challenging as open wounds quickly become colonised and it can be very difficult to distinguish colonisation from infection. Blood cultures can be valuable but are not often positive in this setting. Deep biopsies taken at operation are the most valuable samples, but even in this circumstance, care must be taken to prevent contamination with colonising organisms. For suspected osteomyelitis, it is recommended that five or more samples are taken using separate sets of instruments to minimise the chances of contamination – the same organisms identified from multiple samples are usually associated with genuine infection.

Management of infected traumatic wounds

The management of infection in the setting of traumatic wounds is complex and there is unfortunately a poor evidence base to support much of what is done. There is no doubt that the mainstay of management is timely and rigorous surgical debridement. General principles of antibiotic treatment are that they should only be given when definitely indicated, that the antibiotic should be as narrow spectrum as possible and for as short a duration as possible both to prevent resistance developing in the patient being treated and transmission of resistant organisms to other patients in the same setting. Most hospitals have antibiotic policies based on local epidemiology and these should be adhered to wherever possible. Microbiological advice should be sought in complex cases. **Table 3** gives some suggested regimens for commonly occurring scenarios.

In general, antibiotics should only be used in cases of established infection; however, there are circumstances where pre-emptive or prophylactic antibiotics are indicated because heavy contamination of the wound means that subsequent infection appears inevitable. Good examples of this include open lower extremity fractures and penetrating trauma to the gut.

Table 3 Suggested antibiotic regimens for common conditions associated with trauma

Condition	First-line choice	Penicillin allergy
Fixation of closed fractures	Flucloxacillin single dose only	Teicoplanin single dose only
Open fractures	Co-amoxiclav for up to 72 hours or until wound closure plus co-amoxiclav and gentamicin at first debridement and teicoplanin and gentamicin at definitive soft tissue closure	Clindamycin for up to 72 hours or until wound closure plus clindamycin and gentamicin at first debridement and teicoplanin and gentamicin at definitive soft tissue closure
Simple wound infection/ cellulitis	Flucloxacillin	Clindamycin
Human and animal bites	Co-amoxiclav	Doxycycline and metronidazole or clindamycin and ciprofloxacin
Penetrating trauma to gut	Co-amoxiclav	Ciprofloxacin and metronidazole

Further reading

Anderson A, Miller A, Bookstaver P. Antimicrobial prophylaxis in open lower extremity fractures. Open Access Emerg Med 2011; 3:7–11.

Benedict K, Park BJ. Invasive fungal infections after natural disasters. Emerg Infect Dis 2014; 20:349–355.

Hospenthal DR, Murray CK, Anderson RC, et al. Guidelines for the prevention of infection after combat related injuries. J Trauma 2008; 64:S211–S220.

Related topics of interest

Anticoagulation and thromboembolism

Key points

- In all trauma cases, it is essential to establish whether the patient is on anticoagulants and particular attention must be paid to new less familiar agents (dabigatran and rivaroxaban)
- Established guidelines must be followed in the imaging of anticoagulated trauma patients
- Recommencement of anticoagulation or antiplatelet agents after trauma requires careful review of the risks and benefits

Introduction

This topic focusses on the management of two important issues in trauma care: the management of the injured patient who is already on warfarin and the prevention and management of venous thromboembolism (VTE) in trauma patients. There is minimal evidence to guide decision making in either situation, so retrospective studies, expert opinion, common sense and multidisciplinary decision making are required.

Patients admitted on anticoagulants

The additional risk attributable to anticoagulants and antiplatelet agents in trauma (and how best to investigate and manage these patients) has not been systematically evaluated in prospective studies; however, there are a number of predominantly single centre retrospective studies suggesting worse outcomes. The British Society for Haematology guidelines recommend that patients on a vitamin K antagonist (e.g. warfarin) presenting with head injury should have their international normalised ratio (INR) measured as soon as possible and recommend a lower threshold for performing a head CT scan. Patients on warfarin presenting with a strong suspicion of

intracerebral bleed are recommended to have their anticoagulation reversed even before the results of any investigations. There is evidence to support the intuitive view that warfarin increases the risk of haematoma expansion.

As delayed bleeding can occur in patients on warfarin, it has been suggested that patients with an initial normal CT scan after significant head injury with a supratherapeutic INR have this corrected with vitamin K and maintained as close to 2.0 as possible for 4 weeks. Vitamin K given intravenously will halve the INR within 6 hours. A dose of 5–10 mg is required for full reversal. Oral vitamin K may take up to 24 hours for effective reversal. Prothrombin complex concentrates (PCC) allow rapid and effective reversal of the INR in comparison to fresh frozen plasma.

For patients with multitrauma, without head injury, a pragmatic approach is required and rapid reversal of anticoagulation may be required, especially if there is active bleeding. For patients on the newer direct oral anticoagulants (DOACS), the timing of the last dose (if known) and the renal function can be used to estimate the degree of anticoagulation. Most of these drugs have a half-life of around 12 hours if there is adequate renal function. Basic laboratory tests may be affected by the DOACS (e.g. a prolonged activated partial thromboplastin time and thrombin time for dabigatran and prothrombin time/INR for rivaroxaban) but more specialised tests are required for accurate assay of drug levels and such tests may not be readily available in an emergency situation. Antidotes are undergoing trials at the time of writing. In the interim, many guidelines recommend the use of tranexamic acid and consideration of a PCC, activated PCC (e.g. Factor Eight Inhibitor By-passing Activity, or FEIBA) or recombinant activated factor VII.

Many antiplatelet drugs are irreversible inhibitors of platelets. There is an approximate 10% turnover in platelet mass per day. There is in vitro evidence to suggest that aspirin effects can be reversed by 30% normal platelet mass (3 days or one pooled platelet transfusion) but the P2Y12 inhibitors (such as clopidogrel and prasugrel) may require a higher proportion of normal circulating platelets to reverse the effect and it may take 7 days for normal platelet function to return.

Restarting anticoagulation or antiplatelet agents after trauma requires careful consideration of risks and benefits. In patients with intracerebral bleeding (not specifically trauma related), the American Heart Association and the European Stroke Initiative recommend that in patients with high risk of thromboembolism, anticoagulation should be restarted between 7 and 14 days. Antiplatelet agents are generally considered to be associated with a lower risk of recurrent cerebral bleeding, although the results of prospective studies are awaited.

Venous thromboembolism following trauma

VTE in the lower extremities is common after major trauma. In a study by Geerts et al. using venography, 58% of patients had deep vein thrombosis (DVT) with proximal thrombosis in 18%. Pulmonary embolism (PE) may account for >10% of trauma-related deaths, may be delayed by weeks and can occur despite thromboprophylaxis. The incidence of documented symptomatic VTE after injury is relatively low in some studies however (<1% from one database review).

For major trauma patients, American College of Clinical Pharmacy (ACCP) guidelines recommend pharmacologic prophylaxis [e.g. using low-molecular weight heparin (LMWH)] in combination with mechanical prophylaxis when this is not contraindicated by lower-extremity injury. For major trauma patients in whom LMWH is contraindicated, they suggest mechanical prophylaxis, preferably with intermittent pneumatic compression over no prophylaxis, adding pharmacologic prophylaxis when

the risk of bleeding diminishes. They also recommend that inferior vena cava (IVC) filters should not be used for primary VTE prevention. Although they probably reduce the risk of PE over the short term, complications appear to be frequent, and long-term benefits are unclear. Although retrievable filters have the potential to reduce long-term complications, they often are not removed. A more recent systematic review suggested a number needed to treat between 109 and 962 to prevent one PE. The timing of pharmacological prophylaxis after trauma is often a cause for anxiety. There is some evidence showing that in patients with solid abdominal organ injuries undergoing nonoperative management, early use of LMWH does not seem to increase failure rates or blood transfusion requirements. Using a decision analysis model, Scales et al. showed no clear advantage to providing or withholding anticoagulant prophylaxis for DVT/PE prevention at 24 hours after traumatic brain injury associated with intracerebral haemorrhage (ICH). Further prospective studies are required.

When VTE is diagnosed in the trauma patient, there is little evidence to guide the safe timing and dose of anticoagulation. In patients diagnosed with DVT or PE with a contraindication to anticoagulation IVC filter placement is an accepted alternative. Avoidance of therapeutic anticoagulation for at least 48 hours after high bleeding risk surgery has been recommended and a similar principle could be applied in major trauma requiring surgery. As previously discussed, therapeutic anticoagulation could be delayed for 7 days or more after ICH. LMWH is frequently used for therapeutic anticoagulation due to the short half-life and convenience; however, for patients at high risk of bleeding, unfractionated heparin infusions are an option as they can be quickly reversed and can be used in patients with acute renal injury. From a pragmatic point of view, oral anticoagulation should be delayed till the bleeding risk is sufficiently low and the patient no longer requires invasive procedures.

Further reading

British Committee for Standards in Haematology Writing group (Baglin TP, Brush J, Streiff M). Guidelines on use of vena cava filters. Br J Haematol 2006; 134:590–595.

Eberle BM, Schnüriger B, Inaba K, et al. Thromboembolic prophylaxis with low-molecular-weight heparin in patients with blunt solid abdominal organ injuries undergoing nonoperative management: current practice and outcomes. J Trauma 2011; 70:141–146.

Flibotte JJ, Hagan N, O'Donnell J, Greenberg SM, Rosand J. Warfarin, hematoma expansion, and outcome of intracerebral hemorrhage. Neurology 2004; 63:1059–1064.

Geerts WH, Code KI, Jay RM, Chen E, Szalai JP. A prospective study of venous thromboembolism after major trauma. N Engl J Med 1994; 331:1601–1606.

Gould M, Garcia DA, Wren SM, et al. Prevention of VTE in nonorthopedic surgical patients: antithrombotic therapy and prevention of thrombosis, 9th ed: American College of Chest Physicians Evidence-Based Clinical Practice Guidelines. Chest 2012; 141:e227S–e277S.

Haut ER, Garcia LJ, Shihab HM, et al. The effectiveness of prophylactic inferior vena cava filters in trauma patients: a systematic review and meta-analysis. JAMA Surg 2014; 149:194–202.

Ho KM, Burrell M, Rao S, Baker R. Incidence and risk factors for fatal pulmonary embolism after major trauma: a nested cohort study. Br J Anaesth 2010; 105:596–602.

Keeling D, Baglin T, Tait C, et al. British Committee for Standards in Haematology. Guidelines on oral anticoagulation with warfarin – fourth edition. Br J Haematol 2011; 154:311–324.

Knudson MM, Ikossi DG, Khaw L, Morabito D, Speetzen LS. Thromboembolism after trauma: an analysis of 1602 episodes from the American College of Surgeons National Trauma Data Bank. AnnSurg 2004; 24:490–498.

Li C, Hirsh J, Xie C, Johnston MA, et al. Reversal of the anti-platelet effects of aspirin and clopidogrel. J Thromb Haemost 2012; 10:521–528.

Related topics of interest

- Blood product (1:1:1) resuscitation (p. 42)
- Tranexamic acid (p. 298)
- Viscoelastic assessment of coagulation in trauma (p. 318)

Asphyxiation

Key points

- Asphyxiation is a common cause of death, particularly in younger males
- The resulting hypoxia and hypercarbia cause cell dysfunction, organ dysfunction and death
- Treated firstly by removing the cause, then supplying high flow oxygen and applying cause-specific therapies

Epidemiology

Asphyxia is a common cause of death, particularly in the younger male age group. The United Kingdom Office for National Statistics figures indicate that the category of hanging, strangulation and suffocation is one of the four most common specified mechanisms for injury and poisoning deaths. In 2011, hanging, strangulation, suffocation and poisoning were the most common causes of death in males aged 15–74 years. Most of these deaths were unintentional but a significant proportion were intentional, either suicidal (35% male, 19% female) or homicidal (4.5% male, 3.5% female). Data available from the Centre for Disease Control (CDC) in the United States indicates that between 1999 and 2004 there were approximately 4000 deaths per year attributable to various types of mechanical asphyxiation.

Pathophysiology

Defects involving any of the components of breathing and respiration (ventilation, pulmonary gas exchange, gas transport and cellular oxygen uptake and utilisation) can result in asphyxia. Causes of asphyxiation can be classified as mechanical, interfering with the physical process of breathing, or chemical, when an inhaled substance interferes with the body's ability to use oxygen (**Table 4**).

The final causative pathway is a deficiency of oxygen delivery to the tissues resulting in hypoxia. Asphyxial deaths typically involve respiratory arrest and bradycardia or asystole secondary to hypoxia-induced brainstem dysfunction. Individuals with significant comorbidities such as ischaemic heart disease may be exquisitely sensitive to hypoxia and may suffer exacerbation of these conditions involving myocardial ischaemia and cardiac arrhythmias. The hypoxia will often also be accompanied by hypercarbia and may result in cyanosis, vasodilatation, increased capillary permeability and endothelial disruption and ultimately organ dysfunction and death.

Table 4 Causes of asphyxiation	
Mechanical	**Chemical**
Strangulation	Carbon monoxide
Choking	Cyanide
Environmental (hypoxic atmospheres)	Hydrogen sulphide
Suffocation including smothering	
Traumatic (external pressure)	
Aspiration including drowning	
Postural (positional)	
Hanging	

Clinical features

The clinical features will vary depending upon the underlying causative factors but patients will exhibit signs and symptoms of difficulty breathing with an initially raised respiratory rate until they tire, and gasping as they attempt to increase oxygen uptake. Cyanosis may develop and breathing may be noisy if there is an airway obstruction such as a foreign body. There may be added breath sounds if there is intrinsic lung pathology or a pneumonitic effect from a chemical causative agent. Cardiovascular changes will include initial tachycardia and hypertension followed by a variety of arrhythmias and the neck veins may be distended. Eventually, depending on the degree of hypoxia, the patient will become unconscious and then deteriorate to cardiorespiratory arrest.

Investigations

If asphyxiation is suspected, basic investigations should include venous and arterial blood samples (the presence of a metabolic acidosis may indicate a toxic cause) and a chest X-ray. Venous blood samples should include measurement of urea and electrolytes, and a sample for toxicology. An arterial blood sample will show the level of hypoxia and hypercarbia and most laboratories will be able to measure carbon monoxide levels. A chest X-ray may reveal injuries or lung pathology, X-rays of any other suspected injuries should also be obtained. The value of all these investigations is significantly improved by serial measurements as trends in the values help to show disease progression and the efficacy of interventions.

Diagnosis

Diagnosis of asphyxiation is made clinically supported by observations from simple monitoring and investigations to identify the cause. Basic clinical examination of the cardiorespiratory system combined with the history of the incident and supported by pulse oximetry will make the diagnosis of asphyxia and in the majority of cases indicate the cause. It should be noted that most pulse oximeters cannot distinguish between oxyhaemoglobin and carboxyhaemoglobin which have similar absorption characteristics and will give a misleadingly high reading.

Treatment

A standard approach to the management and treatment of the seriously ill patient should be adopted. A safe approach to the casualty is essential bearing in mind that they may be in a hypoxic environment and the first action required may be extraction to safety. Safety of the rescuer is paramount, eliminating any dangers and minimising risks where possible. If there is a suspicion that cyanide exposure is possible then exhaled air resuscitation must

be avoided and a manual aid such as a bag-valve-mask should be used.

High flow oxygen is essential and respiration must be supported if it is inadequate. If intubation is required to secure the airway and provide ventilation, it should be performed by an appropriately trained individual using a rapid sequence induction technique with full monitoring and trained support personnel. If the cause of asphyxiation is traumatic, strangulation or hanging then there is a risk of cervical spine injury with or without disruption of the larynx and neck structures, potentially making intubation difficult and strategies for failed intubation must be in place.

Once the airway has been secured and ventilation optimised, other injuries and conditions can be identified and treated. Specific treatments and antidotes exist for some of the chemical causes of asphyxia and expert advice should be sought (**Table 5**).

Complications

The duration of hypoxia experienced will determine the degree of neurological damage sustained by the patient from full recovery through worsening levels of hypoxic brain injury to death. There may also be complications of the resuscitation process such as rib fractures, other organ damage such as myocardial injury due to ischaemia and complications specific to the underlying cause (**Table 6**).

Table 5 Treatments for specific causes of asphyxia	
Cause	**Treatment**
Carbon monoxide	100% O_2, hyperbaric oxygen may have a place
Cyanide	Amyl nitrate, hydroxocobalamin, sodium nitrite and thiosulphate
Hydrogen sulphide	Sodium nitrite, hyperbaric oxygen
Sodium nitrite, hyperbaric oxygen	Lung protective ventilation and PEEP
PEEP, positive end-expiratory pressure.	

Table 6 Complications of different causes of asphyxia	
Cause	Complications
Traumatic asphyxia	Other injuries caused by the compression
Hanging and strangulation	Injury to neck structures
Carbon monoxide	Long-term sequelae can include neurological and neuropsychiatric features including irritability, loss of concentration, personality and memory changes and parkinsonism

Further reading

Office for National Statistics (ONS). Injury and
   poisoning mortality in England and Wales, 2011.
   London: ONS, 2013.

Related topics of interest

- Chemical, biological, radiological and nuclear
  environments and trauma (p. 71)

- Epidemiology of trauma (p. 93)

Bariatric trauma

Key points

- The World Health Organization estimates that a global total of 700 million patients were obese in 2015
- Obesity is an independent predictor of mortality in blunt trauma patients and affects the incidence of complications and of multiorgan failure, the length of intensive care admissions, the number of ventilator days and the overall length of hospital admissions
- The injury pattern of obese patients is different to that of those with lower body mass

Introduction

Worldwide, and especially in developed countries, obesity is becoming an increasing problem. The World Health Organization estimates that in 2015 a global total of 700 million people will be obese. Not only does obesity make management more difficult following trauma, but obesity is also an independent predictor of mortality in blunt trauma patients and affects the incidence of complications and of multiorgan failure, the length of intensive care admissions, the number of ventilator days and the overall length of hospital admission. The association between mortality and body mass index (BMI) has not been demonstrated to be linear and so it cannot be assumed that only the super-obese will have the highest rates of complications.

In addition, the injury pattern of obese patients is different to that of those with lower body mass, with sparing of the head but an increased incidence of trunk and lower extremity trauma. Extremity trauma is more likely to result in displaced fractures, such as those of the ankle and elbow.

Pathophysiology of obesity in trauma

The insulin resistance often seen in obese patients has important effects on outcomes and rigorous glycaemic control is required from admission (when dysfunction may be most pronounced). Although the increased body mass has deleterious consequences, it must be supported. Patients in negative nitrogen balance during the early catabolic response to trauma are likely to have especially poor outcomes. Early specialist dietetic advice is essential in order to ensure that this complex metabolic balance is appropriately addressed.

Adipose tissue is not inert and there is increasing evidence to suggest that it has a role analogous to an endocrine organ. The resultant pro-inflammatory state presents challenges in trauma as it causes relative immune compromise and renders already traumatised tissues more liable to damage as well as having implications for infection and thromboembolic events. It has been known for some time that obese trauma patients are prone to venous thromboembolism, but attribution was usually made to the bed-ridden state of these patients. It has now been demonstrated that related to the inflammatory state of obesity, there exists a hypercoagulability which can be measured using thromboelastography/rotation thromboelastometry (TEG/ROTEM). It is therefore advisable to use TEG or ROTEM where available on admission, and to address coagulation issues within the multidisciplinary team. The choice of agent and dose is important as the dose-effect relationship becomes less predictable with rising BMI, and to use standard hospital protocols carries a significant risk of under-anticoagulation.

Patients who have attempted high-speed weight loss may have developed a degree of osteoporosis and so their fracture patterns may appear to be fragility fractures out of keeping with their age. Combining this bone fragility with the high degrees of displacement seen in extremity fractures means that acceptable open reduction and internal fixation require a bespoke operative strategy.

Cuthbertson ebb and flow model of metabolism in trauma outlines an early catabolism-catecholamine surge on injury followed by a high level of cytokine release which results in rapid breakdown of stored energy and the body rapidly losing muscle mass. Negative nitrogen balance has significant consequences for wound healing and oedema. Specialist metabolic advice is required to design a nutritional regime to protect as much as possible against the harmful effects of catabolism.

Practicalities of managing bariatric trauma patients

The trauma team needs to plan for bariatric patients from time and location of injury to discharge home. An acceptable patient journey requires ambulances and their crews to be equipped with uprated equipment and to be trained to use it in such a way as to protect their own and the patient's safety.

Adult trauma patients tend not to be weighed or even have their weight estimated, and not all high BMI patients will be immediately obvious. As dosages, equipment limits and risk stratification all depend on body weight in obese patients, there must be an established means of measuring or estimating body weight.

Trauma teams need to be familiar with the weight limits of beds, operating tables and pneumatic transfer assistance devices. With the advent of the concept of super-obesity, it is advisable for ambulance services to discuss the maximum weight handling ability of trauma centres, as a multiply injured patient who cannot be operated on will inevitable need to be transferred to an alternative centre.

Patients with gastric bands should have them deflated on admission to minimise the risk of aspiration. Centres unused to managing such devices need to seek early telephone advice from bariatric surgical services. Obese patients' relative immobility and high contact pressures make them at high risk of pressure sores. Their ongoing inflammatory response, potentially altered glycaemic control and immune suppression make healing established pressure sores extremely difficult and so meticulous nursing care is required for primary prevention. Early involvement of tissue viability teams is critical if pressure areas threaten to break down.

Adequate imaging is hard to achieve and to interpret in obese patients. In particular, focussed abdominal sonography for trauma is highly unlikely to deliver the four high quality views required to rule out free fluid and trauma teams should have a 'plan B' for these patients.

Surgical considerations

For the surgeon, there are intraoperative challenges including the accessibility of deeper spaces such as the pelvis, difficulty in achieving closed reduction in fractures and preoperative patient positioning in such a way as to afford access without causing or compromising pressure areas.

High degrees of fracture displacement imply significant soft tissue trauma and potentially difficult reduction. In suspected poor bone quality, the use of a locking construct may suggest itself, but this can be complicated by higher profile implants, carrying a higher risk of wound breakdown and infection in poor quality soft tissues.

In abdominal surgery, similar difficulties exist. The lithotomy and supine positions result in abdominal soft tissue compressing viscera and impeding venous return. There is proven increased intra-abdominal pressure in obesity – intraoperatively this may be iatrogenically caused by positioning but it must also be considered as a pre-existing problem when assessing a patient's risk of ischaemic bowel. While not the same entity as abdominal compartment syndrome, it is in some ways analogous, and should be considered as a cause of an unexplained lactate rise. The other potential cause to be excluded is body-weight crush injury: rhabdomyolysis secondary to a heavy and immobile patient traumatising their own muscle mass.

Further reading

Bochicchio GV, Joshi M, Bochicchio K, et al. Impact of obesity in the critically ill trauma patient: a prospective study. J Am Coll Surg 2006; 203:533–538.

Chesser TJS, Hammett RB, Norton SA. Orthopaedic trauma in the obese patient. Injury 2010; 41:247–252.

Liu T, Chen JJ, Bai XJ, Zheng GS, Gao W. The effect of obesity on outcomes in trauma patients: a meta-analysis. Injury 2013; 44:1145–1152.

Related topics of interest

- Metabolic response to trauma (p. 182)
- Viscoelastic assessment of coagulation in trauma (p. 318)

Blast trauma

Key points

- Explosions are complex events and can result in multiple complex injuries
- An understanding of the physics and pathophysiology underlying explosions is essential to anticipating injuries and treatment challenges
- Explosions can result in multiple casualties; each one requiring considerable use of health care resources – anticipating the likely needs of these patients is an essential part of planning for such an incident

Epidemiology

In modern warfare, approximately 80% of injuries result from explosive weapons, making such injuries much more common than gunshot injuries. In the civilian setting, explosive injuries are largely confined to terrorist attacks, which are becoming increasingly frequent. Casualty figures from some recent incidents are given in **Table 7**.

Pathophysiology

An explosion is a rapid, almost instantaneous conversion of chemical energy to kinetic energy and heat as an explosive material is oxidised. There are two components to the explosion: the blast wave and blast wind. The blast wave travels outward from the epicentre of the explosion faster than the blast wind and involves a very rapid, almost instantaneous rise in pressure which lasts for <100 ms. The blast wave travels through the air or water in a manner analogous to a sound wave. The blast wind is a result of the mass movement of gases away from the epicentre of the explosion. The two components of the explosion are shown schematically in **Figure 11**.

Injuries due to explosions

Blast injuries are conventionally classified using the system as follows.

Primary blast injuries

These result from the effects of the blast wave as it strikes and passes ('couples') into the body. Energy is transferred into tissues at the interfaces between gas and tissue.

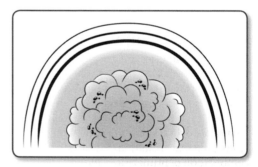

Figure 11 The radial expansion of the blast wave and the explosive products or 'blast wind' moving radially away from the epicentre of the explosion.

Table 7 Recent terrorist attacks with improvised explosive devices		
Attack	**Fatalities**	**Injured**
Nigeria Boko Haram bombing 2015	58	139
Boston Marathon bombing 2013	3	264
Oslo bombing 2011	8	209
7/7 London bombing 2005	52	700
Madrid train bombing 2004	191	1800
Myyrmanni bombing 2002	7	166
Omagh bombing 1998	29	220
Oklahoma City bombing 1995	167	592

Therefore, gas containing organs including the lungs, intestines and eardrums are particularly vulnerable. The energy of the blast wave dissipates rapidly as it moves away from the epicentre of the explosion and therefore significant primary blast injuries are relatively rare as casualties close enough to an explosion to be severely affected by the blast wave are often fatally injured by secondary blast injury.

Secondary blast injuries

These injuries are caused by material accelerated by the expanding explosive products impacting on the casualty's body. These are commonly, but inaccurately referred to as 'shrapnel' wounds. Material accelerated by the blast can be part of the device (e.g. nails or the casing of an artillery shell) or from the environment, including dirt or debris used to conceal an improvised explosive device, foliage, body parts or glass from shattered windows. The former are referred to as primary, the latter secondary fragments.

Tertiary blast injuries

Tertiary blast injuries are caused by the impact of the blast wind on the body and include the effects of impact of an energised body when it strikes other objects or the ground. Tertiary injuries have traditionally included single and multiple amputations, although these actually arise from a combination of primary and tertiary effects in that severing of the limb by the blast wind follows fracture of the bones caused by the blast wave.

Other injuries

Other injuries that do not fit into this classification include burns, crush and psychological injuries. These are sometimes referred to as quaternary injuries, but this lumped together classification of unrelated entities is unhelpful. Burns are common from improvised explosives using 'home-made' explosives, which are often poorly milled and therefore behave more like very rapid combustions rather than true explosions. In these 'explosions', the explosive products are still burning as they are propelled away from the epicentre. Burn injuries also result from secondary fires ignited by the initial explosion. Crush injuries can occur if casualties are caught in buildings that collapse due to a blast.

Clinical features

Casualties from an explosive incident will principally exhibit features of haemorrhagic shock. Secondary blast injuries can result in significant tissue destruction including traumatic amputation resulting in massive blood loss.

Respiratory difficulties occur as a result of blast lung. In severe cases, the blast wave can result in a pneumothorax as shown in the radiograph in **Figure 12**. Blast also causes pulmonary haemorrhage and oedema as shown in the CT scan in **Figure 13**. Intestinal wall haemorrhage and perforation of intestine may also occur and may be delayed in presentation. These are primary blast injuries.

Tympanic membrane rupture is a poor indicator of the risk of primary blast injury in the lungs and intestines. Although the pressure required to injure the lungs and intestines (c.250 kg/m^2) is higher than that at which tympanic membrane rupture occurs (c.50 kg/m^2), the risk of tympanic membrane rupture is related to several factors including the position of the head relative to the explosion. Blast injury to the lung and intestines can occur with intact tympanic membranes and aural examination is a poor screening tool for blast lung with a sensitivity of around 40%.

Investigations

The purpose of investigation is to identify occult bony fractures including spinal injuries and to diagnose primary blast damage to the lung and intestines. For casualties with minor blast injuries, this can be performed with a chest X-ray and plain radiographs of the limbs. In cases of more seriously injured casualties, especially those with extensive external injuries, investigation with spiral CT from head-to-proximal femur is appropriate.

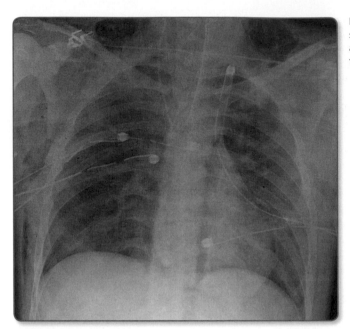

Figure 12 Chest radiograph showing a patient with blast lung and bilateral pneumothoraces treated with bilateral chest drains.

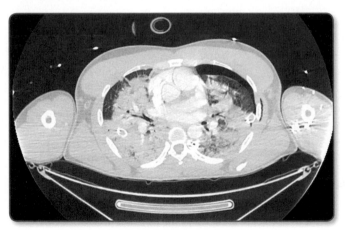

Figure 13 CT scan showing pulmonary contusion and a left-sided pneumothorax in a casualty in close proximity to an explosion.

Soft tissue and bony disruption is not difficult to diagnose. Emerging blast injury to bowel or lung can be more challenging. Blast lung is diagnosed by the presence of pulmonary infiltrates, pneumothorax or pneumomediastinum on imaging. Bowel injury is difficult to diagnose, even on high-resolution CT and may only be detected once perforation occurs and peritonitis develops.

Treatment

The priorities for the treatment of blast casualties are haemorrhage control, ventilatory support and prevention of infection. Haemorrhage should be controlled with the use of pressure dressings, tourniquets or haemostatic dressings. In hospital, surgery should be carried out with simultaneous volume resuscitation with blood products. Massive transfusions may be required and these should consist of appropriate ratios of platelets and plasma to packed red blood cells. Resuscitation may be guided by thromboelastography. Antibiotics and tranexamic acid should be administered as soon as possible.

Initial surgical intervention may well be limited to packing of abdominal organs and shunting of arteries as temporising measures.

Blast injuries can produce grossly contaminated wounds with severe soft-tissue disruption, which require surgical treatment. Grossly contaminated or necrotic tissue should be excised. Myofascial compartments should be released and all wounds irrigated with large amounts of saline delivered at low pressure. Topical negative pressure therapy allows large wounds to be dressed and effectively sealed.

Wounds caused by explosions often evolve over several days and repeated episodes of debridement and irrigation may be required before they can be closed primarily or covered using plastic surgical techniques. Excised tissue should be sent for microbiological culture and histology including staining for fungal infection. Fractures can be stabilised initially with external fixation. Internal fixation of fractures should be delayed until wounds are closed or covered.

Complications

Blast injuries are typically complicated by infection secondary to massive contamination of wounds. The evolution of blast wounds can occur over several days and can frustrate premature efforts to close wounds. Lung protective ventilation is indicated for blast injury patients to reduce the risk of primary blast lung injury being exacerbated by mechanical ventilation.

Further reading

Brooks AJ, Clasper J, Midwinter M, Hodgetts TJ, Mahoney PF. Ryan's Ballistic Trauma, 3rd edn. London: Springer, 2011.

Midwinter MJ. Damage control surgery in the era of damage control resuscitation. J R Army Med Corps 2009; 155:323–326.

Penn-Barwell JG, Bennett PM, Kay A, Sargeant ID. Severe lower extremity combat trauma study

G. Acute bilateral leg amputation following combat injury in the UK servicemen. Injury 2014; 45:1105–1110.

Penn-Barwell JG, Bishop JRB, Roberts S, Midwinter M. Injuries and outcomes: UK military casualties from Iraq and Afghanistan 2003–2012. Bone Joint J 2013; 95-B-Supp 26:1.

Related topics of interest

Blood product (1:1:1) resuscitation

Key points

- The administration of packed red blood cells does not replace clotting factors or platelets
- In patients with significant blood loss, replacement of blood products should aim to replace all the vital elements of whole blood, including clotting factors and platelets
- The term 1:1:1 resuscitation has been given to the practice of replacing blood, plasma and platelets in equal ratios

Introduction

Exsanguinating haemorrhage is the commonest cause of preventable death in both civilian and military trauma, thus control of bleeding in trauma is of critical importance. However, resuscitation that restores a functioning circulating volume is additionally required. Modern resuscitation protocols are based on research that has demonstrated improved patient outcomes with the early use of resuscitation using blood products.

Background

Blood transfusion has been used in the management of trauma since the early 19th century. Since then, lessons learned in times of war have had a significant impact on the development of blood transfusion. The capability to store whole blood for transfusion was developed in 1915 during the First World War. However, the widespread use of whole blood banking did not take place until it was necessitated by the Second World War (1939–1945). During the war in Vietnam (1955–1975), there was a need to transport a vast quantity of stored blood over large distances. This led to the fractionation of whole blood into its component parts (red blood cell units, plasma and platelets) which had a longer shelf life. This also provided a

theoretical advantage in that the patients could be transfused only those components they were deemed to require, thereby avoiding wastage and improving safety. The administration of different blood components was widely accepted as optimal management for all indications where blood transfusion was required without real knowledge of their effectiveness. Subsequent component therapy transfusion guidelines for use in trauma have tended to be based upon expert consensus, data from euvolaemic surgical patients and data from the historical use of whole blood.

Over the past 12 years of conflict in Iraq and Afghanistan, multiple retrospective analyses of combat trauma have demonstrated that replacing lost blood volume with a ratio of component blood products similar to that of whole blood improves survival. This 'balanced' blood product administration is termed '1:1:1' resuscitation: a transfusion ratio one unit of red blood cells, one unit of plasma and one unit of platelets.

Nonblood resuscitation fluids

Traditionally, hypovolaemic trauma patients have initially been treated with 1–2 L of crystalloid (Hartmann's solution or 0.9% sodium chloride). If this did not produce an adequate response, or produced a transient response, red blood cell units were then transfused – the use of plasma, platelets or cryoprecipitate was reserved for those with laboratory evidence of a coagulopathy. The need to assay these laboratory markers caused a significant delay in identifying coagulopathy, and they did not give the complete picture of the impaired coagulation specific to trauma. Multiple studies have demonstrated that 25–30% of major trauma patients have a coagulopathy on arrival at hospital – termed 'trauma-induced coagulopathy' (TIC) – driven by tissue trauma and systemic hypoperfusion. This leads to widespread anticoagulation and fibrinolysis, probably via endothelial activation of protein C. Patients with TIC have up to a sixfold increase in mortality. Exacerbation of TIC is multifactorial but includes a dilutional coagulopathy caused by nonblood product use (such as the use of crystalloid solutions). Crystalloid use in major trauma patients is also associated with a significant increase in bacteraemia, acute respiratory distress syndrome and acute renal failure. Conversely, the early use of plasma has been shown to both prevent and treat this coagulopathy, with the potential to reduce mortality by 50%.

Crystalloids do have some distinct logistical advantages over blood: they are relatively inexpensive, do not require special storage or documentation, do not pose the same infection or transfusion-reaction risks and are not generally in limited supply. However, there is an increasing weight of evidence demonstrating an increase in mortality and morbidity with the use of crystalloids compared to blood products in the management of trauma.

What ratio of component blood products is best?

It is logical that a ratio of component blood products that most resembles whole blood would provide the optimal treatment. Initial retrospective data series did indeed suggest that a ratio of 1:1:1 of red blood cell units to plasma to platelets conferred the greatest survival advantage. However, a number of these studies are adversely affected by survivor bias, in that a significant number of patients died before plasma was available to be given (and therefore had a low plasma to red blood cell unit ratio). In contrast, a single prospective study has shown no benefit of a red blood cell unit to plasma ratio >1:2, and indeed suggested the possibility of superior outcomes (by showing maximal improvement in clotting times and clot strength) at a ratio between 1:2 and 3:4.

Although it is recognised that both platelets and fibrinogen (normally given as cryoprecipitate or fibrinogen concentrate) are needed in balanced resuscitation, the ratios that confer the greatest survival advantage are unknown. The addition of fibrinogen to balanced resuscitation is sometimes termed 1:1:1:1. Point of care testing, such as viscoelastic assessment, enables bespoke resuscitation and helps tailor the specific component needs of trauma patients. Its use in the military setting has led to an increase in the use of plasma, platelets and cryoprecipitate, but not red blood cell units.

Is there a difference between whole blood and balanced component therapy?

1:1:1 therapy does not have the same properties of whole blood, providing only half to two thirds of the oxygen-carrying capacity and clotting function. Typical values include a haemoglobin value of 9.6 g/dL, platelet count of 87,000 and 65% of clotting function. The clinical value of whole blood compared to 1:1:1 resuscitation has only been demonstrated in retrospective analysis of combat trauma patients. Between 2001 and 2007 over 6000 patients received whole blood together with component therapy – these patients had a significantly higher survival rate than those who received component therapy alone. However, another study demonstrated that the use of whole blood showed no benefit over 1:1:1, but both of these studies are likely to be affected by multiple confounders. Fresh whole blood has occasionally been used in patients with ongoing TIC despite their receiving optimal component therapy. Anecdotally this has resulted in remarkable clinical improvement, leading to some calling it 'the elixir of life'.

Pharmacological adjuncts to 1:1:1 resuscitation

Recent civilian and military trials have highlighted the beneficial effects of early (<3 hours after injury) administration of tranexamic acid (TXA) in reducing mortality in the severely injured and, in the UK, this has been widely included in massive transfusion protocols. The mechanism by which TXA confers a survival advantage is not well understood, and is likely to be more complex than inhibition of hyperfibrinolysis alone. In addition, the optimal timing, dosing and indications for treatment are not yet fully understood.

Contemporary and future research

A randomised study comparing ratios of red blood cell units to plasma and to platelets in different ratios (1:1:1 vs. 2:1:1) has recently been carried out in 12 US trauma centres. The results of this research study [Pragmatic Randomized Optimal Platelet and Plasma Ratios (PROPPR)] are now available and demonstrate that more patients in the 1:1:1 group achieved haemostasis and fewer died from exsanguination in the first 24 hours compared to the 1:1:2 group but that there was no difference in all cause mortality between the two groups. Several studies in massive transfusion have highlighted the variability observed between patients in their individual response to ratios of red blood

cell units and plasma. The reason for this is poorly understood and future research might aim to develop tools that can effectively tailor massive transfusion to individual patients' needs, above that provided by current capabilities such as rotational thromboelastogram (which already allows clinicians to move away from predefined ratios after initial transfusion).

The major obstacle to providing balanced blood administration is the availability of products. Development of red blood cell substitutes, in the form of novel oxygen carriers (haemoglobin-based oxygen carriers and fluorocarbon emulsions), has been ongoing for decades without production of a commercially viable product. Lyophilised or freeze-dried plasma is currently being used in some areas, and further research is needed to investigate the feasibility of using freeze-dried platelets in a similar way. The combination of these technologies could theoretically produce a complete freeze-dried balanced resuscitation product, which would have the greatest potential utility in prehospital and military environments.

Further reading

Borgman M, Spinella P, Perkins J, et al. The ratio of blood products transfused affects mortality in patients receiving massive transfusions at a Combat Support Hospital. J Trauma 2007; 63:805–813.

Davenport R, Curry N, Manson J, et al. Hemostatic effects of fresh frozen plasma may be maximal at red cell ratios of 1:2. J Trauma 2011; 70:90–95.

Duchesne J, Heaney J, Guidry C, et al. Diluting the benefits of hemostatic resuscitation. J Trauma 2013; 75:76–82.

Hess J, Holcomb J. Transfusion practice in military trauma. Transfus Med 2008; 18:143–150.

Holcomb JB, Tilley BC, Baraniuk S, et al. Transfusion of plasma, platelets, and red blood cells in a 1:1:1 vs

a 1:1:2 ratio and mortality in patients with severe trauma. The PROPPR randomized clinical trial. JAMA 2015; 313:471–482.

Khan S, Brohi K, Chana M, et al. International trauma research network (INTRN). Hemostatic resuscitation is neither hemostatic nor resuscitative in trauma hemorrhage. J Trauma 2014; 76:561–567;567–568.

Spinella PC, Perkins JG, Grathwohl KW, Beekley AC, Holcomb JB. Warm fresh whole blood is independently associated with improved survival for patients with combat-related traumatic injuries. J Trauma Injury Infect Crit Care 2009; 66:S69–76.

Related topics of interest

Blunt and penetrating cardiac trauma

Key points

- The presentation of cardiac injury is variable and the mortality is high
- Vital signs may underestimate the depth of shock and classical presentations are unreliable. The history is commonly the key factor in diagnosis
- Rapid evaluation and expeditious surgery are essential for survival

Epidemiology

While the true incidence of cardiac trauma cannot be exactly defined, the US National Trauma Data Bank estimates the incidence of penetrating cardiac injury to be 0.16% of all trauma admissions. Approximately two thirds result from gunshot wounds and the remainder from stab wounds. A busy US urban level I trauma centre reported that cardiac injury occurred in 6.4% of those presenting with penetrating thoracic injuries. Not surprisingly, penetrating cardiac injury carries a high mortality, with an overall survival rate of only 19%, which has not demonstrably improved over decades. Mortality is related to the chamber involved, gunshot versus knife wound, and haemodynamics on admission.

The incidence of blunt cardiac trauma is even more difficult to determine with precision. The definition varies widely, some are based on ECG criteria, others rely on cardiac biochemical markers and still others employ echocardiographic findings. Overwhelmingly the aetiology is a motor vehicle collision. The clinical relevance of blunt cardiac injury is limited to patients with significant arrhythmias or new ventricular dysfunction, while the clinical implications of penetrating cardiac trauma are obvious.

The anterior location of the right ventricle makes it the most frequently injured chamber in both blunt and penetrating trauma. With severe blunt force the left ventricle may be compromised. In decreasing frequency, the cardiac chambers injured from penetrating injury are right ventricle, left ventricle, right and left atria.

Pathophysiology

Penetrating cardiac trauma can result in exsanguinating haemorrhage or pericardial tamponade, either of which can be fatal. If tamponade is not present, uncontrolled bleeding into the pleural space demands rapid evaluation and treatment. Vital signs may be maintained in haemorrhagic shock until compensatory mechanisms are exhausted, resulting in death before operative intervention can be performed. The well-defined triad of acidosis, coagulopathy and hypothermia is the result of ongoing blood loss and shock. Therefore, 'normal' vital signs are a poor marker for the depth of shock, which is better determined by base deficit and serum lactate.

Tamponade resulting from penetrating injury may be protective. Although the patient may be in profound shock and markedly hypotensive, exsanguinating haemorrhage will not have occurred. Most published reports confirm the survival benefit of tamponade. Rapid accumulation of as little as 50 m/L of blood causes increased intrapericardial pressure with resultant decreased venous return and cardiac output, hypotension and ultimately death. Beck's triad of muffled heart sounds, hypotension and jugular venous distension is rarely present and precise auscultation of heart sounds is difficult in a noisy trauma bay. Unlike penetrating trauma, there is a wider spectrum of physiologic response to blunt injury including clinically silent, ventricular dysfunction and chamber rupture which may result from direct energy transfer from the chest wall to the heart if it is severe enough. Fortunately this devastating injury, thought to occur at end diastole, is quite rare; however, it is almost uniformly fatal. Myocardial contusion is far more common but its clinical significance is questionable, unless accompanied by ventricular dysfunction or dysrhythmia. The presence of biochemical markers of cardiac injury, specifically troponin, may only be important when combined with echocardiographic findings of right ventricular dysfunction.

Clinical features

Cardiac injury must be suspected with any penetrating injury within the 'cardiac box', defined as the anterior thorax bounded by the clavicles, the costal margin and the midclavicular line. Cardiac injury can result from injury outside the precordium and such injuries are associated with a higher mortality than those within its boundaries, possibly because cardiac injury is not suspected.

Clinical presentation is highly variable ranging from haemodynamic stability to cardiac arrest. Again, the vital signs may be misleading, particularly in younger patients who have better compensatory ability. Shock and depth of shock are characterised by base deficit and lactate. Morality increases with both higher base deficit and the inability to clear lactate. In addition to the standard trauma 'ABCs' a thorough, rapid physical examination is mandatory, identifying the location of wounds, cardiorespiratory status and heart and lung sounds. A portable chest radiograph (CXR) and ultrasound evaluation (focussed assessment with sonography in trauma) of the pericardium and abdomen are essential.

Penetrating injures are generally obvious but smaller puncture wounds, especially in the axilla, may be overlooked. Blunt cardiac injury may not be suspected at first. Blunt trauma may result in other significant injuries, and hypotension, if present, may be thought to be secondary to associated injuries and not ventricular dysfunction. The presence of a sternal fracture, bilateral flail segments or retrosternal haematoma should alert the clinician to the possibility of an associated blunt cardiac injury.

Investigations

A portable CXR is vital; it may be diagnostic of both haemothorax and pneumothorax, but not tamponade. The usefulness of ultrasound cannot be underestimated. Rapid assessment for the presence of haemopericardium and haemoperitoneum can be performed. Blood samples should be sent for full blood count, urea and electrolytes, coagulation profile, lactate and, type and cross. An arterial blood gas is extremely important as it gives vital information regarding oxygenation, ventilation and depth of shock.

The role of ultrasound has been mentioned and is operator-dependent. Formal echocardiography should be reserved for the stable patient with equivocal ultrasound findings. Likewise additional imaging, such as CT scanning, should only be performed in haemodynamically stable patients. This point is crucial; unstable patients need an operation, not additional imaging.

Diagnosis

The combination of physical examination, CXR, ultrasound and haemodynamics will generally confirm the diagnosis. Penetrating cardiac trauma, without tamponade but with an associated haemothorax (which may be indistinguishable from a haemothorax from a noncardiac thoracic injury), will often result in haemodynamic instability. There may or may not be ultrasound evidence of a residual haemopericardium. Tamponade usually presents with some degree of hypotension, ranging from mild to profound, and haemopericardium on ultrasound.

The diagnosis of blunt cardiac injury, especially myocardial contusion, is challenging. Arrhythmias will be seen on a 12-lead ECG and continuous ECG monitoring. Cardiac enzymes are of little value. Formal echocardiography is very useful in determining overall ventricular and valvular function, and regional wall motion abnormalities.

Sudden cardiovascular collapse can occur with either a blunt or penetrating mechanism, but is more commonly seen with the latter. It is, therefore, imperative that the evaluation, workup and diagnosis be performed as rapidly as possible.

A pericardial window remains the gold standard in determining the presence of haemopericardium. The procedure is performed under general anaesthesia. A midline incision is placed over the xiphoid, which is excised, the sternum is elevated, the diaphragm located and using blunt dissection the pericardium is identified. The pericardium is grasped with forceps or Allis clamps and incised. A positive window requires sternotomy. Gentle anaesthetic induction is crucial as patients in tamponade are exquisitely preload dependent, the loss of vasomotor tone on induction can lead to cardiac arrest. A pericardial window is definitive and should be performed if ultrasound is equivocal or unavailable, or if the diagnosis is in doubt.

Treatment

The treatment of penetrating injury is straightforward: operative repair. A comprehensive discussion of the technical details is beyond the scope of this topic. The interested reader is referred to the further reading. Two incisions are used to expose the mediastinum; left anterolateral thoracotomy, which can be extended across the midline as a 'clamshell', and median sternotomy. The advantages of the anterolateral approach are that it is rapid, provides adequate cardiac exposure and is familiar to general surgeons. The main disadvantage is that placing the incision too inferiorly complicates closure and may hinder exposure. The incision should be placed in the inframammary fold. Placing a 20° bump under the back with extension of the ipsilateral arm improves surgical exposure. Median sternotomy is the incision of choice as it provides optimal cardiac exposure. The main determinant of which incision is selected is the surgeon's familiarity with it and confidence in performing it.

Once the mediastinum has been exposed the pericardium is incised; if an anterolateral incision is employed, the pericardium is opened anterior to the phrenic nerve; for sternotomy, the pericardium is opened widely and a pericardial sling constructed. Following evacuation of the haemopericardium the source of bleeding is sought.

There are several techniques for achieving temporary control of cardiac haemorrhage: digital pressure, placement of a Foley catheter and the use of skin staples. The main disadvantage of the Foley is dislodgement thus enlarging the injury. Skin staples have been used to gain temporary control of cardiac wounds until definitive repair can be performed. Digital control is a simple and direct method, and need not completely stop the bleeding but rather decrease it, thereby facilitating definitive repair. It is the author's preferred method.

Atrial injuries can often be controlled with a partial occluding clamp and repaired with 3-0 or 4-0 polypropylene running or horizontal mattress sutures. Injuries to the left atrium are infrequent but challenging given its posterior location. Ventricular injuries are repaired with 3-0 polypropylene, either running or interrupted horizontal mattress. The latter is the author's preference. A larger curve of the needle facilitates engaging the tissue at a right angle and it is essential to drive the needle following its curve. While most injuries can be closed without pledgets, they may be used if the ventricular wall is thin or friable.

Blunt cardiac injuries seldom require definitive treatment. Continuous ECG monitoring for 24 hours may be all that is necessary, and dysrhythmias should be treated using standard therapy. Rarely is the right ventricular dysfunction so severe as to require inotropic support.

Complications

The complications following penetrating cardiac injury are those associated with thoracic surgery for trauma and with mechanical ventilation: pleural effusion, atelectasis, empyema, bacteraemia, wound infection and remote organ failure. Sternal dehiscence and mediastinitis are complications specific to sternotomy. Septal defects and valvular injury are quite rare and diagnosed by echocardiography. Complications are infrequent following blunt trauma; however, postpericardiotomy syndrome can occur with either mechanism.

Further reading

Degiannis E, Bowley DM, Westaby S. Penetrating cardiac injury. Ann R Coll Surg Engl 2005; 87:61–63.

O'Connor JV, Ditillo M, Scalea TM. Penetrating cardiac injury: diagnosis, treatment and outcome. J Royal Army Med Corps 2009; 155:185–190.

O'Connor JV. Cardiac trauma. In: Franco KL, Thourani VH. Cardiothoracic Surgery Review. Philadelphia: Lippincott Williams & Wilkins, 2012.

Wall MJ, Tsai P, Mattox KL. Heart and thoracic vascular injuries. In: Mattox, Moore and Feliciano. Trauma, 7th edition. New York: McGraw Hill, 2012.

Related topics of interest

- Damage control resuscitation and surgery (p. 83)
- Resuscitative balloon occlusion of the aorta (p. 248)
- Thoracic trauma (p. 288)

Brachial plexus injuries

Key points

- Early diagnosis is vital to prevent worsening of the lesion due to axonal cell death and to improve the outcome of surgical repair
- Detailed examination is required to determine the anatomical distribution of the lesion and to ensure that associated injuries are not overlooked
- Early nerve exploration, decompression and repair provide the best opportunity for nerve recovery

Anatomy

The brachial plexus is formed from the anterior primary rami of C5 to T1 (**Figure 14**). The T1 root carries sympathetic outflow to the head, neck and upper limb. The five roots enter the posterior triangle with the subclavian artery between the scalenus anterior and medius muscles. Here C5 and C6 combine to form the upper, C7 continues as the middle and C8 and T1 form the lower trunk. Each trunk has anterior and posterior divisions behind the clavicle and combinations of the divisions within the axilla

form three cords named according to their relationship to the second part of the axillary artery behind pectoralis minor.

The posterior divisions combine to form the posterior cord, the anterior divisions of the upper and middle trunks form the lateral cord and the medial cord is formed by the continuation of the anterior division of the lower trunk. Branches from the cords define the peripheral nerve anatomy of the upper limb. The median nerve is formed by branches from the lateral and medial cords and lies anterior to the third part of the axillary artery.

Epidemiology

Traumatic brachial plexus injuries in young patients are commonly associated with high-energy trauma in motorcycle accidents, pedestrian road traffic collisions, rollover motor vehicle accidents, vehicular ejection and falls from height. Sporting accidents particularly in equine, cycling and alpine sports account for a significant proportion of the remainder in the young adult. In the older patient, lower-energy falls resulting in fractures and dislocations around the

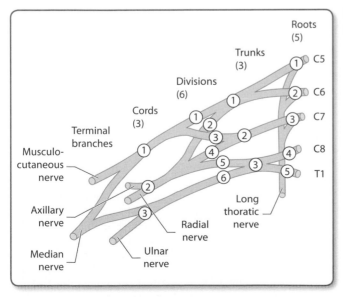

Figure 14 Anatomy of the brachial plexus.

shoulder girdle account for a second peak in incidence. Open injuries are seen as a result of civilian assaults with stab injuries and gunshot wounds and military combat wounds with high energy gunshot wounds, blast injury and fragmentation injury.

Pathophysiology

The upper brachial plexus (supraclavicular) is vulnerable to injury with forced lateral flexion and rotation of the cervical spine and depression of the shoulder girdle. The lower brachial plexus (infraclavicular) crosses the shoulder joint and is prone to injury with fractures and dislocations of the shoulder girdle. Nerves may be injured by compression, traction or laceration.

Nerve compression may result from haematoma associated with concomitant vascular injury, from dislocations or from fracture displacement. Initially there is a temporary conduction block with nerve ischaemia, intraneural oedema or segmental demyelination which may progress to axonal death (axonopathy due to Wallerian degeneration) if the compression is not relieved.

Traction injury results in axonal disruption with either physical continuity of the nerve (axonotmesis) or nerve rupture (neurotmesis). Axonotmesis injuries may vary in severity depending on the degree of disruption of supporting tissues within the nerve (Sunderland classification) with low-grade axonal injury having rapid axonal regrowth at 2–4 mm per day, medium grade less complete and slower regrowth at 1 mm per day and severe grade injury with no regrowth beyond the site of injury resulting in a neuroma-in-continuity due to dense intraneural scarring.

Traction may also result in direct avulsion of nerve roots from the spinal cord. This is termed a preganglionic injury because the site of injury is proximal to the dorsal root ganglion where the sensory nerve cell bodies are located. This spinal cord level injury may involve the long tracts supplying the lower limbs. Nerve laceration may occur from penetrating wounds or from sharp bone fragments.

Failure to promptly diagnose and treat a nerve lesion may result in a worsening of the lesion with axonal cell death. Following injury, the axon cell body upregulates to prepare for axonal regeneration but failure to restore physical continuity of the nerve promptly will result in downregulation of cellular activity and eventually programmed cell death (apoptosis). Early diagnosis and treatment provide more favourable outcomes in nerve surgery.

Clinical features

The nerves within the plexus may be injured at different sites and to different degrees. When a mixed nerve (motor, sensory and vasomotor) has a neurotmesis or axonotmesis injury, there is complete loss of function in the territories supplied by that nerve with flaccid paralysis, areflexia, total loss of sensation and dry erythematous skin due to loss of autonomic function. Patients will also experience pain in the territory of the nerve and tapping over the site of injury will produce unpleasant sensations in the territory of the injured nerve (Hoffmann–Tinel sign). If the nerve is avulsed from the spinal cord the signs of a complete nerve injury will exist but the Hoffman–Tinel sign is absent and the pain experienced is severe deafferentiation pain. Lower degrees of nerve injury with conduction block (demyelination) rather than axonopathy will result in flaccid paralysis and insensate skin in the territory of the injured nerve but there will be preservation of function in small unmyelinated nerve fibres. This was formerly termed neurapraxia with intact autonomic function and preservation of C-fibre activity and deep muscle sensation.

Rupture of the upper trunk will result in loss of biceps, supraspinatus, infraspinatus, deltoid, teres minor, brachialis and brachioradialis. Clinically there is no shoulder abduction or external rotation and elbow flexion is absent. Avulsion of the C5 and C6 nerve roots may result additionally in loss of dorsal scapular nerve, long thoracic nerve and possibly phrenic nerve function. If the C7 root is also involved, there will also be loss of elbow, wrist and finger extension. The lower nerve roots C8 and T1 are less commonly involved in isolation than as a part of a pan-plexus injury. They are susceptible to avulsion injury due to the lack of proximal branches and the direct line of pull to the spinal cord. Avulsion will result in loss of finger flexion, dextrous hand function (intrinsic muscles) and loss of sensation in the medial arm, forearm and hand. In addition, there is a loss of sympathetic outflow to the cervical sympathetic chain with hemifacial anhidrosis, partial ptosis and miosis (Horner's sign).

Injury at the infraclavicular level to the cords or their branches will clinically resemble proximal peripheral nerve injury rather than the radicular pattern seen in the supraclavicular lesions.

Examination

A thorough neurological examination should be performed and documented as part of the secondary survey. Muscle charting should be used to record the Medical Research Council (MRC) grade of muscle strength. Sensation should be recorded as normal, altered or absent in all cutaneous territories. Autonomic dysfunction should be recorded and note made of any features of a Horner's syndrome. Lower limb examination to establish long tract dysfunction (clonus, hyper-reflexia and dissociated sensory loss) is essential.

Vessels, bones and joints in the injured limb must be examined because there is a high incidence of compartment syndrome and concomitant musculoskeletal injury without pain due to the brachial plexus injury. Early diagnosis is not always possible because patients may be ventilated due to associated head, chest and abdominal injuries but often a patient will be noted to have a unilateral brachial paresis on reversing paralysis and reducing sedation during weaning. A careful examination at this stage may help establishing an early diagnosis.

Investigations

The trauma chest radiograph may identify phrenic nerve paralysis and rib, clavicle and shoulder girdle fractures. The trauma computed tomography (CT) scan may identify cervical spine, first rib and scapula fractures which are associated with brachial plexus injuries. CT angiography may identify major proximal upper limb vessel disruption. Skeletal survey of the paralysed limb will often identify occult fractures and dislocations.

MRI of the cervical spine and brachial plexus is useful in identifying established pseudomeningoceles in nerve root avulsions arising from tearing of the dural coverings around the exiting nerve root at the foramen and consequent cerebrospinal fluid leak. There may be evidence of epidural bleeding around the spinal cord, cord oedema and fractures and ligamentous injuries in the cervical spinal. MRI has replaced the former gold standard of CT myelography to identify avulsed nerve roots.

Neurophysiological tests confirm the clinical suspicion of brachial plexus injury and provide information on the site and degree of nerve injury. In postganglionic ruptures, there is absent motor and sensory conduction in the injured nerve after Wallerian degeneration has occurred and needle electromyogram will confirm denervation changes in the muscles. In preganglionic avulsions, there is absent motor conduction but intact sensory conduction as the sensory cell body in the dorsal root ganglion is still attached to the peripheral nerve axon, although the patient cannot perceive a sensory stimulus as there is no central connection. Somatosensory-evoked potentials, when recordings are made from the sensory cortex during peripheral stimulation, are absent. Neurophysiological studies are useful in monitoring reinnervation following injury or surgery.

Management

The role of the specialist brachial plexus surgeon is in establishing a diagnosis, grading the severity of the nerve injury, providing a prognosis for the patient, accessing support services, managing patient expectations and restoring function. Systematic repeated clinical examination is essential in defining a nerve injury and any potential for recovery without surgery. The Hoffmann–Tinel sign is useful for gauging the rate and extent of neurological recovery. Deep muscle pain is an early sign of motor reinnervation. Early exploratory surgery may be necessary to establish an accurate diagnosis in some cases.

Open injuries, vascular injury, evidence of at least some complete injury on initial examination, deteriorating function under observation or failure to progress in line with expectation are all indications for prompt surgical exploration. Later surgery may be required when associated injuries precluded early diagnosis and surgery, with deteriorating pain due to perineural fibrosis and for reconstruction or salvage procedures.

Early nerve exploration and decompression provide the appropriate environment for nerve recovery. Simple lacerations may be primarily repaired if undertaken acutely. Nerve ruptures may be bridged with reversed, autologous sensory cable nerve grafts taken from the injured limb or using the sural nerves from the lower limbs. Nerve grafting in proximal mixed (motor, sensory and autonomic) nerve injuries is unpredictable. There is often apoptosis and the regeneration potential of the proximal nerve stump cannot be accurately predicted. There is potential for neuroma-in-continuity formation at proximal and distal ends of the nerve grafts, poor revascularisation of long grafts, axonal misdirection (sensory and motor cross wiring with no functional gain), cocontraction of agonist–antagonist muscle groups when a single nerve root is used for grafting multiple distal nerves (mixed avulsion and rupture injury) and long reinnervation times for proximal injuries to distal muscles resulting in motor end-plate deterioration and poor functional gains. In addition, avulsion injuries are not amenable to grafting.

Nerve transfer surgery uses intact extraplexal nerves (e.g. spinal accessory nerve, phrenic nerve or intercostal nerves) or fascicles from a functioning intraplexal nerve (ulnar fascicle to biceps; triceps branch to axillary) to reinnervate important muscles by direct coaptation close to the motor end-plate. This reduces reinnervation times and restores early function. It can provide reconstructive options when patient's present late and proximal nerve surgery has failed. Nerve surgery may be combined with arthrodeses, tendon transfers and functioning free muscle transfers.

Further reading

Birch R. Surgical disorders of the peripheral nerves, 2nd Edition. London: Springer-Verlag Limited, 2011.

British Orthopaedic Association (BOA). Standards for Trauma (BOAST), BOAST 5: Peripheral Nerve Injury. London: BOA, 2012.

Shin A. Late reconstruction for brachial plexus injury. Neurosurg Clin North Am 2009; 20:51–64.

Related topics of interest

Brain stem death and organ donation

Key points

- In the UK, around 1000 people die each year while waiting for an organ transplant
- In the UK, only about one-third of the population is registered organ donors
- In the UK, the potential donor rate is estimated at 65 per million people, the actual donor rate currently stands at 19.6

Introduction

The demand for solid organ transplantation continues to far-outstrip supply (**Figure 15**). In the UK, despite a 50% increase in donation rates between 2008 and 2013, it is estimated that about 1000 people a year still die while waiting for an organ transplant. Organ donations can be life-saving (heart, lung and liver) or life-enhancing (kidney and pancreas) and are of financial benefit to healthcare systems. Healthcare professionals have a duty of care to facilitate the wishes of patients to donate organs.

The total potential donor rate can be defined as the number of patients per million population who are on a ventilator, have no contraindication to donation and who are having life-sustaining treatment withdrawn. In the UK, the potential donor rate is estimated at 65 per million people and the actual donor rate currently stands at 19.6. In the UK, about one third of the population is registered organ donors although surveys demonstrate a strong desire on the part of a majority of the population to donate organs at the end of life. The reasons for the loss of potential donors include failure to identify

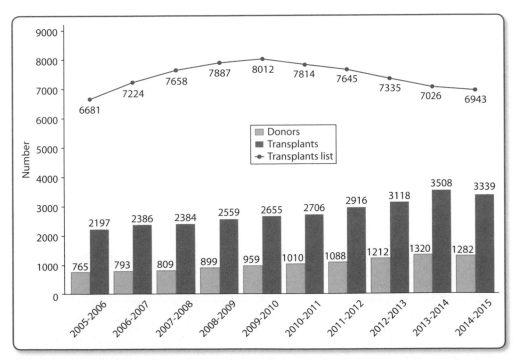

Figure 15 Deceased donors and transplants in the UK 2005–2015, and patients on the active transplant list. With permission from NHS Blood and Transplant Organ donation and transplantation. Activity report 2015/15. Watford: NHS Blood and Transport, 2015.

potential donors, failure to carry out brain stem testing, family refusal and Coroner refusal (**Figure 16**). There is considerable international variation in retrieval and donation practice and actual donor rates vary accordingly (**Figure 17**).

Defining the end of life

While the majority of organs are retrieved from patients who have fulfilled the criteria for brain stem death, an increasing number are obtained from patients who are not brain dead, but are having treatment withdrawn for other reasons. After a period of asystole, so-called donation after cardiac death (DCD) can proceed, usually for abdominal organs. The shortage of thoracic organs for transplant has led to attempts to retrieve heart and lungs from some of these patients also. In the USA, this has been termed donation after circulatory determination of death (DCDD).

Confirming brain stem death

The death of a trauma victim in intensive care is often sudden and unexpected, raising the possibility of organ donation. Acting in the best overall interests of the patient can be challenging for clinicians, as this involves balancing compassion and sensitivity for the relatives' needs, the requirements of the law relevant to the potential for organ donation and any expressed wishes of the patient. As a consequence, the situation will inevitably be emotionally charged and raising the subject of donation difficult. Brain stem death is often the mode of death for trauma victims in critical care. Once the diagnosis of brain stem death is considered, all patients should be stabilised for neurological assessment of brain stem function.

Testing for the presence of brain stem function should be undertaken in accordance with the Academy of Medical Royal Colleges' code of practice for the diagnosis and

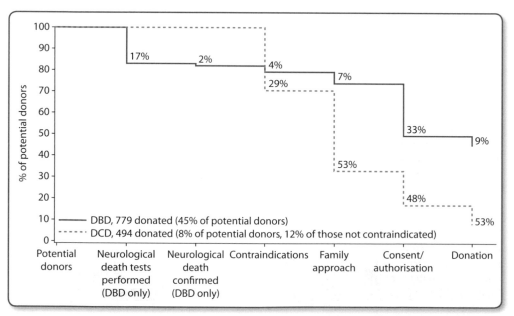

Figure 16 Causes of loss of donated organs. A potential donor after brain death (DBD) is one who meets all four criteria for neurological death testing and has not had cardiac arrest despite resuscitation, is not a neonate <2 months post term and has not had a return of brain stem reflexes. A potential donor after cardiac death (DCD) is one who had treatment withdrawn and death was expected within 4 hours. With permission from NHS Blood and Transplant. Organ donation and transplantation. Activity report 2014/15. Watford: NHS Blood and Transplant, 2015.

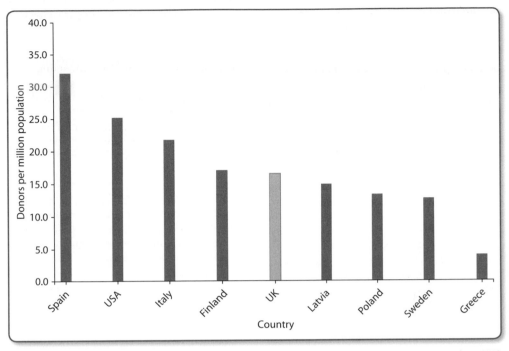

Figure 17 International organ donor rates from Europe and the United States, 2010. With permission from NHS Blood and Transplant Council of Europe – Transplant Newsletter.

confirmation of death (AMRC, 2008), and the Working Party Report on the Diagnosis of Brain Stem Death in Infants and Children (1991). Guidance from the General Medical Council and British Medical Association states that brainstem testing of all appropriate patients, whether there is the potential for organ donation or not, should be a part of normal end of life care practice, as this is in the patient's best interests. The main prerequisite for proceeding with brain stem death tests (assessing for the irreversible loss of brain stem function) is the presence of irreversible structural brain damage and the presence of irreversible coma. Structural damage is usually confirmed by CT or MRI imaging. Clinicians also have to be satisfied that there are no confounding factors or exclusion criteria present, these include:

- Sedative drugs
- Muscle relaxants
- Primary hypothermia (temperature <34°C)
- Metabolic and endocrine disorders which can mimic brain stem death

Patients who develop brain stem death may display severe physiological derangements, therefore stabilisation of organ function prior to brain stem death testing is required in order to ensure that tests are performed accurately. Deterioration in cardiovascular function associated with intracranial hypertension is often characterised by two phases. A sympathetic storm resulting in neurogenic myocardial dysfunction and intense vasoconstriction is followed by sympathetic depletion, receptor downregulation and vasodilatation. Hypothermia is a common phenomenon and neurogenic pulmonary oedema can also be seen. Reduced production of antidiuretic hormone causes diabetes insipidus (DI); this occurs in approximately 65% of brain stem dead patients and needs to be identified early, the effects reversed and its progress arrested. Judicious fluid administration is essential to ensure an adequate circulation without causing pulmonary oedema. Vasopressin is the vasopressor of choice to maintain vascular tone and also helps to reduce DI. In addition, bolus dosing with desmopressin acetate (DDAVP) may be necessary to control urine output. Lung recruitment manoeuvres (according to local intensive care unit policy) are required to optimise gas exchange and maintain lung volumes. Active warming is also often necessary.

Brain stem death tests

In the UK, confirmation of brain stem death is a clinical process. Two clinicians, one of whom has to be a consultant, perform a series of tests assessing for the absence of brain stem (cranial nerve) reflexes and the presence of irreversible apnoea. Retrieval and transplantation teams are not involved with brain stem death testing or with the decision to withdraw active treatment. At least two sets of tests are performed and the findings should be clearly documented in the notes:

- The pupils are fixed and do not respond to light
- The corneal reflexes are absent
- The oculovestibular reflexes are absent. (There are no eye movements following the slow injection of at least 50 mL of ice-cold water into each ear in turn (the caloric reflex test).
- There are no motor responses in the cranial nerve distribution in response to stimulation of the face, limbs or
- The cough and gag reflexes are absent
- There is no observed respiratory effort in response to disconnection of the ventilator for a period sufficient to ensure an arterial partial pressure of carbon dioxide to at least 6.0 kPa (6.5 kPa in patients with chronic carbon dioxide retention) after adequate oxygenation,
- Where clinical examination cannot confirm the diagnosis with safety, ancillary tests can be used. Situations that limit clinical brain stem death testing include severe facial trauma, ongoing haemodynamic or respiratory instability and where the residual presence of active metabolites of long-acting sedatives cannot be excluded. These ancillary investigations include a four-vessel angiogram (considered the gold

standard), CT or MRI angiogram or evoked potentials. The choice of test depends on local availability and expertise and their interpretation should be carried out in conjunction with the clinical findings.

Following confirmation of brain stem death, or prior to the withdrawal of treatment, trauma cases have to be reported to and discussed with the Coroner or Procurator Fiscal (in Scotland) to obtain agreement for organ retrieval and transplantation. Information that the Coroner or Procurator Fiscal may require includes:

- Confirmation of time, date and place of death
- An accurate description of the circumstances surrounding the death and detail regarding the trauma
- Whether there is suspected alcohol or drug involvement
- If there has been criminal activity in relation to the death or if a Health and Safety inquiry is required
- Whether there is a possibility of neglect during treatment
- Whether appropriate consent or authorisation has been obtained from the deceased or the next of kin

Where the Coroner/Procurator Fiscal is unable to agree to the donation process, a full explanation regarding the reasoning is considered best practice, as refusal can cause distress to donor families.

Approaching relatives regarding potential organ donation requires careful preparation and teamwork. It is essential that the specialist nurse (organ donation) or transplant coordination team are involved as early as possible in the process, as they play a vital role in communicating with the family, coroner and retrieval teams and managing the donation and retrieval process.

There are few absolute contraindications to organ donation and transplantation; these include:

- HIV-positive status with an AIDS defining illness
- Known new variant Creutzfeldt–Jakob disease (CJD) or a family history of new variant CJD
- Active disseminated malignancy

Absolute and relative exclusion criteria are constantly under review, and individual cases always need to be discussed with the specialist nurse or transplant coordinator for clarification. Following confirmation of brain stem death and consent for organ donation, donor optimisation ensures that the organs are maintained in the best possible physiological state. In addition to the aspects mentioned earlier, methyl prednisolone is administered and the donor managed using a standardised care bundle.

Approaching relatives for organ donation is often a joint process between the transplant coordinators and treating clinicians, although there is some variation in practice across the UK. Once consent has been obtained, the coordinator organises the retrieval operation and continues to liaise with the relatives and clinical staff regarding donor optimisation and timing of the retrieval surgery. The retrieval surgery is done following identification of recipients, especially for cardiothoracic organs.

Further reading

Academy of Medical Royal Colleges (AMRC). A code of practice for the diagnosis and confirmation of death. London: AMRC; 2008.

General Medical Council (GMC). Treatment and care towards the end of life: good practice in decision making. London: GMC; 2010.

Organ Donation Taskforce. Organs for Transplants: A report from the Organ Donation Taskforce. London: Department of Health; 2008.

British Paediatric Association. Diagnosis of brain-stem death in infants and children: a working party report of the British Paediatric Association. London: British Paediatric Association; 1991.

Related topics of interest

Burns

Key points

- Specialist multidisciplinary management is essential for optimal outcome in burns
- Burns involving >30% total body surface area (TBSA), will trigger the systemic inflammatory response syndrome (SIRS) causing profound physiological derangement
- Burns over 15% TBSA in adults and 10% in children require administration of prophylactic intravenous fluids

Background

Burn injury is a common experience with up to 150,000 cases of burn injury presenting to UK emergency departments per year, although fewer than 10% of these require hospitalisation. Only about 500 severe burns are admitted to the UK burn centres each year. The majority of those admitted are children. A higher prevalence of burn injury is seen in patient groups at the extremes of age, and in the presence of psychiatric disorders, substance misuse and epilepsy. There is also an association with reckless behaviour in young adults and teenagers, mainly males. Severe burns are challenging and complex. Definitive care is best provided by large multidisciplinary teams working in centres of excellence.

The burn wound and systemic effects

Skin has a role in immune function, thermoregulation, fluid balance, metabolic function and sensory perception. A burn wound disrupts all of these, as well as being aesthetically and psychologically damaging. Heat causes cell death as well as sublethal cell damage. Injured cells release cytokines, initiating an inflammatory reaction. In small burns, this effect remains local to the injury. Above a certain threshold of burn size, the amount of intravascular fluid lost because of inflammatory capillary leakage exceeds compensatory mechanisms and

hypovolaemia becomes evident. This is known as burn shock. Burn size is the percentage of the TBSA burnt. With burns involving >30% TBSA, the SIRS is triggered causing profound physiological derangement.

Causes of thermal injury to the skin include flame, scald, steam, electric current and contact burns. Scalds are the most common cause in children and flame in adults. Contact burns typically occur in the very young and the elderly as a result of inability to move away from a hot object.

The depth of a burn has a direct influence on how it will heal and, therefore, how it is treated. The most superficial of burns cause inflammation to the epidermis only, which resolves within a day or two. Slightly deeper burns cause a minor degree of cell death in the epidermis and deeper inflammation. The keratinocytes lining the skin adnexal structures, such as sweat glands and hair follicles, provide an ability for the epidermis to regenerate within a couple of weeks without scarring. These burns are described as superficial partial thickness. Deep partial thickness burns significantly damage these reservoirs of keratinocytes and alter the structural elements of the dermis. Healing is slower and often leaves scars. Full-thickness burns destroy all elements of the skin and healing can only be by re-epithelialisation from the wound edges: scarring is inevitable. Areas of inflammation can progress to necrosis over many hours thus causing the burn to deepen. Poor management of the wound and the patient's general condition contribute to this progression. Circumferential deep burns cause constriction and can impede respiratory excursion of the torso and distal perfusion in the limbs. This may require surgical incision of the constriction (escharotomy).

Inhalation injury

When the hot and toxic products of combustion are inhaled, injury can be caused by three mechanisms: direct damage to the upper (supraglottic) airways by heat, potentially leading to oedema; chemical damage to the lower airways from toxic products of combustion and absorption of toxic products into the circulation through the alveoli causing systemic intoxication. Examples of the latter include carbon monoxide and cyanide poisoning. In large burns, pulmonary sequelae of SIRS will cause further insult to the lungs.

General management of burn injury

A systematic approach is essential. Aspects of the primary survey related to burn injury are as follows:

Airway

The possibility of airway obstruction due to upper airways burns must be identified. Risk factors include:

- Exposure to fire or smoke in an enclosed space
- An altered level of consciousness at any time
- Change in voice, hoarseness or coughing
- Signs of burns to the face including singed nasal hairs or carbonaceous sputum

Arterial gases and carboxyhaemoglobin levels should be measured, both blood gases and chest X-ray findings may initially be normal. If there is already evidence of evolving airway obstruction, the patient should be intubated leaving the endotracheal tube uncut. It is important to remember that airway closure due to inhalational oedema is relatively rare and usually of gradual onset.

Breathing

Humidified 100% oxygen must be given and respiration monitored clinically and with blood gases. Circumferential torso burns may cause reduced respiratory excursion requiring escharotomies.

Circulation

Burn shock develops over several hours. If a patient is hypovolaemic soon after sustaining the burn, other causes such as haemorrhage from other injuries, must be identified. Calculating fluid requirements to prevent burn shock takes time and is not part of the primary survey. Ideally vascular access lines should not be inserted through burnt skin.

Disability

If a patient has a reduced level of consciousness, causes of hypoxia and cerebral hypoperfusion should be sought and corrected, and head injury and intoxication should also be excluded.

Environment

Burn patients are at significant risk of hypothermia and must be kept warm.

Other initial interventions

Early adequate analgesia is essential. Prolonged cooling of the burn wound can reduce the degree of inflammation but this effect may be restricted to the first half hour or so after injury. Domestic cold tap water is appropriate for this; there is no evidence of added benefit in using sterile fluids or proprietary cooling gels. Prophylactic antibiotics are not required for isolated burn injury.

A nasogastric tube and urinary catheter should be inserted in burns over 20% TBSA.

Specific burn management

For burns over 15% TBSA in adults and 10% in children, administration of prophylactic intravenous fluids to reduce burn shock is established practice. The amount required is proportional to the size of burn so it is necessary to calculate this. The physiological response to fluids must be monitored. The depth of burn has less of an impact than area.

Assessment of burn size

Accurate assessment of a burn can only take place after a surgical scrub of the wound. For anything other than small burns, this should only take place within a special burns unit where it will normally be performed under general anaesthetic. An estimate can be made by using a Lund and Browder chart (**Figure 18**). Some areas have letters rather than numbers and these correspond to parts of the body

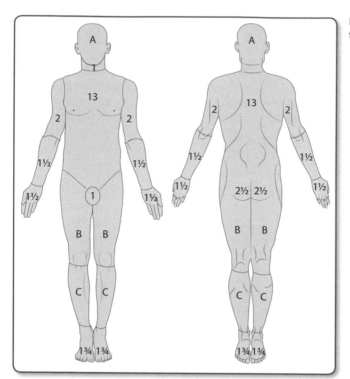

Figure 18 Lund and Browder chart for the assessment of burn size.

that change in relative proportion according to age.

The palmar surface of the patient's hand with the fingers and thumb fully adducted can be used to represent 1% TBSA.

Assessment of fluid requirements

Several formulae are available and advice should be sought from the local burn service as to which is to be used. A common formula in the UK practice is:

$$2 \times \%\text{TBSA burned} \times \text{patient's weight in kg}$$

This volume is the amount of intravenous crystalloid, ideally Ringer lactate/Hartmann, that is expected to be required above normal in the first 24 hours since the burn. Half should be given in the first 8 hours and the second half in the subsequent 16 hours. Using normal saline risks the development of hyperchloraemic acidosis. The calculated amount does not factor in other causes of hypovolaemia such as haemorrhage from other injuries. The adequacy of fluid administration is most easily determined by urine output. A target range of 0.5–1.0 mL/kg/h is appropriate. While it is understood that fluid administration needs to be increased when the urine output is low, it is equally important to reduce fluid administration if the urine output is high.

Assessment of burn depth

Simple erythema is not included when calculating the size of a burn. Superficial partial-thickness burns exhibit marked erythema which blanches with pressure and there is blistering with watery exudate. Deep partial-thickness burns are whiter with some redness which does not blanche and are generally dry. Full-thickness burns are leathery, waxy, firm and dry and there may be charring.

Monitoring

With burns over approximately 30% TBSA, the physiological manifestations of the SIR will become evident and managing the patient in a critical care environment will be essential.

Dressings

The wound should not be disturbed unnecessarily and there is no indication for the application of antiseptic ointments or creams. Burns may be loosely covered with cling film, laid on rather than wrapped around. Smaller burns may be dressed with Vaseline-based dressings.

Chemical burns

Both domestic and industrial chemicals may cause burns. Information is available from the online database of the UK's National Poisons Information Service or industrial data sheets. Alkali burns are frequently more severe as penetration is deeper due to their liquefactive action. Most common acids cause a coagulative necrosis which retards deeper penetration. Immediate management is focussed on removal of the causative agent, normally by dilution with copious amounts of water. Specific antidotes are rarely indicated. Once the burn process has been stopped, the burn is treated in a similar manner to thermal burns.

Electrical burns

There are three categories of electrical burns which are as follows:

Normal mains (240 V) and industrial (440 V) electricity

Alternating current can produce tetany of muscles causing the patient to hold on to the electrical source. Deep local burns may occur at the entrance and exit points. Significant tissue damage is uncommon. If the current passes through the thorax, cardiac arrest or dysrhythmias may occur. Prolonged attempts at cardiopulmonary resuscitation are indicated in cardiac arrest due to electrocution. If the patient is asymptomatic

and ECG normal at the time of presentation, there is no evidence that prolonged cardiac monitoring is indicated.

High-voltage (>1,000 V) electricity

High-voltage electricity is found mainly in transmission cables. Full-thickness entrance and exit wounds will be visible and there may what appears to be a blast element. Extensive deep tissue damage may have occurred under normal looking skin. Muscle damage can develop into compartment syndrome requiring fasciotomies and surgical debridement and rhabdomyolysis may precipitate acute renal failure. More aggressive fluid resuscitation may therefore be required. Current may 'flash-over' a burns patient causing a flash burn to the skin without necessarily affecting deeper tissues.

Lightning

A lightning strike generates a very high temperature causing burns and the effects are usually immediately fatal. Most survivors have suffered an indirect strike from an adjacent object. The current often travels across the skin but exit wounds are common in the soles of the feet. Cardiorespiratory arrest can be reversible so resuscitation should be attempted.

Burn networks and referral criteria

The National Burn Care Review (2001 and subsequent revisions) stratified the provision of burn services in the National Health Service (NHS). There are supraregional burn networks that manage and provide care within three tiers of service: burn facilities are those in hospitals with standard plastic surgery wards for simple burns, burn units have a separate burns ward and specialist staff for the care of moderate injuries, and burn centres are tertiary referral centres for complex injuries with full access to all critical care services. The following should be referred for specialist care:

- All burns ≥2% TBSA in children or ≥3% in adults

- All full-thickness burns and all circumferential burns
- Any burn with suspicion of nonaccidental injury should be referred to a burn unit/centre for expert assessment within 24 hours
- Any burn that has not healed in within 2 weeks

The following cases should be discussed with a burns service as they may require transfer to specialist care:

- All burns to hands, feet, face, perineum or genitalia
- Burns to skin associated with chemical, electrical or cold injury
- Unwell children with a burn or possible toxic shock syndrome
- Patients with comorbidities that may affect treatment

Further reading

Herndon DN (Ed). Total burn care, 4th Edition. London: Saunders Elsevier, 2012.

Australia and New Zealand Burn Association Ltd. Emergency management of severe burns course manual. Albany Creek: UK Edition, 2012.

National Network for Burn Care (NNBC). National Burn Care Referral Guidance. Version 1, Approved February 2012. London: NNBC, 2012.

National Health Service (NHS) England. NHS standard contract for specialised burn care (all ages). London: NHS England, 2013.

Related topics of interest

- Chemical, biological, radiological and nuclear environments and trauma (p. 71)
- Penetrating neck injury (p. 227)
- Systemic inflammatory response syndrome (p. 279)

\<C>ABCDE resuscitation

Key points

- Historically, the paradigm of trauma management has been to assess and treat patients according to the ABCDE sequence, this should be replaced by \<C>ABCDE where \<C> is control of exsanguinating external haemorrhage
- In patients with massive external haemorrhage, the priority in management must be control of this haemorrhage
- Preventing blood loss is always preferable to blood transfusion

Introduction

The assessment and management of trauma patients has followed the primary survey ABCDE system since the introduction of the advanced trauma life support (ATLS) course in the late 1970s. This involves the assessment and management of Airway, with cervical spine control, Breathing, with administration of high flow oxygen, Circulation with control of haemorrhage, Disability and Exposure with control of environment. However, in some patients with massive external haemorrhage (\<C>), the priority must be to primarily address the control and management of bleeding, before addressing other issues. As a consequence a new paradigm \<C>ABCDE has been proposed which addresses exsanguinating external haemorrhage (if present) first.

History

The establishment of the ATLS system, with agreed priorities for assessment and management, has led to very significant advances in trauma care. ATLS originated from the personal experiences of James Styner and the care available to his family after a plane crash in the 1970s, and led to the establishment of the ATLS programme run by the American College of Surgeons. This has been adopted worldwide as the standard and language of trauma care. However, advances in trauma care are often related to conflict, and over the last decade it has become apparent from military experience that in some patients, priority should be given to control of massive haemorrhage.

Background

The mechanism of injury seen in recent conflicts in Iraq and Afghanistan has been predominantly blast, with a lower proportion of high-velocity gunshot wounds, blunt injuries and burns. Advances in personal protection have meant that the head and torso have been relatively protected, while the limbs have remained exposed, particularly to blast, causing devastating peripheral injuries resulting in massive haemorrhage.

Unless this massive haemorrhage is dealt with promptly, the patient will exsanguinate. It has been estimated that 10% of all deaths on the battlefield are caused by exsanguination from limb injuries. The precise incidence of massive external haemorrhage amenable to prehospital control in civilian medicine is less clear. However, the National Confidential Enquiry into Patient Outcome and Death (NCEPOD) report on trauma in 2007 recognised that control of haemorrhage is 'crucially important'. Between 30% and 40% of early trauma deaths are attributable to haemorrhage, and hypotension from blood loss is a major factor in the development of secondary brain injury, as well as significantly contributing to later deaths from multiorgan failure. The deaths referred to in the NCEPOD report included both internal and external bleeding; however, controlling external haemorrhage, in comparison to internal, can be rapidly affected by simply measures.

The NCEPOD report also stressed the importance of early effective control of the airway. While an obstructed airway must undoubtedly be rapidly managed, significantly mortality and morbidity may be averted by first promptly controlling massive haemorrhage, hence the use of the \<C>ABC paradigm.

Techniques of haemorrhage control

Advances in the techniques of haemorrhage control in the last decade have made control of exsanguinating external haemorrhage a realistic and practical option when managing trauma patients. Control of exsanguinating external haemorrhage is achieved by the use of dressings, either with or without novel haemostatic agents and limb tourniquets. The application of these methods of haemorrhage control must be rapid in order to prevent ongoing blood loss and to allow timely assessment and life-saving airway and breathing interventions.

Dressings and haemostatic agents

Compression and elevation have been the mainstays of treatment of bleeding peripheral wounds for decades. Modern first field dressings incorporating some elasticity, and therefore enabling compression, have been developed in the last few years. The UK Defence Medical Services and some civilian prehospital services have adopted the emergency care bandage which is supplied in sizes suitable for both limb and abdominal application.

The latest generation of dressings has been developed alongside technology for controlling haemorrhage using compounds that facilitate normal coagulation, such as QuikClot, HemCon and Celox. These compounds either concentrate intrinsic clotting ability by rapid absorption of water from blood, or are mucoadhesive agents that seal the wound. QuikClot is an example of a clotting factor concentrator – composed of a rayon/polyester gauze that is impregnated with kaolin. HemCon and Celox are mucoadhesive agents, in which deacylated chitosan acetate is the active ingredient (a compound derived from crustacean shells). On contact with red blood cells, the chitosan cross-links and strongly adheres to the wound surface. All three of these products are available as a packing-gauze which can be used to exert direct pressure in addition to the actions listed above. These haemostatic packing-gauzes have particularly utility in junctional wounds in the neck, groin or axilla.

Tourniquets

After the Second World War concern was raised that the benefit of a limb tourniquet was out-weighed by its potential to cause irrecoverable tissue damage and as a result they were no longer routinely used. Retrospective data from the Vietnam War (1955–1975) suggest that failure to use limb tourniquets was responsible for 9% of fatalities. However, more recently, the use of limb tourniquets has undoubtedly been responsible for significant improvements in combat survival: the combat application tourniquet (CAT) bears little resemblance to the unwieldy rubber tubing of 20 years ago. Additionally, the CAT is applied with the knowledge that it is being used to save life, which may well indicate that the limb is nonsalvageable anyway. Having relearnt the lessons of conflict, the development of a simple, light and easy to use tourniquet has revolutionised the management of devastating peripheral limb injuries. This allows buddy or even self-aid to apply the tourniquet to stop catastrophic bleeding, allowing maintenance of circulation and time for definitive procedures to be carried out.

Haemostatic resuscitation

Effective, early haemorrhage control with CATs and haemostatic dressings (and the concept of <C>ABCDE) has had a significant positive effect on combat outcomes over the past 10 years. It is, however, difficult to tease-out the exact effect of this paradigm shift in practice owing to the other simultaneous advances in combat casualty care. It should be remembered that early effective external haemorrhage control with <C>ABCDE is only one small but important part of haemostatic resuscitation (HR). The term HR describes the use of effective haemorrhage control together with early balanced blood product administration. In summary, the use of <C>ABCDE will allow the provider to address the highest lethality first and improve outcomes in their trauma patients. Preventing blood loss should always be regarded as preferable to blood transfusion.

Further reading

Gruen RL, Brohi K, Schreiber M, et al. Haemorrhage control in severely injured patients. Lancet 2012; 380:1099–1108.

Hodgetts TJ, Mahoney PF, Russell MQ, Byers M. ABC to <C>ABC: redefining the military trauma paradigm. Emerg Med J 2006; 23:745–746.

Kragh J, Walters T, Baer D, et al. Practical use of emergency tourniquets to stop bleeding in major limb trauma. J Trauma 2008; 64:S38–S50.

Mahambrey T, Pendry K, Nee A, Bonney S, Nee P. Critical care in emergency department: massive haemorrhage in trauma. EMJ 2013; 30:9–14.

Rossaint R, Bouillon B, Cerny V, et al. Management of bleeding following major trauma: an updated European guideline. Critical Care 2010; 14:R52.

Related topics of interest

- Blood product (1:1:1) resuscitation (p. 42)
- Tourniquets (p. 295)

- Traumatic amputation (p. 304)

Cervical spine injuries

Key points

- Cervical spine injury is relatively common in patients following major trauma, with an incidence of between 3% and 4%
- Cervical spine injuries carry the potential for significant morbidity and mortality
- Current best practice recognises that cervical spine immobilisation is not without the potential for harm and therefore should only be employed in patients at high risk of cervical spine injury

Epidemiology

Cervical spine injury occurs in between 3% and 4% of major trauma cases. Fortunately, the incidence of cervical cord injury is noticeably less – about 0.8%. Cervical spinal cord injuries account for nearly half of all cord injuries following major trauma. Thoracic cord injuries account for approximately 30% and lumbar cord injuries 25%. In the UK the most common cause of spinal injury, accounting for a third of all injuries, is road traffic collision. Falls from >2 m contribute to approximately 30%, with falls of <2 m about 20%. Injuries following sporting and leisure activities such as horse riding, although less common, display a strong association with actual cord injury.

The likelihood of a spinal injury having been sustained increases as the patient's Glasgow coma score (GCS) decreases. In patients who were unable to be clinically evaluated due to a head injury, 7.7% were found to have a cervical spine injury compared to an incidence of 2.8% in alert patients. When considering all spinal injuries, 70% of patients will have a GCS of 15.

Pathophysiology

Primary neurological damage is direct damage to neural tissue due to trauma. Abnormal flexion, extension and rotation directly disrupt the nerves or bony fragments and fractures cause injury to the cord. This neural damage is irreversible. Secondary neurological damage caused by hypoxia, hypoperfusion and further mechanical disruption can be minimised.

Clinical features

A conscious patient may report pain or demonstrate a neurological deficit. In the unconscious patient, suspicion is raised based on the presenting mechanism of injury and clinical findings before confirmation by imaging. Current best practice is aimed at appropriate targeting of spinal immobilisation for selected patients. Spinal immobilisation is not without the potential for negative sequelae and significant cost. The ability of immobilisation to prevent further deterioration of neurological deficit has also been called into question.

Examination

Examination of the trauma patient for a cervical spine injury is tailored to the overall clinical situation. Injuries are not infrequently identified during radiological imaging such as CT scanning, as part of a trauma series of images. Suspicion of an injury may be heightened by findings from clinical examination. A conscious patient may complain of pain at a specific level and examination of the spine may identify tenderness or deformity. The conscious patient may also be able to identify a deficit as part of a neurological assessment. In the unconscious patient, there may be signs that are associated with spinal cord injury:

- Flaccid areflexia with loss of anal tone
- Diaphragmatic breathing
- Priapism
- Neurogenic shock – hypotension and bradycardia in the absence of hypovolaemia

In the conscious patient, an assessment of motor function, sensory level, proprioception and autonomic function can be made.

Neurological assessment

Motor function

The ability of the patient to voluntarily contract specific muscle groups is assessed on both sides of the body (**Table 8**). In the semiconscious patient, lack of involuntary movement in response to pain may also indicate a deficit.

Sensation

An assessment of the patient's ability to detect pin-prick and temperature sensation in each dermatome, on each side of the body will identify the level of loss of sensation (**Figure 19**).

Proprioception

In the conscious patient, this is the ability to identify the position of fingers or toes with the eyes closed.

Table 8 Motor spinal levels and muscle movement	
Motor spinal level	Key muscles
C5	Elbow flexors
C6	Wrist extensors
C7	Elbow extensors
C8	Finger flexors
T1	Finger abductors
L2	Hip flexors
L3	Knee extensors
L4	Ankle dorsiflexors
L5	Long toe extensions
S1	Ankle plantar flexors
Score	Classification
0	Total paralysis
1	Palpable or visible contraction
2	Active movement, gravity eliminated
3	Active movement, against gravity
4	Active movement, against some resistance
5	Active movement, against full resistance
NT	Not testable

Autonomic function

Loss of bladder or rectal control, or the presence of priapism may indicate loss of autonomic function.

Complete and incomplete lesions

Injury to the cord can result in complete transection with total loss of function below the level of the injury, or incomplete injury with some residual neurological function. The final outcome of injury may not be known for a significant length of time.

Clinical features

Neurogenic shock

Neurogenic shock is the term given to hypotension with associated bradycardia and classically peripheral vasodilatation, which can be seen after a high (above T6) cord injury. Disruption of the descending sympathetic pathways removes sympathetic innervation to the heart, resulting in the bradycardia, and loss of tone from the vasculature, leading to uninhibited vasodilatation and a redistributive shock. Neurogenic shock is a diagnosis of exclusion; other causes of shock must be considered and excluded first. In addition, a spinal injury may mask tachycardia, and falsely reassure clinicians regarding haemodynamic instability and haemorrhage.

Spinal shock

Spinal shock is the complete loss of all neurological functions immediately after injury. A period of flaccid paralysis together with areflexia lasts from a few days to weeks precluding full assessment of the extent of the injury and deficit. Full recovery can be seen after periods of profound paralysis; in areas without recovery, flaccid paralysis is replaced by spasticity.

Respiratory compromise

Innervation of the diaphragm is from the C3–5 region. If cord injury is below this in the lower cervical or upper thoracic region then

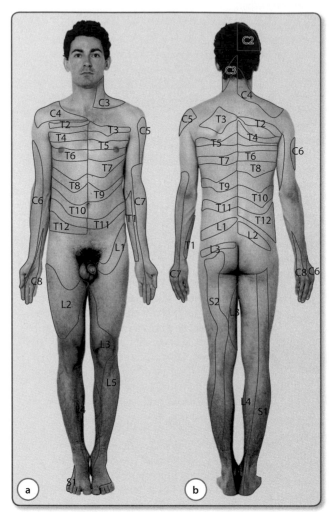

Figure 19 Dermatomes (a) front, (b) back. Photograph © 2012 by Sam Scott-Hunter. Reproduced from Tunstall R, Shah N. *Pocket Tutor Surface Anatomy*. London: JP Medical, 2012.

a classical breathing pattern, reliant on the diaphragm, may be seen.

Investigations

Seriously injured patients may well undergo C-spine imaging as part of their imaging protocol, usually in the form of 'whole body' CT scans. These images may confirm expected or demonstrate unexpected spinal injury. For alert, less injured patients, the need for imaging, and which modality, has to be decided. Significant research has been undertaken in an attempt to avoid unnecessary X-ray imaging in patients following injury. The NEXUS (National

Emergency X-ray Utilization Study) and Canadian C-spine rules aim to identify patients in whom significant injury to the cervical spine can be excluded without the need for imaging. The NEXUS observational study describes five low-risk criteria which, if all are met, can reliably exclude significant injury:

- No midline cervical tenderness
- No focal neurological deficit
- Normal alertness
- No intoxication
- No painful distracting injury

The Canadian C-spine rule asks three questions:

1. Is there any high-risk factor present that mandates radiography?
- Age ≥65 years
- Dangerous mechanism of injury
- Paraesthesia in the extremities
2. Is there any low-risk factor present that allows safe assessment of range of motion?
- Simple rear-end motor vehicle collision
- Sitting position in the emergency department
- Patient ambulatory at any time since injury
- Delayed onset of neck pain
- Absence of midline C-spine tenderness
3. Can the patient actively rotate their neck 45° to the left and right?

If no, high-risk factors are present, coupled with the presence of any low-risk factor then rotation can be assessed. The mechanisms considered to be dangerous are as follows:
- A fall from >1 m or five stairs
- An axial load to the head (e.g. from diving)
- A high-speed motor traffic collision (combined speed >100 km/h)
- A rollover motor vehicle accident
- Ejection from a motor vehicle
- An accident involving motorised recreational vehicles
- A bicycle collision

The Canadian C-spine rules importantly exclude certain groups of patients including those <16 years, patients with a GCS of <15, patients with abnormal vital sings (systolic blood pressure <90 mmHg, respiratory rate <10 or >24 breaths per minute) and patients with known vertebral disease such as ankylosing spondylitis.

The two most common forms of radiological imaging readily available are plain radiographs (lateral, anteroposterior and odontoid peg views) and computerised tomography. MRI is the gold standard for imaging soft tissue structures but availability and practicability in the trauma situation is variable. CT is far superior for identifying injury when compared to plain films and as such should be used as the primary imaging modality in:
- Patients with a GCS of ≤13 on initial assessment
- Intubated patients
- Patients undergoing scanning for head or multiregion trauma
- Patients in whom there is suspicion or certainty of injury on plain films or in whom the plain film series has been inadequate

MRI should be used in patients:
- Who have neurological signs and symptoms attributable to the cervical spine
- In whom there is suspicion of vertebral injury
- Who require assessment of ligamentous and disc injuries suggested by plain films or CT

Treatment

Management of patients with cervical spine injuries initially involves addressing immediate life-threatening injuries while minimising further movement of the spinal column. Minimising secondary neurological damage caused by hypoxia, hypoperfusion and potentially further mechanical disruption is essential. Patients may be globally hypoxic and hypoperfused from concomitant injuries following major trauma. Adequate resuscitation will not only improve overall survival but may lessen final spinal injury as well.

Efforts to improve oxygenation and perfusion should not be hampered by spinal immobilisation.

Ongoing management requires complex, skilled multidisciplinary care, again aiming to prevent further deterioration in injury and associated loss of function. Benefits have been demonstrated when patients are treated in specialised centres especially when caring for patients with spinal cord injuries.

Paediatric considerations

Fortunately spinal injuries are even rarer amongst the paediatric population. Up to two thirds of injuries seen in children under the age of 8 years can be defined as spinal cord injury without radiological abnormality. This arises as the result of the increased hypermobility and laxity of the paediatric bony spinal column which can withstand trauma without fracturing. Underlying cord damage can be demonstrated by MRI scanning.

Whiplash-associated disorder

This is the term given to a group of clinical manifestations seen after an acceleration–deceleration mechanism, most commonly after a road traffic collision. It is a common occurrence with over 1,500 claims for whiplash made to insurers each day resulting in over £2 billion worth of insurance claims per year, though the incidence of whiplash injury varies significantly from country to country.

The symptoms reported commonly include neck pain, headache and neck stiffness as well as shoulder pain, arm pain or numbness, paraesthesia, weakness, visual and auditory symptoms, dizziness and concentration difficulties. Neck pain can be classified into four grades, with whiplash-associated disorders (WAD) coming under grades 1–4:
1. Neck pain with little or no interference with daily activities
2. Neck pain that limits daily activity
3. Neck pain accompanied by radiculopathy
4. Neck pain with serious pathology such as tumour, fracture and infection

The recovery of WAD is prolonged with half of patients reporting pain 1 year after the injury. This should be viewed, however, in the light of 20–40% of the general population reporting neck pain in the previous month. A number of prognostic factors have been investigated including demographical, societal, prior health, psychological, health behaviours and litigation, though strong associations are yet to be clearly defined.

Exclusion tools should be used to avoid unnecessary imaging for patients with grade 1 and 2 neck pain. Patients should then be encouraged to remain active with the reinforcement that a positive attitude to recovery is important, as is return to normal daily activities. Self-management of pain with over-the-counter analgesia as needed is often sufficient.

Further reading

Arnold H. Trauma Care Manual, 2nd Edition. In: Greaves I, Porter K, Garner J. 2009. Boca Raton: Taylor & Francis, 2008.

Holm LW, Carroll LJ, Cassidy JD, et al. The burden and determinants of neck pain in whiplash-associated disorders after traffic collisions. Results of the Bone and Joint Decade 2000–2010 Task Force on Neck Pain and Its Associated Disorders. Spine 2008; 33:S52–S59.

Kwan I, Bunn F, Roberts IG. Spinal immobilisation for trauma patients (review). The Cochrane Collaboration. New Jersey: John Wiley & Sons Limited, 2009.

Moss R, Porter K, Greaves I. Minimal patient handling: a faculty of pre-hospital care consensus statement. Trauma 2015; 17:70–72.

The College of Emergency Medicine Clinical Effectiveness Committee. Guideline on the management of alert, adult patients with a potential cervical spine injury in the emergency department. London: College of Emergency Medicine, 2010.

Related topics of interest

Chemical, biological, radiological and nuclear environments and trauma

Key points

- In a chemical, biological, radiological or nuclear (CRBN) environment, trauma remains a priority for casualty management
- The level of casualty care will depend on the type of environment and presence of any hazard
- The priorities for CBRN and trauma casualty treatment are the management of catastrophic haemorrhage, basic airway management, antidote administration, breathing and circulatory support, decontamination and evacuation to a more permissive environment

Introduction

The term CBRN is generally used to describe the deliberate release of hazardous materials. While traditionally developed for use on the battlefield, these agents have also been used by terrorists against civilian populations and during ethnic conflict. Rarely, release of toxic materials will occur as a result of industrial errors of malfunctions. The use of such agents will complicate trauma casualty care especially in the context of combined injuries (CBRN and trauma). A generic approach can be applied to the management of any casualty in a CBRN environment including trauma.

CBRN agents

Chemical agents

These agents are usually grouped into classes based on their mechanism of action. They include nerve agents, cyanides, blistering agents (vesicants), pulmonary (lung-damaging) agents and incapacitants (mental and physical). The term toxic industrial chemicals is also used; however, there is significant overlap with some of the chemical agent classes (e.g. chlorine and phosgene are pulmonary agents).

Biological agents

These agents are split into live biological agents (bacteria, viruses and fungi) and toxins (chemical agents of biological origin). Live agents that are transmissible from person-to-person will cause a contagious hazard while toxins may be a contamination hazard.

Radiological hazards

Radiological agents are radioisotopes (unstable isotopes) that emit ionising radiation as α- or β-particles or as X-ray or gamma electromagnetic radiation (or a combination). Radiological hazards will cause irradiation ranging from levels insufficient to cause any clinical effect through to acute radiation syndrome (ARS); there may also be contamination with radioactive matter. These hazards may be used overtly as a 'dirty bomb' (radioactive material combined with conventional explosive) or covertly, either released into the environment, possibly in food or water, or as a potent gamma source causing irradiation only.

Nuclear weapons

These weapons are associated with nuclear fission and the splitting of the atom. This yields an enormous amount of energy in the form of blast, thermal and ionising radiation including neutrons.

Implications of a CBRN incident

A CBRN incident has a number of implications for both the types of casualties and the impact on casualty care. These include:

- Differing casualty types (four Is) including intoxicated (chemical), infected (biological) and irradiated (radiation and nuclear) as well as injured (trauma).

- Casualty hazards (two Cs) from CBRN exposure including contamination and contagious.
- The requirement to manage contaminated wounds.
- The potential presentation of many psychological casualties.

In addition, the requirement to wear additional personal protective equipment (PPE) will compromise medical dexterity and be a potential hazard due to heat and psychological stress. This may compromise casualty assessment and the provision of life-saving trauma interventions. Initially the incident must be contained until a formal assessment of the casualty hazard risk has been carried out. Effective decontamination processes must be established and isolation facilities are likely to be required if the agent is contagious. There is also the risk of compromise of medical facilities due to contaminated or contagious self-referring patients.

Principles of CBRN casualty management

The underpinning principles of CBRN casualty management are:

- Recognition
- Safety. This includes hazard avoidance and use of appropriate PPE
- Self-aid and first-aid management
- Triage
- Assessment of the casualty supported by scene assessment with detection equipment
- Life-saving interventions (T1 casualties only)
- Casualty hazards management
- Advanced medical care. This is divided into supportive management (including critical care) and definitive management (including antidotes, antibiotics and surgery), both in a hospital environment
- Rehabilitation

Priorities for CBRN casualty treatment

The priorities for casualty care in a CBRN environment follow the conventional <C>ABCDE sequence with some modifications. These are:

- Management of catastrophic haemorrhage (<C>)
- Basic airway management (A)
- Antidotes (a)
- B – breathing support (B)
- C – circulatory support (C)
- D – decontamination (Decon) as well as disability (d)
- E – evacuation to a more permissive environment (Evac)

The priorities depend on the type of hazard present and risk from patients. The CBRN functional response zones are defined as:

Hot zone

This is a nonpermissive area where there is a direct hazard to the responder from the environment. Casualty management in this area is limited to enhanced first aid with a focus on trauma and chemical life-saving interventions (<C>AaB) including the use of antidote autoinjectors. The priority for all casualties remains evacuation from the hot zone.

Exclusion zone

This is a type of hot zone where despite protective measures such as PPE, there remains a significant hazard. Examples include a zone around an explosive device or a potent radiation source.

Warm zone

The warm zone is a semipermissive buffer area where there is a secondary contamination hazard due to contaminated casualties or equipment, or a contagious casualty. Casualty management is limited by PPE but includes intravenous or intraosseous antidote administration and decontamination (<C>AaBC–Decon–Evac).

Clean (cold) zone

This is the area beyond the clean/dirty line (inner cordon) with optimal access to the casualty. There may be a residual hazard from wound and internal contamination as well as from a contagious patient.

Triage of CBRN casualties

Conventional triage categories are used in a CBRN environment. Triage is used for the prioritisation of treatment, medical evacuation and decontamination. The criteria are:

- T1 (immediate) – the presence of a life-threatening condition requiring a life-saving intervention. This includes catastrophic haemorrhage, airway compromise, unconsciousness or fitting.
- T2 (urgent) – the nonambulatory or incapacitated (not obeying commands) casualty not meeting the T1 criteria.
- T3 (delayed) – the walking casualty who is obeying commands.
- T4 (expectant) – this category is only used if there is an overwhelming demand on finite resources and where the continuing management of a casualty will be detrimental to casualties with greater survivability.

Management of combined injuries

The combined casualties will be complex both to assess and to treat. The presence of trauma may mask the effects of chemical agents and vice versa. The effects are also likely to be synergistic with multiple challenges for oxygen delivery. The presence of chemical agents may also complicate any anaesthetic procedure which may be required, e.g. nondepolarising muscle relaxants are recommended in cases of nerve agent exposure. Combined casualties with traumatic injuries are likely to require surgery and in some cases the wounds may still be contaminated. Full wound decontamination of devitalised tissue will require surgical debridement. Patients should be managed in well-ventilated areas to prevent any accumulation or off-gassing. However, the risk to a surgical team from CBRN contaminated wounds is likely to be at a very low level once external decontamination has been carried out. Surgical precautions should include the use of double nitrile gloves and changing of the outer sacrificial layer, the use of forceps to avoid any direct physical contact, and the rapid removal of any potentially contaminated foreign bodies and their safe disposal.

In conventional incidents, biological wound contamination is assumed and prophylactic broad-spectrum antibiotics are given routinely during initial resuscitation.

For a radiological incident with trauma, the management of the trauma must take priority. For patients who have received a radiation dose high enough to cause ARS, any surgery should be prioritised during the window of opportunity of the first few days before bone marrow suppression occurs, leading to immunosuppression and coagulopathy.

Radioactive fragments may present a continuing but quantifiable hazard to the surgeon. A high-dose rate fragment may have already caused sufficient tissue damage to make a limb nonviable. A similar fragment to the torso may be nonsurvivable. For low-dose exposures, standard precautions will provide adequate protection and significant contamination can be monitored with appropriate radiological equipment. Alpha-emitting sources may not be a significant radiological hazard once fibrosis has occurred due to poor tissue penetration, as long as the compound remains chemically and biologically inert. Antidote therapy (decorporation) may be an adjunct to the removal of any residual radiological material and exploits the compound's chemical properties. Specialist advice should be sought with details of the isotope and any dose rate reading, if known.

Further reading

Departments of the Army, Navy and the Air Force. NATO handbook on the medical aspects of NBC defensive operations. AMedP-6(B). Brussels: NATO, 1996.

Greaves I, Hunt P. Responding to terrorism: a medical handbook. Edinburgh: Churchill Livingstone, 2011.

Health Protection Agency (HPA). CBRN incidents: clinical management & health protection. London: HPA, 2006.

Related topics of interest

- Blast trauma (p. 38)
- Psychological aspects of trauma (p. 239)
- Triage (p. 312)

Commonly missed injuries

Key points

- Inadequate assessment or failure to suspect a fracture based on the examination and mechanism of injury results in missed injuries
- Inadequate radiographs increase the risk of missing a fracture
- There is a significant level of missed injury in multiple trauma patients, the more seriously the patient is injured, the more likely other injuries are to be missed

Introduction

Certain injuries have a reputation for being missed on initial presentation. This may be due to the inexperience of the doctor assessing a patient, failure to follow accepted practices or some specific feature of the injury or of the circumstances of the presentation that make errors more likely. This topic is a summary of the most important of these injuries.

Bony injuries

As well as difficulty in assessing the patient because of age, communication issues or mental status, fractures can be missed when:

- There is an inadequate history or examination
- There is failure to appreciate the mechanism of injury and possible associated injuries
- There are errors when requesting radiographs or clinical information is missing (e.g. suspecting a scaphoid fracture and requesting a wrist radiograph, or failing to request a foot radiograph in a patient with a fifth metatarsal fracture)
- The radiographs or views obtained are inadequate (e.g. failure to obtain C1–T1 on a lateral C-spine film)
- There is failure to interpret a radiograph correctly

These problems are exacerbated when patients are being seen in the emergency department under considerable time pressure. Therefore, prior to requesting radiographs a full accurate history and detailed examination are mandatory. A clinical question, as well as clinical information on the radiological request form will increase the utility of the imaging. The side, site and required views (with an adequate justification) should be clearly stated.

When reviewing radiographs it is essential to ensure that patient identifiers concur and that the correct side has been investigated. When computer image retrieval systems are used, it is essential to ensure that the images being viewed are those from the current attendance and not from an earlier attendance when radiographs of the same region were requested. The views and images must be reviewed for adequacy and the required films requested if they have not been done. There should be no hesitation in requesting further films if these are necessary or in seeking a second opinion from a radiologist, senior colleague or specialist clinician. Compromise leads to error. It is important to be conversant with the normal radiographic anatomy of the region in question and to know of the common variants likely to be encountered.

The multiply injured patient

The <C>ABCDE protocol is devised to rapidly identify and treat life-threatening traumatic injuries. Despite this systematic assessment, a proportion of patients' injuries escape detection. A higher incidence of initially unnoticed injuries is found in patients with higher injury severity scores, altered consciousness and prolonged admissions. The evolution of rapid CT assessment and the tertiary survey recognise this risk and have reduced the incidence of missed injuries.

Specific injuries – fractures and dislocations

Cervical spine injuries

Historically, plain radiographs were hindered by inadequate views and difficulty in interpretation. The incidence of missed injuries has decreased with the increased availability of, and familiarity with, CT scanning. However, C-spine injury should be excluded in all polytrauma patients. In an unconscious patient, hypotension in the presence of a relative bradycardia failing to respond to fluid challenges may be an early sign of spinal cord trauma. A thorough neurological assessment should be performed, considering ligamentous injury in the absence of a fracture in children or adults with persistent neck pain.

Salter–Harris fractures

In children, Salter–Harris 1 or 5 growth plate injuries are easily missed, risking growth disturbance or arrest, particularly in type 5 injuries. Intra-articular fractures are also difficult to diagnose and characterise.

Posterior dislocation of shoulder

Posterior shoulder dislocations (**Figure 20**) are rare injuries and prone to late presentation. The patient will hold their arm internally rotated and adducted with inability to externally rotate their shoulder or supinate their forearm. A posterior dislocation should be particularly suspected in epileptic patients with shoulder pain, patients following an electrocution injury or in those with a history of alcohol abuse. The diagnosis may be missed on anteroposterior (AP) radiographs, where the humeral head is said to resemble a light bulb. Additional axillary and lateral scapula views often reveal a dislocation and associated reverse Hill–Sachs lesion, a humeral head compression fracture caused by impaction on glenoid. The humeral head can be difficult to relocate, and treatment is often determined by the duration of injury and size of Hill–Sachs lesion.

Fractures of the radial head and neck

Radial head and neck fractures may be missed on the initial radiographs. Contributing factors include confusion with overlying bones and the fact that the only abnormality may be a minor change in the angle of the cortex of the neck. The history, location of the pain and relation to elbow movement are clues to the diagnosis. The

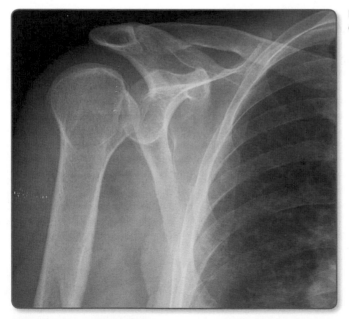

Figure 20 Posterior shoulder dislocation.

presence of a positive fat pad should lead to a diagnosis of presumed fracture and to appropriate follow up. Fractures may be more clearly visible on a delayed film.

Forearm fracture dislocations

Forearm fractures, particularly in children can be difficult to interpret with growth plates and ossification centres to consider. Even in the adult, fracture dislocations can be missed when the proximal and distal radioulnar joints are not assessed on both AP and lateral radiographs. Radial head reduction becomes more difficult where there is a delay in diagnosis, often requiring more invasive surgery. Secondly, although a fracture of the distal radius is unlikely to be missed, radiographs should be evaluated for associated Galeazzi distal radioulnar joint dislocation.

Scaphoid fracture

With better understanding of the mechanism of injury, increased awareness of occult fractures and implementation of diagnostic pathways, the number of missed scaphoid fractures has reduced. Paralleling this is a decrease in morbidity with delay in diagnosis which raises risk of avascular necrosis and nonunion. A fracture should be suspected in all patients complaining of wrist pain following a fall onto outstretched hand with anatomical snuffbox or scaphoid tubercle tenderness and pain on axial loading of thumb (Chen test). Standard scaphoid views in wrist injuries specifically look for thin cortical breaks in the distal pole and waist of the scaphoid. Immobilisation and re-evaluation at 2 weeks should follow if an occult fracture is suspected and the initial films are normal.

Lunate dislocation

The lunate dislocates in a volar direction out of the radiocarpal joint (**Figure 21**). Despite considerable pain and swelling following high-energy trauma, the dislocation can be overlooked on plain radiographs by inexperienced clinicians. Urgent reduction may be necessary to relieve median nerve compression and minimise cartilage damage. The AP radiographs may show changes in shape (quadrangular lunate to triangular)

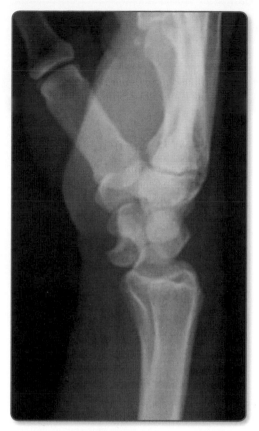

Figure 21 Lunate dislocation.

and reduced joint space between the lunate and scaphoid. The injury is best visualised on lateral wrist views, when the normal alignment of the lunate with the capitate is lost.

Maisonneuve fracture

The Maisonneuve fracture is a spiral fracture of the proximal third of the fibula associated with a fracture of the distal tibia. This injury is missed because the patient fails to complain of proximal fibula pain or the clinician fails to appreciate the mechanism of injury and dissipation of forces in external rotation type injuries. The ankle is often radiographed in isolation as this is the focus of pain. However, the finding of a transverse medial malleolus fracture should raise the possibility of a fibula fracture proximal to the distal talofibular joint and should prompt closer inspection of the ankle mortise and fibula.

Calcaneal fractures

Avulsion fracture of the anterior process of the calcaneum may present as ankle pain, typically following a forced inversion plantar-flexion injury and causing confusion with an ankle sprain. The injury is missed when the anterior process is not scrutinised on lateral ankle radiographs. Calcaneal stress fractures present with chronic heel pain, and should be considered as a diagnosis in osteoporotic patients. Lateral calcaneal views may show lucent lines and subtle vertical sclerotic lines which may be missed or occult on radiographs, but distinctly visible on MRI.

Slipped capital femoral epiphysis

This injury occurs in children and is prone to delayed or missed diagnosis. The child may present with knee pain distracting an inexperienced clinician. Early radiographs can be subtle and difficult to interpret, becoming more obvious as symptoms develop and the slip progresses. In 25%, the injury is bilateral. More advanced slips alter surgical management and long-term outcome. In a limping child, with hip or knee pain examination for leg length discrepancy is essential as is close scrutiny of the AP pelvis (Klein's line) and frog leg laterals for epiphyseal displacement.

Specific injuries – soft tissue injuries

Achilles tendon rupture

Athletic individuals report sudden pain, akin to being kicked in the heel while pushing off, often with an audible pop. However, patients often self-diagnose an ankle sprain and present late to emergency departments. Absence of a palpable gap and negative Thompson calf squeeze test give false reassurance in partial tears or delayed presentations with functional haematomas. Inability to heel raise should prompt further investigation with dynamic ultrasound. Large tendon deficits with the ankle in plantar flexion or delayed presentations may require operative intervention.

Anterior cruciate ligament rupture

The tendon either ruptures, is partially torn, or in children can avulse its insertion into the tibial eminence. The patient gives a history of the knee giving way, often an audible pop or tear and inability to continue with the current activity. In addition to pain, a tense haematoma develops which obscures initial assessment. The Lachman's test is most sensitive; anterior draw and pivot shift tests confirm diagnosis. The efficacy of these examinations is operator-dependent and proportional to experience. Undiagnosed, the patient will have persistent instability and pain, while increased knee translation causes accelerated degenerative change and damage to menisci. Initially there is likely to be sufficient pain to prevent an adequate diagnostic examination and arrangement of appropriate follow up for reassessment is essential when a diagnosis of significant intra-articular injury is suspected but cannot be confirmed.

Ulnar collateral ligament rupture

This ligament resists valgus deformity of the first metacarpophalangeal joint, offering stability when gripping objects and in pincer movements. It is injured when the thumb is forcefully abducted. The patient must be examined for focal tenderness and asymmetrical instability (>30° valgus deviation). Radiographs may identify a bony avulsion and valgus stress views highlight laxity. Early intervention (<2 weeks) produces superior surgical outcomes.

Further reading

Apley AG, Solomon L. Apley's system of orthopaedics and fractures, 9th edn. USA: CRC Press, 2010.

McRae R, Esser M. Practical fracture treatment, 5th edn. Edinburgh: Churchill Livingstone, 2008.

Segal LS, Shrader MW. Missed fractures in paediatric trauma patients. Acta Orthop Belg 2013; 79:608–615.

Related topics of interest

- Nonaccidental injury (p. 205)
- Spinal cord injury without radiological abnormality (p. 273)
- Tertiary survey (p. 282)

Compartment syndrome

Key points

- Acute compartment syndrome is a limb-threatening surgical emergency
- The diagnosis is clinical in most cases, but compartment pressure measurement may be required
- Untreated compartment syndrome results in significant disability

Pathophysiology and consequences

Compartment syndrome is characterised by muscle ischaemia caused by an increase in pressure above the local capillary closing pressure within a muscle compartment. The muscle compartment can be made up of a single muscle or several, and is surrounded by unyielding inelastic tissues such as bone and fascia. If muscle ischaemia persists, irreversible changes occur in the muscle with potentially severe functional consequences. Compartment syndrome can occur in any muscle but is particularly common in the leg and less so in the forearm, hand, foot and thigh. Compartment syndrome can be acute, often associated with trauma or chronic, transiently associated with exercise. This is not considered further here.

The source of the increased pressure can be thought of as endogenous, from within the compartment, or exogenous from outside:
Endogenous causes include:

- Bleeding from local trauma as a result of damage to local vessels, muscle tears or from fractured bone ends. This may be exacerbated by anticoagulants or other causes of increased bleeding
- Local oedema with a multiplicity of causes including surgical trauma (e.g. after reaming a long bone for insertion of an intramedullary nail), swelling associated with injury (particularly crush injury and burns) or following ischaemia and subsequent reperfusion. Less common causes include reperfusion after repair of a blocked artery, after the release of a tourniquet (following prolonged

application), toxins such as in snake envenomation and isolated limb perfusion chemotherapy.

Exogenous causes include:

- Tight encircling dressings or splints such as plaster casts
- Pressure from positioning under anaesthetic for operative procedures, or prolonged lying on a limb, e.g. after drug intoxication or a medical procedure or illness
- Tight circumferential eschar or contracted scar after burns

In practice, the cause is often multifactorial, e.g. a patient may suffer bleeding from a broken bone and injured muscle following a tibial fracture, leading to swelling, and the consequent pressure increase may be potentiated by the use of plaster splintage.

Once established, irreversible changes in the muscle can be seen histologically from about 4 hours after the onset of complete ischaemia. Clinically, the time of onset is uncertain so the situation may have already progressed by the time of diagnosis. This emphasises the need for rapid diagnosis and intervention.

Consequences of compartment syndrome are local and systemic.
Local:

- Muscle necrosis leading to contractures and weakness
- Ischaemic nerve damage
- Distal ischaemic changes if traversing arteries become occluded
- Sepsis resulting from infection in necrotic muscle especially if decompression is late
- Scarring from fasciotomy

Systemic:

- Renal failure as a result of rhabdomyolysis

Clinical features

The hallmark symptom of compartment syndrome is pain. The pain characteristically has a burning or tight character and is extremely severe, generally perceived as being in excess of that anticipated. It may not be adequately controlled even by opiate analgesia and will increase when the affected muscles are stretched passively: this is the only consistently helpful clinical sign. When associated with trauma, application of casts, splints, and bandages may result in the pain increasing rather than decreasing.

Other features tend to occur late or are unreliable and so play no part in excluding the diagnosis of compartment syndrome. These include tenderness and tightness on palpation of the compartment, altered function of nerves which traverse the compartment and loss of distal pulses (a very late finding because compartment syndrome occurs and can persist at pressures which occlude capillaries but leave traversing veins and arteries open).

There is no reassurance if a fracture is an open injury. The soft tissue injury cannot be relied upon to decompress the muscle compartments.

Diagnostic difficulty may occur if there are factors which affect the patient's appreciation of pain, these include:

- An altered conscious level
- Spinal cord or peripheral nerve injury
- Drug or alcohol intoxication
- Sedation
- Anaesthesia including regional blocks, epidurals and spinal anaesthetics as well as general anaesthesia
- Prolonged tourniquet times during surgery

In such cases, it may be necessary to measure the pressure within the muscle compartments. This is usually done with commercially available handheld devices or by using a line connected to a pressure transducer attached to a monitor. Measurements should be taken from all potentially affected compartments. In the leg, there are four compartments: anterior, lateral (or peroneal), superficial posterior and deep posterior. The deep posterior compartment is difficult to measure as other compartments overlie it. Measured pressures should be subtracted from the diastolic blood pressure. This difference is termed the delta-P (ΔP). The ΔP should be over 30 mmHg, if not, compartment syndrome should be diagnosed. There is little evidence to support an absolute pressure value as the threshold for decompression. In selected high-risk individuals, continuous monitoring of the compartment pressure with an indwelling catheter placed in the anterior compartment of the leg may be justified.

Treatment

Once compartment syndrome is diagnosed, intervention is required urgently. All circumferential dressings must be released completely. Plaster casts must be split along their whole length, including padding, so that skin can be seen. In some cases, this will lead to rapid resolution of symptoms, but further close observation will be needed to ensure recovery. The affected limb must be elevated to the level of the heart in order to optimise venous drainage without compromising arterial inflow to the compartment.

If spontaneous improvement has not occurred, urgent surgery will be needed. Fasciotomy of the affected compartments is performed as soon as possible after diagnosis. The exact technique depends on the location, but care must be taken to ensure complete release including fascia and skin over the full extent of the compartment. In the lower leg, this is generally done with long medial and lateral incisions through which all four compartments are released.

Fasciotomy will usually make any fracture present more unstable. As a consequence appropriate fracture stabilisation at the time of release will be necessary. This will often be external fixation in order to reduce the risk of infection associated with internal fixation. The wounds must be left open, usually for at least 48 hours, in order to allow swelling to settle, and appropriate sterile dressings must be applied. The use of topical negative pressure dressings or "shoe-lace" closure with vascular loops may reduce the time before closure can be achieved.

In some cases, split skin grafting will be required. In all cases, there will be prominent scars. Renal function must be monitored carefully to identify acute kidney injury secondary to myoglobinuria.

In very rare cases, where compartment syndrome has been diagnosed very late, fasciotomy may be associated with the risk of severe infection. In such cases, a carefully considered decision not to perform fasciotomy may need to be made by clinicians with extensive experience of this condition.

Further reading

Frink M, Hildebrand F, Krettek C, Brand J, Hankemeier S. Compartment syndrome of the lower leg and foot. Clin Orthop Relat Res 2010; 468:940–950.

McQueen MM, Court-Brown CM. Compartment monitoring in tibial fractures. The pressure threshold for decompression. J Bone Joint Surg Br 1996; 78:99–104.

Nanchahal J Nanchahal J, Nayagam S, Khan U, et al. Standards for the management of open fractures of the lower limb. London: Royal Society of Medicine Press Ltd, 2009.

Related topics of interest

Damage control resuscitation and surgery

Key points

- The primary aim of damage control resuscitation is to prevent coagulopathy and minimise ongoing haemorrhage
- Damage control surgery prioritises physiology over anatomical injury
- Damage control surgery is a component of damage control resuscitation

Introduction

This approach to managing severely injured patients arose following an observation that definitive surgery for every injury at first operation appeared to be associated with a high mortality. Such patients were often found to have developed the lethal triad of hypothermia, acidosis and coagulopathy. This compounded their acquired anatomical injury and impacted on their physiological ability to compensate.

The term 'damage control' was taken from the process of the same name used by the Royal Navy to keep afloat battle damaged warships while reducing the disruption to battle fighting to a minimum.

Similarly, in damage control surgery, concentrated efforts are made to minimise the duration of the operative intervention. This allows further resuscitation on the intensive care unit until such time that the patient is sufficiently stable to endure more prolonged but definitive surgery.

While the damage control concept was initially described in the management of life-threatening abdominal haemorrhage, its principles have now been extended across all surgical specialities.

The process of damage control

Four stages of damage control have been described:

DC0

The first stage takes place prehospital or in the emergency department and consists of:

- Early rewarming
- Use of topical haemostatics
- Tourniquet application
- Circumferential compression of pelvic fractures
- Administration of tranexamic acid

DC1

Following initial assessment in the emergency department, damage control surgery is carried out. If sufficient prehospital information is available, usually because of the presence of a prehospital doctor, the decision may be taken to take the patient directly to the operating theatre without emergency department assessment. Damage control abdominal surgery aims to:

- Control haemorrhage
- Minimise peritoneal contamination
- Achieve temporary abdominal closure

DC2

This stage begins in theatre and continues after surgery on the intensive care unit and consists of:

- Management of hypothermia and prevention of further heat loss
- Correction of coagulopathy
- Correction of acidosis

DC3

Following physiological optimisation, the patient will return to theatre within 72 hours of DC2 (above), for:

- Definitive surgery
- Creation of stomas, feeding access
- Closure of fascial layers

Damage control resuscitation

Damage control resuscitation represents an extension of the damage control philosophy. While damage control surgery is focussed on managing the major trauma patient who has developed the lethal triad, damage control resuscitation is focussed on preventing its development. Measures include the use of permissive hypotension, limiting or avoiding crystalloid infusions and optimising blood product replacement ratios. The use of tranexamic acid, (an antifibrinolytic), is strongly advocated. Damage control surgery should be seen as part of the continuum of damage control resuscitation. Indeed damage control resuscitation may be so successful as to permit some patients who previously would have only been considered for damage control surgery to undergo earlier definitive operative management.

Indications for damage control surgery

Only a select few patients will require this approach to managing their injuries; sound clinical judgement must be applied to identify those most likely to benefit. Indications include:

- Heart rate >120 bpm
- Systolic blood pressure <90 mmHg
- Positive focussed assessment with sonography for trauma
- Multiple life-threatening injuries
- pH <7.2
- Hypothermia
- More than 10 units of packed red blood cell transfusion during resuscitation
- Coagulopathy on laboratory evaluation
- Operative time >90 minutes
- Lactate >5 mmol/L
- Appropriate clinical experience and resources available at the receiving centre

A damage control laparotomy differs from the standard approach in that the focus is on obtaining haemorrhage control and minimising peritoneal contamination and the use of temporary abdominal closure devices. A damage control approach to a bleeding solid organ involves either removal or compression, e.g. intra-abdominal haemorrhage from the liver surface is best managed by using packs to compress the source of bleeding, while massive haemorrhage associated with splenic injury warrants splenectomy. In order to minimise contamination of the abdominal cavity, nonviable bowel is resected and urinary and biliary diversion are prioritised. Ideally injuries to major blood vessels are repaired; however, if necessary, ligation of the vessel or a temporary vascular shunt may be considered as alternatives. At the end of the procedure, the abdomen is closed using a temporary device; the aim being to prevent visceral adherence to the abdominal wall and help drain oedema in addition to bringing the incisional edges together. Fascial closure of the abdomen is not recommended due to the risk of developing intra-abdominal hypertension.

Increasingly, interventional radiology is also being used, either as a primary method of achieving haemostasis or as an adjunct to the surgical procedure. Primary sites of embolisation include areas where surgical access and repair may be technically difficult or prolonged, such as vessels supplying the pelvis, liver, retroperitoneum or spleen. Other endovascular procedures which may be considered for traumatic vascular injury include stenting and the use of balloon catheters. These devices provide proximal vessel occlusion, which can control continued bleeding until operative repair or more distal control can be obtained.

Intensive care management

The focus of care on the intensive care unit is to restore the patient's physiological parameters to normal. This is achieved by the correction of coagulopathy, reversal of acidosis and continued resuscitation with the preferential use of blood products over crystalloid infusions. Physiological targets include normothermia, systemic lactate <2.0 mmol/L and a urine output of 0.5–1 mL/kg as an indicator of end target-organ perfusion.

Return to theatre

This should usually occur within 12–48 hours of damage control surgery and definitive surgical management of the injuries can now be considered. The abdominal packs are removed and a thorough re-examination of the abdominal structures is undertaken. Fluid collections are drained, necrotic tissue is debrided and feeding access established. If major bleeding reoccurs, the abdomen can be repacked and the patient returned to the intensive care unit for further attempts at a later date. Formal closure of the abdomen may be achieved if oedema has resolved, alternatively temporary closure may continue until formal closure is possible. If vascular shunts have been inserted, definitive bypass procedures may be considered.

Complications

In addition to the increased resources required to manage these patients, not all patients need to undergo damage control surgery in the first instance, as the damage control approach is not without risk of exposing the patient to significant morbidity. This can include the development of intra-abdominal hypertension and abdominal compartment syndrome and the risk of wound complications or intra-abdominal abscess formation, which can occur in up to 25% of patients. Complications associated with vascular damage control surgery may include distal ischaemia requiring subsequent revascularisation or amputation, sepsis, chronic pain and malunion of fractures. It is therefore critical that the 10% of polytrauma patients most likely to benefit from this method of management are correctly identified early in the course of their resuscitation.

Further reading

Chovanes J, Cannon JW, Nunez TC. The evolution of damage control surgery. Surg Clin North Am 2012; 92:859–875.

Germanos S, Gourgiotis S, Villias C, et al. Damage control surgery in the abdomen: an approach for the management of severe injured patients. Int J Surg 2008; 6:246–252.

Lamb CM, MacGoey P, Navarro AP, et al. Damage control surgery in the era of damage control resuscitation. Br J Anaesth 2014; 113:242–249.

Related topics of interest

- Abdominal trauma (p. 1)
- Blood product (1:1:1) resuscitation (p. 42)
- <C>ABCDE resuscitation (p. 63)

Elbow injuries

Key points

- The 'pink pulseless' hand in displaced paediatric supracondylar fractures of the humerus requires accurate neurovascular assessment
- The 'terrible triad' describes a combination of an elbow dislocation with coronoid and radial head fractures
- Comminuted fractures of the distal humerus in the elderly may benefit from primary total elbow arthroplasty rather than fixation

Elbow injuries in children

Supracondylar fractures of the humerus

Supracondylar fractures normally result from a fall onto the outstretched hand. Ninety-five per cent are extension type fractures with the distal fragment displaced posteriorly, the remainder flexion-displacement fractures. The extension types are classified according to the Gartland classification (**Figure 22**).

Gartland I fractures are managed conservatively in a collar and cuff or Softcast for 2 or 3 weeks. Gartland II fractures are managed according to the degree of displacement. If there is angulation but the anterior humeral line is maintained, they can be managed conservatively. If the anterior humeral line passes in front of the capitellum, the fracture may be reduced by flexing the elbow beyond 90°. If this is not tolerated, manipulation under general anaesthesia may be required, sometimes with Kirschner wire fixation. If there is angulation and rotation (Gartland IIb), the fracture must be manipulated and stabilised with Kirschner wires (**Figures 23** and **24**).

Grade III injuries necessitate careful assessment of the neurovascular status. The radial pulse and capillary refill should be assessed. The peripheral nerves should be examined individually. The anterior interosseous nerve (AIN) is the most commonly injured nerve.

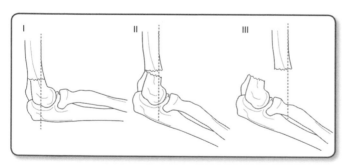

Figure 22 Gartland classification for extension type supracondylar fractures of the humerus [I. undisplaced, II. posterior angulation (a – no rotation, b – rotated), III. off ended].

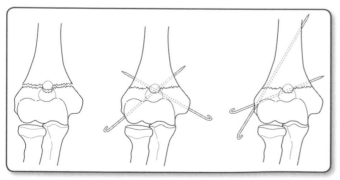

Figure 23 Kirschner wire configuration in supracondylar fracture management.

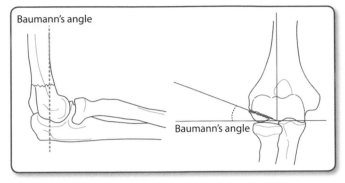

Figure 24 The radiographic parameters indicating a satisfactory reduction are the anterior humeral line passing through the capitellum (lateral view) along with adequate restoration of Baumann's angle (anteroposterior view).

If the neurovascular status is not compromised, the fracture requires closed or open reduction supplemented with Kirschner wires. There is controversy regarding management of the 'pink, pulseless' hand (where the radial pulse is not palpable but the hand well perfused). The author's practice is to splint in a position of comfort (usually extension), inform the vascular surgeons, look for signs of brachial artery injury, such as bruising over the medial elbow and seek evidence of AIN injury (**Figure 25**). This is important, as where there is no deficit, if the radial pulse does not return following reduction on table; it is probably due to vasospasm and does not require exploration. If however there is pre-existing AIN deficit, where the pulse does not return immediately

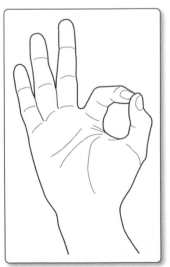

Figure 25 The 'OK' sign to assess anterior interosseous nerve function.

following reduction, exploration of the vessel should be considered even if reduction appears satisfactory. The risks of surgery include infection, nerve injury (ulnar nerve when the medial wire is passed), malunion and growth disturbance. The wires require removal at 3–4 weeks.

Medial and lateral condyle fractures of the humerus

Medial epicondylar fractures are due to avulsion of the attached common flexor origin. They may be associated with elbow dislocations and should be excluded following reduction. If the joint is not congruent after reduction, there should be a high index of suspicion that a bony fragment is trapped in the joint, in which case open reduction and fixation of the fragment will be required. In the case of elbow dislocation, stability should be assessed (see below).

Lateral condyle fractures are classified according to the Milch classification (**Figure 26**). Undisplaced fractures (<2 mm) can be managed conservatively. Regular radiographic assessment is required for 3 weeks to ensure that there is no displacement. This can be difficult to assess on plain radiographs, which do not adequately demonstrate the large cartilaginous components of such fragments. Displaced fractures require open reduction and internal fixation, often with crossed Kirschner wires.

Lateral condyle fractures, if missed, can result in cubitus valgus and tardy ulnar nerve palsy in later life, as it stretches on the medial side.

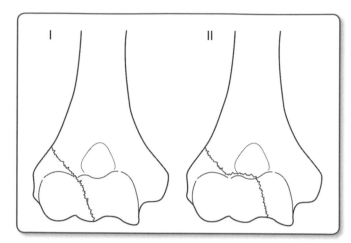

Figure 26 Milch classification of lateral condylar fractures: Type I – Fracture through the capitellum. Type II – transtrochlear – lateral metaphyseal fracture.

The adult elbow

Fractures of the distal humerus

These are common in elderly patients with osteoporotic bone. All patients should undergo careful assessment of their neurovascular and soft tissue status before and after application of an above elbow backslab. In younger patients with intra-articular fractures, the AO principles of anatomical reduction, rigid fixation and early mobilisation should be applied. A CT should be obtained to delineate the fracture and aid operative planning. Plates are usually applied medially and posterolaterally, resulting in an orthogonal configuration. Postoperatively, the patient will gradually increase the range of movement.

In older patients with good bone quality, a similar management strategy is employed. In very infirm patients, if significant comminution or bone loss is present, a conservative approach may be taken, the 'bag of bones' strategy. The fracture is treated with cast immobilisation for 3–4 weeks followed by mobilisation. Alternatively, if fixation is not possible, a primary total elbow arthroplasty may be considered. This has been shown to have a better functional outcome if performed de novo, rather than following previous fixation attempts.

Elbow dislocation

Elbow dislocations most commonly occur posterolaterally. A simple dislocation requires reduction in the emergency department after examination of the neurovascular status, which must be repeated after reduction (**Figure 27**). A post-reduction radiograph is required to ensure joint congruency. A hinged brace can be applied, allowing flexion and extension in a stable arc of movement. This can be increased at 2 weekly intervals until left unlocked, and removed 6–8 weeks after injury.

The 'terrible triad' describes a radial head and coronoid fracture with elbow dislocation. This injury configuration is very unstable

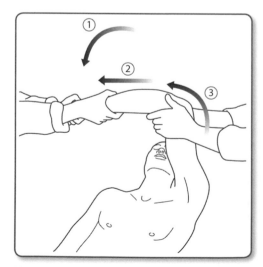

Figure 27 Technique for reducing posterolateral elbow dislocations.

Table 9 Stabilisers of the elbow	
Primary stabilisers	**Secondary stabilisers**
Ulnar collateral ligament	Radiocapitellar joint
Ulnohumeral joint (coronoid, olecranon)	Elbow capsule and lateral ligament complex
	Traversing muscles

and requires treatment of the injured elbow stabilisers (**Table 9**) once reduced. It often follows a fall on the outstretched hand with the elbow extended. Immediate management includes neurovascular assessment, and radiographs to confirm the dislocation and identify any associated fractures. The elbow is reduced and splinted in 90° flexion. If the reduction is performed on an anaesthetised patient, the stability of the elbow can be assessed by applying a varus force throughout flexion and extension (to assess the lateral ligament complex) and a valgus force in 30° and 90° flexion (assesses the ulnar collateral ligament and radial head). After reduction, the neurovascular status should be reassessed.

Radial head fracture

Radial head fractures may occur in isolation after a fall on the outstretched hand. They may also represent part of an Essex–Lopresti type lesion, where the interosseous membrane between ulna and radius is injured, resulting in proximal shear of the radius in relation to the ulna. This results in radial head fracture and subluxation of the distal radioulnar joint, indicated by tenderness in this region.

Radial head fractures are classified using the Mason classification (**Figure 28**). Mason I injuries are managed conservatively, with mobilisation as pain allows. Mason II injuries may be managed nonoperatively if the articular step is <2 mm. If greater than this, open reduction internal fixation may be indicated if there is a block to supination/pronation. Mason III and IV injuries are often managed operatively. Radial head replacement may give a better outcome than fixation if the radial head is in three or more parts.

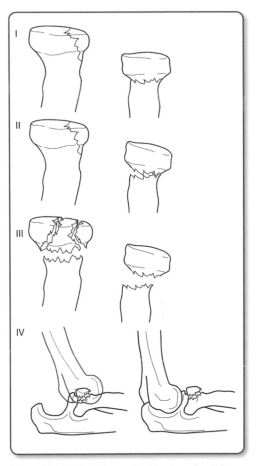

Figure 28 Modified Mason classification of radial head and neck fractures, type I–IV.

Coronoid fractures

The coronoid is a primary elbow stabiliser. These fractures are classified according to the Regan and Morrey system (**Figure 29**). They may occur in isolation or in conjunction with a dislocation.

Type 1 fractures are managed conservatively with early mobilisation once the acute symptoms have settled. Types 2 and 3 fractures often require open reduction and internal fixation to restore elbow stability. Postoperatively, the patient is mobilised in a hinged brace within the arc of stability. This is gradually increased over time.

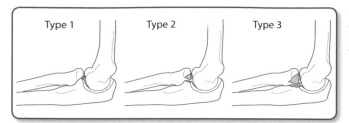

Figure 29 Regan and Morrey classification of coronoid fractures (type 1 tip only, type 2 <50% and type 3 >50%).

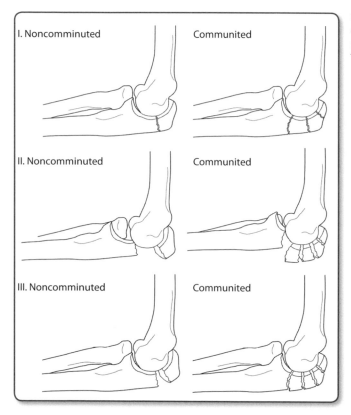

Figure 30 Mayo classification of olecranon fractures. Type I – undisplaced. Type II – displaced. Type III – unstable.

Olecranon fractures

These follow a fall on to the apex of the elbow. The Mayo classification is used (**Figure 30**). Type 1 (undisplaced) fractures are treated nonoperatively, with cast immobilisation for 3 weeks. Weekly radiographs are performed to ensure that no displacement occurs. Type 2 (displaced, >3 mm and forearm stable) and type 3 (displaced, >3 mm and forearm unstable) fractures are treated operatively using a tension band wire construct or plate fixation (**Figure 31**).

Monteggia fracture-dislocations

Such injuries involve a fracture of the proximal ulna with concomitant dislocation (or fracture) of the radial head. They occur from a fall backwards on the outstretched hand. They are classified according to the Bado classification (I–IV, see **Figure 32**). Bado I–III fractures require fixation of the proximal ulna fracture, resulting in reduction of the radiocapitellar joint. Intraoperatively, radiocapitellar joint stability is assessed

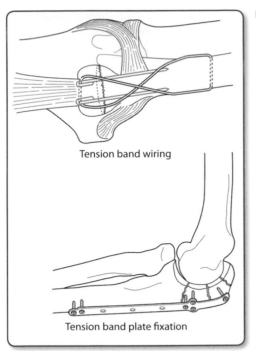

Figure 31 Methods of olecranon fixation.

Tension band wiring

Tension band plate fixation

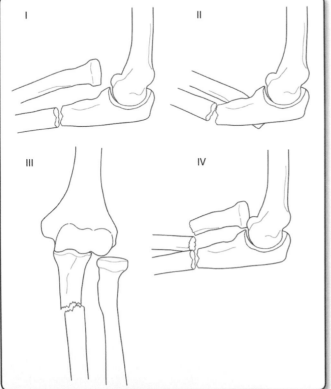

Figure 32 Bado classification of Monteggia fractures (type I anterior dislocation of radial head, type II posterior, type III lateral and type IV proximal radius fractured also).

I

II

III

IV

through supination and pronation. The elbow is immobilised in a stable position, often at 90° of flexion with the forearm midprone, for 3 weeks. Bado IV fractures require fixation of both radius and ulna.

Further reading

Edwardson SA, Murray O, Joseph J, et al. Paediatric supracondylar fractures: an overview of current management and guide to open approaches. Orthop Trauma 27; 303–311.

McRae R, Esser M. Practical Fracture Treatment, 5th Edition. Edinburgh: Elsevier, 2008.
Modi C, et al. Elbow instability. Orthop Trauma 2012; 26:316–327.

Related topics of interest

Epidemiology of trauma

Key points

- 1 in 10 deaths globally is caused by trauma
- Road traffic collision and self-harm are the commonest causes of fatal injury
- Trauma is the most common cause of death in children and adolescents

Introduction

Opening the newspaper at the time of writing (December, 2014), the headlines are dominated by news of mass casualties, either war-related or the result of civilian terrorism; 'Taliban murdered 132 children in school', or 'Sydney mourns two hostages killed in the kidnapping drama.' Inside pages have another type of news: '18-year-old lost control of his car while driving under the influence of narcotics, and was seriously injured.'

While the former events make headlines, it is the everyday accidents on the road or at home that cause the greatest number of deaths and the most disability resulting from trauma. For this reason, trauma has been called the 'silent epidemic of the 21st century.'

Global mortality statistics

Of the estimated 52.8 million deaths worldwide in 2010, about 5.1 million were caused by injuries, and the total number of deaths from injuries exceeded that of human immunodeficiency virus, tuberculosis and malaria combined (3.8 million). At the top of the global list of causes of death were ischemic heart disease (about 7 million), cerebrovascular disease (5.9 million) and chronic obstructive pulmonary disease (2.9 million). About 69% of fatal injuries are unintentional, 26% intentional and 4% caused by nature, war and legal intervention (**Table 10**).

The total number of road injury deaths in 2010 was 1.3 million (an increase of 46% from 1990). The second most common cause of death from trauma was self-harm (0.88 million, an increase of 32% in 20 years) followed by falls (0.54 million, an increase of

Table 10 Causes of injury-related deaths globally in 2010*

Cause of death	No. of deaths/100,000 persons	Percentage of injury-related deaths
Unintentional injuries	3520	69.4
Transportation-related injuries	1397	27.5
Falls	541	10.7
Drowning	349	6.9
Injuries from fire, heat and hot substances	338	6.7
Poisonings	180	3.5
Intentional injuries	1340	26.4
Self-harm	884	17.4
Interpersonal violence	456	9.0
Forces of nature	196	3.9
Collective violence and legal interventions	18	0.4
Other	715	14.1

*Modified from Norton R, Kobusingye O. Injuries. N Engl J Med 2013; 368:1723–1730.

55% over the same period) and interpersonal violence (0.46 million, 35% up over 20 years). Overall, the number of deaths from trauma increased by 24% in the period from 1990 to 2010.

Geographical considerations

In terms of trauma epidemiology, continents are not equal. More specifically the death rates are much higher in low- and middle-income countries compared with high-income countries. The estimated death rate from road-traffic collisions was highest in Africa (20.9/100,000) followed by the Americas (17.6). Falls were the most common reason in Southeast Asia (12.0) and drowning in Western Pacific Region (5.7). Europe dominated in poisoning (18.1) and self-harm (16.9), while interpersonal violence was most the common cause in the Americas (24.1). In view of the many persistent conflicts in the Middle East, it is not surprising that the estimated death rate from war and conflict was highest in the Eastern Mediterranean Region (17.7/100,000 people). Overall, estimated death rates from trauma (2008 figures) in high-income countries vary from 0.1 (war and conflict) to 13.4 (self-harm) per 100,000 people.

Europe

Trauma is a major cause of disability and hospital admissions. Over the years 2010–2012, the average annual fatality rate from trauma in the 28 European Union (EU) countries was 238,000. The number of hospital admissions was 5.4 million with 35.7 million trauma-related outpatient visits. Home, leisure and sports injuries accounted for 74% of all injures receiving hospital treatment.

The evidence demonstrates great variation in the proportion of deaths caused by injuries in different countries, with the highest rates in Lithuania (11%), Slovenia (8%) and Finland (8%), and the lowest in United Kingdom, Spain and Greece (all 3%). The EU average is 5%. The highest proportions of trauma-related hospital admissions were seen in Malta (15.0%), Austria (12.4%) and Poland (12.0%), the lowest in Portugal (4.0%), Bulgaria (5.2%) and Romania (5.2%), with an EU average of 8.3%.

Children and adolescents

Unlike degenerative diseases, trauma affects all age groups including children and adolescents. According to the Injuries in the EU 2010–2012 report, injury was the most common cause of death (28%) in children and adolescents followed by malignant neoplasms (19%) and congenital malformations (11%). In the age group of 15–24 years, 62% of all deaths were as a result of trauma.

Risk factors and prevention

Individual risk factors for road accidents, falls or self-harm include environmental factors (road and street design, speed limits, safety features in modern cars, helmet use among motorcyclists and bicyclists, safety considerations among the elderly and the availability of small arms) as well as individual factors such as alcohol and drug abuse and mental health issues. As a result, unlike cardiovascular disease, where there is a small number of accepted risk factors (including hypertension and smoking), addressing remediable causative factors for traumatic injuries and deaths is complex.

Nevertheless, prevention of injuries is likely to have the greatest effect in reducing the global trauma burden, and it is achievable with concerted effort, as shown by the halving of death rates from road-traffic collisions in the last 30 years in countries such as Australia, Canada and the United States. Prevention requires a multisectorial approach including both legislative and nonlegislative initiatives. Accessible and affordable health care including prehospital and hospital management as well as appropriate rehabilitation services are essential in reducing the global burden of trauma on populations, especially in developing countries. A recent emphasis on promoting the principles and essential requirements of trauma care in low- and middle-income countries is a laudable effort to change the projected trends in increases in deaths from transport-related injuries, self-harm, falls, burns and interpersonal violence over the next 20 years. Trauma care professionals are in a key position not just in managing individual patients with injuries, but also in promoting knowledge and influencing decision makers to make a priority of trauma prevention and the creation of trauma systems which will better serve our communities.

Further reading

Bikbov B, Perico N, Remuzzi G. Mortality landscape in the Global Burden of Diseases, Injuries and Risk Factors Study. Eur J Intern Med 2014; 25:1–5.

Injuries in the European Union. Summary of injury statistics for the years 2010–2012; Amsterdam, European Association for Injury Prevention and Safety Promotion (EuroSafe), 2014.

Leppäniemi AK. Update on global trends in trauma. Trauma 2009; 11:37–47.

Norton R, Kobusingye O. Injuries. N Engl J Med 2013; 368:1723–1730.

Related topics of interest

Fat embolism syndrome

Key points

- Fat embolism syndrome (FES) is an uncommon consequence of fat embolism
- The diagnosis of FES is largely clinical and a high degree of suspicion must be maintained
- Treatment of FES is supportive and the majority of those developing the syndrome recover fully

Epidemiology

Fat embolism may occur in the majority of major trauma patients; however, the associated syndrome may be unrecognised due in part to inconsistencies in the method of diagnosis and also to wide variations in the severity of presentation. Although associated with long bone fractures, FES has been recorded following soft-tissue injuries, burns and some nontraumatic conditions. Fat embolism also occurs following trauma-related procedures and elective arthroplasty. It likely occurs in the majority of long bone fractures and pelvic fractures, yet most patients remain asymptomatic or will develop subclinical mild hypoxia. The fully established syndrome is associated with a mortality of 10–15%. In a large series of patients suffering fatalities due to major trauma, there was a 100% incidence of fat embolism and an incidence of fat embolism in 3.4% of tibial fractures, 9% of femoral fractures and 20% of patients with both tibial and femoral fractures has been reported.

Pathology

The following 'mechanical' and 'metabolic' theories have persuasive supporting features and it is likely that there is overlap in the degree to which they are responsible for the development of FES.

The mechanical theory

This suggests that bone marrow and fat enter the bloodstream through torn-open venous channels. Fat embolism can occur in the absence of trauma and certainly in the absence of long bone fractures and it has been demonstrated by transoesophageal ultrasonography that showers of emboli occur during intramedullary nailing without producing clinical signs or symptoms. However, procedures producing higher volumes of emboli demonstrate a higher incidence of FES. The fat may then enter the arterial circulation either via a patent foramen ovale secondary to increased pressures on the right side of the circulation, or as microemboli passing through the lungs.

The metabolic theory

This theory postulates an alternative aetiology, and suggests that circulating chylomicrons aggregate as a secondary effect of trauma. Possible initiating factors include the release of lipase from damaged tissues. It is suggested that the clinical manifestations begin with the release of free fatty acids by pulmonary lipase or lipase released by the injured tissues, which in turn initiate the inflammatory and clotting cascades and the complement system. Tissue damage is increased by oxygen free-radicals and activated proteases. As a result of this, capillary leakage occurs, with local oedema and haemorrhage, alveolar collapse and consequent ventilation–perfusion mismatch leading to hypoxia. This theory may offer a persuasive explanation for the tendency of FES to present 24–72 hours after the initial insult.

Clinical presentation

There is considerable debate as to the clinical manifestations which accurately define FES. The following list gives an outline of the features which may raise suspicion of the diagnosis.

Major features

Respiratory

The major respiratory features are dyspnoea, tachypnoea and hypoxaemia suggestive of acute respiratory distress syndrome. Although various radiographic abnormalities (see below) are described, none are diagnostic for FES. Routine analysis of blood gases following major long bone fractures in the absence of associated chest injuries or any clinical evidence of FES shows deranged gases in up to one third of patients. The likelihood of FES following intramedullary nailing is suggested by intraoperative pyrexia.

Neurological

Major neurological features include confusion and reduced level of consciousness. In the head-injured patient, the onset of confusion is an indication for cranial computerised tomography (CT) scanning in order to exclude any intracerebral pathology directly due to trauma. Neurological symptoms are usually transient and rarely focal in their presentation. Seizures have been described.

Skin

A petechial rash may occur on the trunk and limbs, and occasionally the conjunctivae and oral mucosa. More than six petechiae can be regarded to be pathological.

Minor features

Minor features include pyrexia, renal insufficiency and retinal changes. These features are relatively nonspecific and must be used alongside a clinical picture which is congruent with a diagnosis of FES. Schonfeld has proposed a set of criteria with several of the above features being attributed weighted scores in order to offer a semiquantitative means of diagnosing FES. However, high importance is attributed to features which are very nonspecific, thus allowing room for doubt.

Investigations

FES is a clinical diagnosis but imaging and biochemical investigations may be of use to support this.

Imaging

The chest radiograph is often normal in the early stages. Bilateral fluffy infiltrates may develop as well as signs consistent with alveolar oedema or haemorrhage. Ventilation/perfusion scans may show perfusion defects with a normal ventilatory pattern. CT of the chest can show areas of ground glass opacification and septal thickening. Lymphadenopathy may also be present as a result of the inflammatory response resulting from ischaemia and toxic metabolites. Magnetic resonance imaging of the brain may show varying degrees of high-intensity T2 signal, depending on the degree of neurological impairment present.

Blood tests

Arterial blood gas analysis will demonstrate hypoxaemia consistent with ventilation–perfusion mismatch and the diagnostic partial pressure of oxygen will be <8 kPa. Thrombocytopaenia may occur, with platelet counts being <150,000/mm^3. The main cause of platelet consumption is in pulmonary aggregates. Coagulopathy varies from mild to disseminated intravascular coagulation.

Other diagnostic tests

Fat may be demonstrated in sputum and urine; however, this may occur in the trauma victim in the absence of FES. Bronchoalveolar lavage may show fat globules within alveolar macrophages, but the sensitivity and specificity of this are unknown.

Treatment

Treatment is largely supportive with oxygen therapy and mechanical ventilatory support with a focus on lung protective strategies if required. Monitoring should include regular blood gas analysis, chest radiographs, blood and platelet counts. The patient's neurological state should be reviewed regularly. Neither heparin nor corticosteroids have been proven to be of any clear benefit.

Prevention

Rigorous attempts should be made to prevent the development of FES. Fractures should be rapidly reduced and immobilized. Early surgical intervention rather than conservative management can further reduce the risk. Attempts should be made to minimise increases in intramedullary pressures which can lead to the development of fat embolus. The use of prophylactic steroid therapy may cause more harm than good to most patients recovering with supportive therapy alone.

Further reading

Eriksson EA, Pellegrini DC, Vanderkolk WE, et al. Incidence of pulmonary fat embolism at autopsy: an undiagnosed epidemic. J Trauma 2011; 71:312–315.

Mellor A, Soni N. Fat embolism. Anaesthesia 2001; 56:145–154.

Peltier LF. Fat embolism – a current concept. Clin Orthop Relat Res 1969; 66:241–253.

Related topics of interest

- Acute respiratory distress syndrome (p. 9)
- Long-bone fractures (p. 171)
- Metabolic response to trauma (p. 182)

Foot fractures – hindfoot

Key points

- Hindfoot fractures are commonly missed resulting in avoidable disability
- Computed tomography (CT) scanning is the imaging modality of choice for planning treatment
- Avascular necrosis of the talus is a significant complication of talar fractures

Introduction

Hindfoot fractures are frequently missed and often mismanaged due to incomplete understanding of the mechanics of the injury, incomplete history-taking and inadequate radiological investigation. Incorrect treatment of these injuries may lead to long-term disability and pain.

Fractures of the talus

Talar fractures are rare and usually associated with high-velocity trauma. The talus is a complex structure (**Figure 33**); 60% of its surface is covered with articular cartilage and it receives its blood supply from anterior tibial, posterior tibial and peroneal vessels. Interosseous blood supply to the body of the talus is from the anastomotic artery of the tarsal sinus and tarsal canal running in an anteroposterior direction making the body vulnerable to avascular necrosis in fracture of the neck of the talus. Fractures may involve the head, neck or body of the talus.

Talar head fractures are uncommon and frequently missed. CT is required for diagnosis and characterisation and displaced fractures require operative fixation. Talar neck fractures account for 50% of all talar fractures. This fracture was first described in 1919 by Anderson as aviator's fracture or aviator's astragalus (astragalus is a largely obsolete name for the talus) caused by a hyperdorsiflexion mechanism from a decelerating type injury when the rudder bar of an early aircraft was driven forcibly against the sole of the foot.

These fractures may be associated with osteonecrosis of the talus due of interruption of the blood supply. Hawkins' classification (1970) provides guidelines for treatment and prognosis regarding the development of osteonecrosis (**Table 11**).

Type 1 fractures can be treated in plaster with the foot plantigrade for 8 weeks. Type 2, 3 and 4 fractures require early open reduction and internal fixation usually approached anteriorly using a single or double incision (anteromedial/anterolateral). Fixation is achieved with compression screws or modern talar neck plates. Medial comminution should be addressed to prevent varus malalignment.

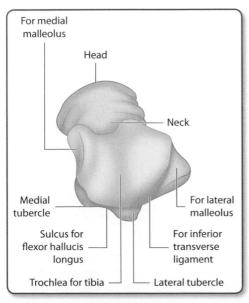

Figure 33 Anatomy of the talus.

Labels: For medial malleolus · Head · Neck · Medial tubercle · Sulcus for flexor hallucis longus · Trochlea for tibia · For lateral malleolus · For inferior transverse ligament · Lateral tubercle

Table 11 Hawkins' classification of talar neck fractures	
Type 1	Minimal or no displacement
Type 2	Displaced fracture with subtalar subluxation/dislocation
Type 3	Displaced fracture with subtalar and ankle dislocation
Type 4	The above with talonavicular dislocation (later added by Canale and Kelly)

The higher the grade of fracture, the poorer is the prognosis due to the severity of vascular compromise. Hawkins' sign seen as an osteoporotic lucent line at 8–12 weeks is an important prognostic indicator (**Figure 34**).

Talar dome fractures are high-energy injuries. If displaced they are associated with a poorer prognosis and require early open reduction and fixation to avoid skin breakdown and osteonecrosis. Lateral process fractures are usually due to a dorsiflexion and inversion mechanism, commonly in snowboard injuries. Posterior process fractures are hyperplantar flexion injuries. If displaced these fractures need operative fixation. Osteochondral fractures occur in the anterolateral and posteromedial talar dome and can be dealt through arthroscopy of the ankle. Most of these fractures are associated with ankle injuries and may be dismissed as ankle sprains. CT or magnetic resonance imaging is required to diagnose and characterise these injuries.

Complications of talar fractures

Avascular necrosis occurs in 50% of talar neck fractures and a significant percentage of displaced body fractures. Treatment is by long periods of protected weight bearing. Malunion, especially varus malunion in communited neck fracture, causes pain on weight bearing and predisposes to secondary osteoarthritis. Secondary osteoarthritis may occur as a consequence of malunion and fractures involving the articular surface and also following avascular necrosis.

Fractures of the calcaneum

Calcaneal fractures account for 60% of tarsal bone fractures and 2% of all fractures. About 75% of calcaneal fractures are intra-articular. The calcaneum supports the subtalar joint consisting of anterior, middle and posterior facets. It articulates distally with the calcaneocuboid joint through the anterior process. Pain, heal tenderness and inability to weight bear are common. Bruising to the sole of the foot and flattening and widening of the heel may also occur.

The initial diagnosis is by X-ray which should include lateral and axial views of the calcaneum and Broden's view (40° internal rotation of the ankle). Bohler's angle in the lateral view gives some indication of fracture displacement, an angle of <20° suggesting a fracture (**Figure 35**). However, Bohler's angle may be normal even in the presence of a fracture.

CT scanning is essential to demonstrate the anatomy of the fracture and to assess the

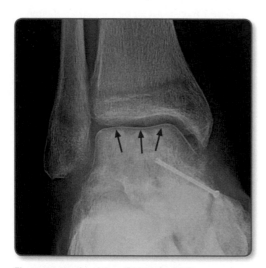

Figure 34 Hawkins' sign. Copyright 2015, Dr Matt Skalski. Image courtesy of Dr Matt Skalski and Radiopedia.org. Used under license.

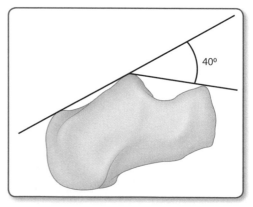

Figure 35 Bohler's angle. With permission from Greaves I, Johnson G (eds). Practical Emergency Medicine (Arnold Publication). Oxford: CRC Press, 2002.

displacement especially prior to operative treatment. It must include coronal, axial and sagittal scans.

Intra-articular fractures are commonly caused by axial loading due to a fall from a height onto the heel. They are associated with spine (10% of patients) and hip fractures. The calcaneus is driven upwards against the lateral process of the talus which acts as a splitting wedge causing the primary fracture line and separating the calcaneus into anteromedial and posterolateral fragments. A continued axial load results in collapse of the calcaneus into a varus position causing a secondary fracture line. This second fracture line extends backwards into the posterior facet and forwards into the calcaneocuboid joint making a three part fracture. The lateral wall expands as the posterior facet of the calcaneus is driven into the body resulting in a short wide heel.

Essex-Lopresti classified calcaneal fractures based on the secondary fracture line seen on lateral radiographs as the 'tongue' type with the fracture line running posteriorly to reach the body below the insertion of the Achilles tendon and 'joint depression' type with the fracture line passing down the lateral side of the calcaneum behind the posterior articular facet. Eastwood and Atkins produced a classification based on the appearance of the lateral wall on coronal CT, dividing fractures into three types. In type 1, the lateral wall is formed by lateral joint fragment, in type 2 by the lateral joint and body fragment and in type 3 by the body fragment alone. Sanders classified the fracture based on coronal CT into types 1, 2, 3 and 4 fractures (**Table 12**) depending on the number of fracture fragments and subclassified them into A, B and C according to the location of the primary fracture line.

Extra-articular fractures include extra-articular body fractures, avulsion or beak fractures at the insertion of tendo Achilles, anterior process fractures at calcaneocuboid joint and sustentacular fractures.

The aim of fracture treatment is to restore the height, length and width of the calcaneum. Undisplaced intra- and extra-articular

Table 12 Sanders classification of calcaneal fracture (simplified, types 2 and 3 are further subdivided)	
Type 1	Undisplaced posterior facet (irrespective of the number of fracture lines)
Type 2	One fracture line in the posterior facet (two fragments)
Type 3	Two fracture lines in the posterior facet (three fragments)
Type 4	Comminuted with more than three fracture lines in the posterior facet (four or more fragments)

fractures are treated with initial application of ice packs and elevation followed by 6 weeks of nonweight bearing mobilization.

The treatment of intra-articular fractures varies depending on the fracture anatomy and patient factors including age and comorbidities. Sanders types 2 and 3 fractures do better with open reduction and internal fixation. Type 4 fractures can be treated with open reduction or immediate arthrodesis depending on the experience of the surgeon. An extended lateral approach to expose and reduce the fracture fragments and fixation with a specific calcaneal plate followed by nonweight bearing cast or mobilization for 6–8 weeks is usually employed.

Surgery should be undertaken after the swelling has settled (which may take up to 2 weeks of elevation and ice packs) to avoid the complication of wound breakdown. Percutaneous fixation with screws has become popular recently as the operation can be undertaken earlier and before the swelling goes down. Displaced beak and sustentacular fractures require closed or open reduction and internal fixation.

Complications of calcaneal fractures

Complications include malunion causing alteration in gait pattern, peroneal tendon or sural nerve impingement due to valgus heel and post-traumatic osteoarthritis of the subtalar or calcaneocuboid joints.

Further reading

Canale ST, Kelly FB Jr. Fractures of the neck of talus: long term evaluation of 71 cases. J Bone Joint Surg 1978; 60A:143.

Eastwood DM, Gregg PJ, Atkins RM. Intra-articular fractures of the calcaneum. J Bone Joint Surg 1995; 7SB:183–188.

Sanders R. Current concepts review: displaced intra-articular fractures of the calcaneus. J Bone Joint Surg Am 2000; 82-A:225–250.

Related topics of interest

- Ankle injuries (p. 22)
- Foot fractures – midfoot and forefoot (p. 103)
- Fracture classifications (p. 107)

Foot fractures – midfoot and forefoot

Key points

- Injuries to the midfoot are uncommon, but are easily missed
- The commonest fracture is the Lisfranc fracture (**Figure 36**), a displacement of one or more metatarsals from the tarsus
- In suspected midfoot fractures, additional imaging including computed tomography (CT) scanning or magnetic resonance imaging (MRI) should be requested

Introduction

The midfoot comprises the tarsal navicular, the cuboid, the cuneiforms and their associated joints and stabilising ligaments. These bones are strategically located between the flexible forefoot composed of the metatarsals and phalanges and the rigid hindfoot composed of the calcaneum (os calcis) and the talus. Injuries to the midfoot are often missed on initial radiographs. A high index of suspicion and more detailed investigations are warranted in order to make a diagnosis.

Lisfranc injuries (tarsometatarsal joint injuries)

These injuries in which one or more of the metatarsal bones are displaced from the tarsus at the level of the tarsometatarsal joint were first described by Jasques Lisfranc (1790–1847), a Napoleonic field surgeon. Lisfranc injuries are rare and commonly missed on routine radiographs.

The second metatarsal forms the keystone of the transverse metatarsal arch which is wider on the dorsal aspect than the plantar. The arch is stabilised by the strong plantar tarsometatarsal ligament. The crucial Lisfranc ligament connects the medial cuneiform and the medial base of the second metatarsal. The transverse ligament from the second through to fifth metatarsal provides additional stability. Because of the strong plantar stabilizers, dorsal dislocation is common.

Mechanism of injury

The possible mechanisms of injury include axial loading and twisting encountered during football or simply descending a curb. In these scenarios, the toes are planted on the ground while the heel is being axially loaded by the body weight. Sometimes direct trauma such as a fall from height or heavy objects falling onto the dorsum of the foot may result in a Lisfranc injury.

Presentation

Patients present with pain and swelling on the midfoot and are unable to bear weight on their affected foot. A tell-tale sign for these injuries is the presence of central plantar ecchymosis. Examination should also exclude

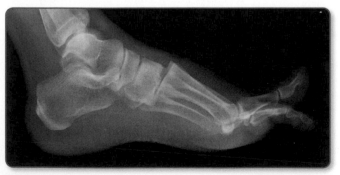

Figure 36 A Lisfranc fracture.

neurovascular injuries and compartment syndrome.

Classification

Hardcastle classified these injuries into three groups:

- Type A – total incongruity (homolateral) with entire lateral or medial tarsometatarsal dislocation
- Type B – partial incongruity with medial first metatarsal or lateral four metatarsal subluxation or dislocation
- Type C – divergent with first metatarsal deviating medially and lateral four deviating laterally

Investigations

The interpretation of radiographs can be difficult due to the complex anatomy of the midfoot. Comparison films with the contralateral limb as well as weightbearing radiographs are useful.

Important radiological findings include avulsion at the base of medial border of the second metatarsal and a >2 mm widening in this area and/or an impaction fracture of the distal cuboid at the lateral metatarsal base. CT scan and MRI have proven invaluable in the diagnosis of Lisfranc injuries when radiographs show equivocal findings. The disadvantage is that they are static modalities and unlike stress radiographs, will not demonstrate instability.

Management

The initial management of these injuries includes analgesia, splinting, elevation and measures to control swelling. Definitive management will depend on whether the injury is a stable simple sprain injury that can be managed by cast and nonweight bearing for 6 weeks or an unstable injury which requires open reduction and internal fixation. Post-traumatic arthrosis is a late complication which requires tarsometatarsal joint arthrodesis.

Navicular fractures

The navicular bone constitutes an important part of the medial longitudinal arch of the foot. Fractures can involve the dorsal lip, tuberosity or the body of the navicular. Stress fractures are common among athletes and military recruits and are often missed. Foot radiographs may show an accessory navicular which can be misdiagnosed as a fracture.

Dorsal lip fracture accounts for 50% of navicular fractures and are due to a hyperplantar flexion and inversion mechanism due to avulsion of the dorsal ligaments. Tuberosity fractures constitute 25% of navicular fractures and generally result from avulsion of the tibialis posterior tendon, frequently confused with an accessory ossicle.

Fractures of the body of the navicular account for 25% of fractures and are caused by direct crushing from the dorsal surface or by indirect compression between cuneiforms and talus in a nutcracker type injury. Sangeorzan et al. classified these fractures into types 1, 2 and 3 fractures with 2 and 3 being complex injuries.

Management

The aims of treatment are to maintain the length of the medial column and to restore articular congruity. X-rays and CT scans are required to diagnose these injuries. Dorsal lip and tuberosity fractures require fixation only if the fragment is large, otherwise they can be treated conservatively in plaster. Excision is sometimes needed for displaced fragments that cannot be fixed. Types 2 and 3 body fractures require open reduction and internal fixation and are associated with avascular necrosis in up to 30% of cases.

Navicular stress fractures

Stress fractures are a subset of navicular fractures seen among athletes due to repetitive microtrauma. Patients usually report a recent increase in the intensity of their activity and present with pain and a variable degree of swelling. Initial radiographs may be equivocal, late radiographs may show evidence of periosteal reaction. MRI can be useful in early cases before abnormalities are seen on plain radiographs. Management is usually conservative with rest and a period of nonweight bearing followed by a gradual return to activity.

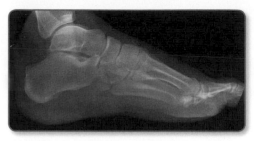

Figure 37 A nutcracker fracture of the cuboid. With permission from Mr Michael Fuller.

Fractures of the cuboid

The cuboid forms part of the lateral longitudinal arch. Fractures of the cuboid are rare and are usually associated with other fractures and dislocations across the midfoot and hindfoot. They are commonly referred to as nutcracker injuries (**Figure 37**) because the cuboid is fractured by being crushed between the fourth and fifth metatarsals and the calcaneum in a plantar flexion type injury.

These are high-energy injuries leading to compression failure on the lateral side and tensile failure on the medial side. The aim of the treatment is to restore the lateral column and displaced fractures require open reduction and internal fixation and in specific instances, bone grafting.

Midtarsal (Chopart's joint) dislocation

The midtarsal joint (Chopart's joint) is composed of the talonavicular joint and the calcaneocuboid joint. Low-energy mechanisms such as a foot twisting injury as well as high-energy road traffic collisions may be responsible for this rare injury. Neurovascular compromise and compartment syndrome can occur. A common mistake is failure to recognise that the injury occurred at the level of the foot, erroneously requesting X-rays of the ankle instead. Satisfactory results can be expected with prompt diagnosis and anatomic reduction with or without internal stabilization.

Metatarsal fractures

Metatarsal fractures are often the result of direct blow from an object dropped onto or running over the dorsum of foot. These fractures may alter the weightbearing distribution of the forefoot. Isolated neck and shaft fractures can be treated nonoperatively if the adjacent metatarsals are intact to provide stabilisation. Displaced fracture of the first metatarsal and multiple displaced or angulated metatarsal fractures require open or closed reduction and fixation.

Stress fractures are a subset of fractures occurring in the second and third metatarsals (the immobile segment of the forefoot). Stress fracture is often seen in military recruits, high-level athletes, ballet dancers and gymnasts. It also occurs in perimenopausal females and as a complication of metabolic bone disease and rheumatoid arthritis. Patients present with gradual onset of pain and occasional swelling in the forefoot usually a few weeks after commencing the athletic activity. An initial radiograph is usually negative and bone scan and MRI assist in the diagnosis. Management is conservative with reduction of activity and immobilization.

Jones fracture occurs about 1–2 cm distal to the tip of the fifth metatarsal tuberosity. Because of the poor blood supply to this area of metaphyseal and diaphyseal anastomosis, these fractures are prone to delayed or nonunion. Acute fractures can be treated conservatively in a plaster cast. However delayed or nonunion, if symptomatic, requires open reduction and internal fixation; bone grafting may be necessary.

Phalangeal fractures

Phalangeal fractures are typically toe stubbing injuries resulting in condylar fractures. They are usually stable and treated with buddy strapping. Displaced intra-articular fractures require reduction and cross Kirschner wire fixation and sometimes primary fusion of the involved joints.

Further reading

DiGiovanni CW. Fractures of the navicular. Foot Ankle Clin 2004; 9:25–63.

Panchbhavi VK, Vallurupalli S, Yang J, Andersen CR. Screw fixation compared with suture-button fixation of isolated Lisfranc ligament injuries. J Bone Joint Surg Am 2009; 91:1143–1148.

Woodward S, Jacobson JA, Femino JE, et al. Sonographic evaluation of Lisfranc ligament injuries. J Ultrasound Med 2009; 28:351–357.

Related topics of interest

- Ankle injuries (p. 22)
- Foot fractures – hindfoot (p. 99)
- Long-bone fractures (p. 171)

Fracture classifications

Key points

- Classification systems allow the comparison of treatment centres and modalities as well as prediction of outcomes by injury type
- Classification systems may be anatomical, injury specific or generic
- The most comprehensive and widely used system is the AO (Arbeitsgemeinschaft für osteosynthesefragen) classification

Introduction

Traumatic injuries have generic features related to the mechanism of injury and specific characteristics unique to each particular soft tissue wound and each of the individual 206 bones comprising the adult skeleton. The predictability of traumatic injuries suggests the use of classification systems. This topic discusses the role of classification systems in trauma.

Attempts to classify skeletal injuries date back as far as ancient Egyptian times from which papyrus documents have been found which divide fractures into open and closed injuries, recognising that the former have poorer outcomes. In the 18th century, in the absence of clinical imaging, classification relied on pattern recognition where a particular deformity would raise suspicion of a recognised underlying fracture, e.g. the dinner fork deformity from a fall onto an outstretched hand, seen in distal radius fragility fractures (Colles fracture). With the advent of plain radiographs and computed tomography (CT), classification systems have evolved considerably. Their role in trauma care is predominantly to identify and describe injuries in a transferable manner which is essential if injuries and their outcomes are to be compared for research purposes and when educating trainee healthcare professionals. Classification systems can also facilitate decision-making when planning treatment and can be used to predict outcomes.

The majority of classifications rely upon an observer interpreting plain radiographs, utilising their clinical knowledge and applying an understanding of bony anatomy to judge the severity of a fracture, taking into account the location and fracture lines, degree of displacement and comminution. Thus the main limitation is usually interobserver variability, where one observer will decipher and classify the same radiograph differently to another. Classification systems are now assessed using a universal statistical method, the Kappa or weighted Kappa statistic. This quantifies the reliability and validity of a classification system. Further limitation results from the inadequacy of radiographs, exacerbated by osteopenic bone and measurement error when quantifying the displacement or angulation of fracture fragments. Although CT has enhanced image quality, its role is predominantly in surgical planning for the management of intra-articular fractures to aid reconstruction of the articular surface: Sander's classification of calcaneal fractures using semicoronal sequences underlines the advantages of CT images and is used in clinical practice. The remainder of this topic describes examples of generic and site-specific classification systems.

Open fractures

During the initial patient assessment, it is important to identify whether a fracture is open, exposed to the outside environment (technically compound) or closed with complete soft tissue cover. The Gustilo–Anderson classification of open fractures first described in 1976 has stood the test of time and is still widely used although it has been modified. Not only does it standardise the assessment of wounds and treatment, the classification has sufficient external validation to allow prediction of the likely outcome of individual injuries with regard to risk of infection.

The Gustilo grade (**Table 13**), an ordinal classification, is dependent upon a number of factors including the mechanism of injury (low vs. high-energy) and associated bony

Table 13 Gustilo classification of open fractures	
Grade	**Definition**
I	Open fracture, clean wound, wound <1 cm in length
II	Open fracture, wound >1 cm but <10 cm in length without extensive soft-tissue damage, flaps and avulsions
III	Open fracture with extensive soft-tissue laceration (>10 cm) damage, or loss or an open segmental fracture. This type also includes fractures requiring vascular repair, or fractures that have been open for 8 hours before they are treated
IIIA	Type III with adequate periosteal coverage of the fracture bone despite the extensive soft-tissue laceration or damage
IIIB	Type III with extensive soft-tissue loss, periosteal stripping and bone damage. Usually associated with massive contamination
IIIC	Type III associated with an arterial injury requiring repair

comminution and periosteal stripping, the dimensions of any associated soft tissue injury, the requirement for reconstructive surgery and the presence of neurovascular injury. For example, a Gustilo grade I is a low-energy injury with a clean wound <1 cm in size and little comminution and a 0–12% risk of infection. Gustilo grade III injuries, however, are associated with high-energy mechanisms with significant fracture comminution and periosteal stripping and the potential for contamination. They often require plastic reconstruction. They are reported to have a 30–55% risk of infection. Although critics state that there is high interobserver variability, the classification has been fundamental to the development of, and enhancements in, open fracture care. Gustilo grading is usually only possible following surgical exploration.

The AO/Orthopaedic Trauma Association (OTA) classification system

It is important to describe a fracture using transferable language in order to facilitate accurate communication with other health professionals and to maintain consistent definitions in research. There is a multitude of fracture classification systems in use today, each system having its own merits. Some further systems are described in the appropriate key topic. Perhaps the most widely used by clinicians in modern-day practice is the system established by the AO Foundation for Trauma.

The AO/OTA classification system provides a comprehensive way of stratifying fractures based on radiographs. An alphanumeric code is obtained in a structured stepwise manner to illustrate fracture personality and guide treatment. Firstly, the injured bone is identified and numbered, followed by the region within that bone. Each long bone is divided into a central portion (diaphysis), or the most proximal or distal region (metaphyses). As the region within each bone has unique fracture patterns, healing potential and requirement for operative fixation, they are treated differently. Fractures at the end of long bones will often involve the articular surface and need to be addressed surgically. Intra-articular fractures must be reduced anatomically and fixed rigidly to promote primary bone healing. The goal of fixation of diaphyseal fractures is to restore alignment, length and rotation with relative stability at the fracture site to promote secondary bone healing and callus formation.

Fractures are then grouped and subgrouped, this provides specific descriptive details and key features of any given bone. For example, diaphyseal fractures are discriminated by the fracture configuration including whether they are simple or compound and by the number of bony fragments. For example, two bone fragments – type A, complex with either a butterfly or wedge segment, type B or type C comminuted with no contact between the main bone fragments. Type A shaft fractures are subgrouped by the fracture pattern; spiral (type A1) due to a torsional force at the time of injury; oblique (type A2) where the fracture line is >30° to the long axis of the bone or transverse (type A3) where the fracture line is <30° to the long axis of bone. Subgrouping is often site-specific, differing from bone-to-bone, allowing specific features to be incorporated and improving precision of the system. The system is necessarily complex.

Fracture-specific classification systems

There are certain classifications which are fracture specific and frequently used in orthopaedic practice. These systems categorise fractures in a hierarchical manor based on severity. The following commonly used classifications are described for illustrative purposes, demonstrating the clinical correlations of different fracture patterns.

Weber classification

This system (see pages 22–25) is useful when assessing the fibula component of ankle fractures and syndesmosis integrity. It differentiates injuries according to the fibula fracture site in relation to the tibial plafond (syndesmosis). Weber A fractures are distal to the syndesmosis, B fractures are at the level of the syndesmosis and C fractures are located proximal to this. Disruption to the syndesmosis implies ankle instability, there may or may not be talar shift apparent on the X-ray. Type B or C injuries are considered unstable and require operative fixation to restore bony alignment and ankle stability.

Neer classification

Proximal humeral fractures (see pages 264–269) predominately affect elderly patients with poor bone density. Neer devised a classification based on the number of fracture fragments (humeral head, greater and lesser tuberosity and humeral shaft). Each fragment by definition must be displaced by 1 cm or misaligned by 45° relative to its original anatomical location. The majority of injuries are two-part through the surgical neck of the humerus and are treated conservatively. Grossly displaced fractures are considered for internal fixation taking into account patient factors and pain intensity. Three-part fractures will require fixation and patients with four-part fractures are appropriate candidates for arthroplasty procedures. In practice, it is difficult to distinguish the number of fragments and reproducibly assess displacement. In additional to patient factors, clinicians may use CT reconstructions to facilitate decision-making.

Salter–Harris growth plate injuries

Injuries of this kind (see pages 322–326) which are unique to the immature skeleton cannot be addressed by a generic classification, reinforcing the need for specific systems. Defining the severity of a growth plate injury generates prognostic estimates and allows reasonably accurate advice to be offered to patients and their families with regard to premature closure and subsequent limb shortening or abnormal growth. Growth potential is a vital consideration in the management of paediatric injuries and defines treatment.

Further reading

Gustilo RB, Anderson JT. Prevention of infection in the treatment of one thousand and twenty-five open fractures of long bones: retrospective and prospective analyses. J Bone Joint Surg Am 1976; 58:453–458.

Orthopaedic Trauma Association Committee for Coding and Classification. Fracture and dislocation compendium. J Orthop Trauma 1996; 10:v–ix, 1–154.

Dirschl D. Classification of fractures. In: Bucholz RW, Heckman JD, Court-Brown CM (eds) Rockwood and Green's fractures in adults, vol. 1, 6th edn. Philadelphia: Lippincott Williams and Wilkins 2006: 43–58.

Related topics of interest

Fragility fractures

Key points

- Osteoporosis should be considered in all elderly patients sustaining a fracture and any risk factors should be identified
- Patients sustaining fragility fractures of the hip often have multiple comorbidities requiring optimisation before surgery which should be performed within 36 hours unless it is medically contraindicated
- Secondary prevention of osteoporotic fractures is essential in all fragility fractures and is often facilitated by a nurse led fracture-liaison service

Epidemiology

A fragility fracture occurs from a low-energy mechanism that would not produce a fracture in healthy bone. The World Health Organisation (WHO) defines this as a fracture that occurs from a standing height. The UK National Hip Fracture Database recorded that 64,838 patients sustained a hip fracture in 2013. A 50-year-old woman in the United Kingdom has a lifetime risk of hip fracture of 11.4% and a risk of distal radius fracture of 16.6%. The management of these patients not only involves orthopaedic treatment to allow early mobilisation and maximise functional recovery but also the identification and management of the underlying cause of the fragility fracture so that measures can be undertaken to reduce the risk of further fractures.

Pathophysiology

The chief determinant of peak bone mass is genetic. During childhood, there is a gradual increase in bone mass which accelerates around the time of puberty. Peak bone mass is achieved between the ages of 20 and 30 years. This is followed by a gradual decline in bone mass with increasing age. Excessive loss of bone mass results in osteoporosis. The WHO definition of osteoporosis is a bone mass of 2.5 standard deviations or more below that of a healthy young adult, the so-called T-score.

Nutrition and bone loss

The main nutritional factors in the development of osteoporosis are deficiency in calcium, vitamin D and protein. Calcium is a major component of the extracellular matrix of bone and is found in dairy products and green vegetables. Vitamin D is produced in the skin by the action of ultraviolet light, with further activation following hydroxylation in the liver then the kidneys, it is also found in some foods, notably fatty fish. Vitamin D regulates calcium absorption in the duodenum and its deficiency therefore results in loss of bone mass. Combined calcium and vitamin D supplements have been shown to be a cost-effective means of treating osteoporosis.

Protein is another important component of the extracellular bone matrix and maintaining adequate dietary protein intake has been shown to correlate with bone mass and outcome following hip fracture.

Postmenopausal bone loss

Following the menopause, there is a period of rapid bone loss in relation to oestrogen deficiency, this lasts around 5 years and is followed by a period of slower decline. Reduced circulating oestrogen results in disruption of osteoclast–osteoblast coupling during bone remodelling with a resultant net bone loss. Oestrogen replacement therapy reduces the risk of hip and vertebral fractures; however, continuous hormone replacement therapy can increase the risk of cardiovascular disease, venous thromboembolism and certain cancers and consequently its use to reduce the risk of fragility fractures is only recommended in patients at significant risk or in whom other treatments are unsuitable.

Other factors

Lack of exercise, specifically load-bearing exercise, has also been implicated as a risk factor in the development of osteoporosis, as has smoking, both by its direct effects on bone and by lowering oestrogen and testosterone levels (**Table 14**). Many medical conditions are associated with osteoporosis. These include diabetes mellitus, chronic lung disease, thyroid disease and hyperparathyroidism where an increase in circulating parathyroid hormone directly leads to increased bone resorption. Medicines linked to osteoporosis include anticonvulsants, antidepressants and benzodiazepines.

Table 14 Risk factors for osteoporotic fractures	
Nonmodifiable risk factors	**Modifiable risk factors**
Genetic	Smoking
Fragility fracture in first-degree relative	Excessive alcohol consumption
Caucasian race	Low body mass
Female	Nutrition (low intake of calcium/vitamin D)
Age	Falls
	Lack of exercise
	Oestrogen deficiency

Common types of fragility fractures

Hip fractures

Fractures of the proximal femur occur as low-energy injuries in elderly patients who often have multiple comorbidities (**Figure 38**). To enable effective pain control and allow early mobilisation, the majority of these injuries are managed surgically with either internal fixation, with a sliding hip screw or intramedullary nail, or with hemiarthroplasty to replace the femoral head in fractures where the femoral head blood supply has been disrupted. Current UK guidelines emphasise the importance of early surgery, within 36 hours of injury, to avoid the complications of prolonged bed rest, particularly pressure sores, and there is some evidence suggesting that this reduces mortality. The guidelines also stress the need for a multidisciplinary approach to the management of these patients involving orthogeriatricians, anaesthetists and surgeons.

Distal radius fractures

Injuries to the distal radius occur when a fall is broken by an outstretched hand (**Figure 39**). These injuries are managed initially by manipulation in the emergency department where indicated and application of a plaster backslab. Surgical treatment of the injury involves reduction and fixation with either

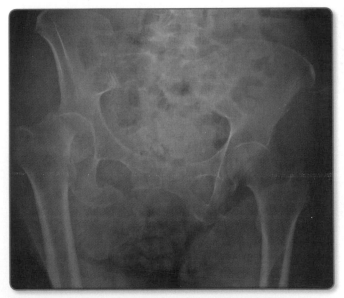

Figure 38 Right intracapsular neck of femur fracture.

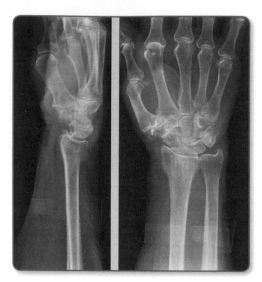

Figure 39 Distal radius fragility fracture with characteristic shortening and dorsal angulation.

Kirschner (K) wires or open reduction and fixation with plates, the recent Distal Radius Acute Fracture Fixation Trial (DRAFFT) trial suggests the majority of distal radius fractures can be effectively managed with K-wire stabilisation. The goal of surgery is to restore radial length, inclination and tilt; however, the evidence that improving these anatomical parameters improves functional outcomes in elderly patients is lacking.

Vertebral fractures

Fragility fractures of the spine follow low-energy injuries. They characteristically produce a wedge compression pattern of injury and are generally stable injuries. As they occur in an elderly population of patients, it is important to exclude other pathological causes of fracture such as malignancy; however, the majority can be managed with analgesia and early mobilisation. There is no conclusive evidence to support the use of spinal bracing in these patients. In those patients with persistent symptoms, intervention options include the use of vertebroplasty, involving the injection of polymethyl methacrylate bone cement into the vertebral body to stabilise the fracture, or kyphoplasty where a balloon is inflated in the vertebral body to restore the vertebral height before cement stabilisation is performed. There is conflicting evidence regarding the efficacy of these procedures although in the UK, National Institute for Care and Health Excellence (NICE) currently endorses their use in selected patients.

Prevention of fragility fractures

Assessment of risk of fragility fractures involves taking a history regarding the risk factors outlined above. The fracture risk assessment tool allows estimation of fragility fracture risk in patients aged between 40 and 80 years from the history and demographic factors alone. Further investigation of bone mass is usually performed with dual energy X-ray absorptiometry (DEXA) scanning to produce a T-score of bone mass.

In patients who have sustained a fragility fracture, secondary preventative measures are indicated to reduce the risk of further fracture. These should involve assessment of the risk of such a fracture together with further investigation of bone mass where indicated.

Prevention of osteoporosis includes lifestyle advice such as cessation of smoking, moderation of alcohol intake and weight-bearing exercise as well as ensuring adequate nutrition. Medical management includes supplementation of vitamin D and calcium. Other medical therapies include bisphosphonates, selective oestrogen receptor modulators such as raloxifene and parathyroid hormone (teriparatide).

The current NICE guidelines on secondary prevention in patients who have sustained a fragility fracture include calcium and vitamin D supplementation, in patients aged over 75 years bisphosphonates are advised without further investigation. In those between the ages of 64 and 74 years further investigation is performed in the form of DEXA scanning. Raloxifene or teriparatide are used in those patients where bisphosphonates are contraindicated. The most up-to-date NICE guidelines can be reviewed online.

Further reading

Dell R, Greene D, Anderson D, Williams K. Osteoporosis disease management: what every orthopaedic surgeon should know. J Bone Joint Surg Am 2009; 91:79–86.

Hiligsmann M, Ben Sedrine W, Bruyère O, et al. Cost-effectiveness of vitamin D and calcium supplementation in the treatment of elderly women and men with osteoporosis. Eur Public Health 2015; 25:20–25.

National Institute for Health and Care Excellence (NICE). Secondary prevention of osteoporotic fragility fractures in post-menopausal women. London: NICE; 2004.

Marsh D, Currie C, Brown P. The care of patients with fragility fractures. London: British Orthopaedic Association, 2007.

Related topics of interest

- Hip fractures and dislocations (p. 129)
- Metabolic response to trauma (p. 182)
- Pathological fractures (p. 219)

Genitourinary trauma

Key points

- Trauma to the genitourinary tract is rarely life threatening but can result in significant morbidity if it is not recognised and treated promptly
- Modern cross-sectional imaging allows accurate diagnosis, classification and management
- In the most commonly injured organ, the kidney, minimally invasive techniques have resulted in a reduction in comorbidity and an improvement in organ preservation

Epidemiology

Trauma of the urinary tract has been shown to occur in approximately 10% of trauma cases. Renal injuries are the commonest, while injuries to the ureters are rare and are usually associated with pelvic surgery. Bladder and urethral trauma is typically associated with pelvic fractures. Testicular trauma is often associated with sporting injuries. In Europe, urinary tract injury results predominantly from blunt trauma associated with road traffic collisions, although the incidence of penetrating injuries is increasing with the rise in inner city violence.

Clinical features

The important details to be obtained from any evaluation following genitourinary trauma are the mechanism of injury, any history of recent pelvic surgery, whether there is an associated pelvic fracture, the presence of haematuria (visible or microscopic), the location of bruising and tenderness and (if possible) whether there is difficulty voiding urine.

Kidney

The kidney can be injured by direct trauma, e.g. crushing of the organ between vertebrae and ribs or against a hard object, or by deceleration. Deceleration injuries may result in hilar vascular injury or ureteropelvic

disruption. Thus, the mechanism of injury and presence of haematuria (visible or microscopic) are particularly important as is the presence of loin bruising, loin tenderness and haemodynamic instability.

Ureters

Risk factors for ureteral injury include advanced malignancy, prior surgery and irradiation. Traumatic injury is rare and associated with penetrating abdominal trauma. Unrecognised ureteric injuries are well described. They present with excessive postoperative drain output, urinoma, ureteric obstruction, abscess formation or fistula formation.

Bladder and urethra

Pelvic fracture, blunt or penetrating trauma to the distended bladder and iatrogenic injury (associated with lower abdominal and pelvic surgery) are the commonest causes of bladder and urethral trauma. A history of pelvic fracture (or pelvic surgery) and the presence of frank haematuria, lower abdominal pain and difficulty voiding are signs of bladder injury. A urethral injury may present with blood at the penile meatus, urinary retention, perineal bruising and a distended bladder.

External genitalia

Testicular injury is not common and is generally associated with sporting injuries and motorcycle accidents. There has been a recent rise in genital injury in armed forces personnel due to blast from improvised explosive devices. Pain, scrotal swelling and bruising are common findings following trauma. Extrusion of testicles through a scrotal rupture may also be apparent.

Investigations

Urine dipstick, routine blood tests, cross-sectional imaging, cystography, retrograde urethrography and ultrasound are the investigations of choice in genitourinary trauma.

Kidneys

Frank haematuria or dipstick haematuria associated with a drop in systolic blood pressure (<90 mmHg) is an indication for contrast-enhanced CT with delayed phase (10 minutes). This demonstrates vascular and parenchymal injuries (**Figure 40**). The delayed phase may identify pelviureteric junction or collecting system injuries.

If a renal injury is suspected intraoperatively, then a one-shot intravenous urogram (IVU – contrast bolus followed by abdominal X-ray at 10 minutes) to check for functioning kidneys as well as extravasation can be considered. Unfortunately, the images are usually of poor quality and palpation of the contralateral kidney is considered a more 'reliable' option.

Ureters

The choice of investigation for ureteric injuries is governed by the clinical situation. For intraoperative injuries, a retrograde ureteropyelogram is the investigation of choice and can allow stenting. The delayed phase of a contrast CT is performed in situations where diagnosis is delayed.

Bladder and urethra

Conventional or CT cystography is used to evaluate bladder injuries. This requires the bladder to be filled to at least 350–400 mL with contrast via a urethral catheter followed by anteroposterior and postdrainage films. Retrograde urethrography is the standard investigation for evaluating urethral injury (**Figure 41**). Gentle urethral catheterisation prior to imaging may be performed by a urologist if the situation does not allow urethrography.

External genitalia

Ultrasound scanning will assist the diagnosis of intrascrotal pathology. Loss of homogeneity is highly suggestive of testicular rupture.

Classification

Injuries to the kidneys are classified using the American Association for the Surgery of Trauma (AAST) renal trauma severity scale (**Table 15**).

Ureteric injuries can be classified using the AAST scale for ureteric injury (**Table 16**).

Bladder injuries can be divided into bladder contusion, intraperitoneal rupture, extraperitoneal rupture or combined intra-

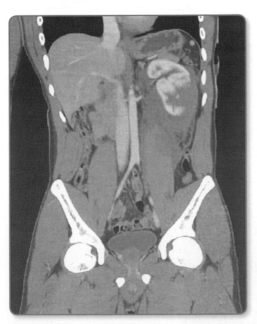

Figure 40 Grade 3 left renal laceration with large retroperitoneal haematoma.

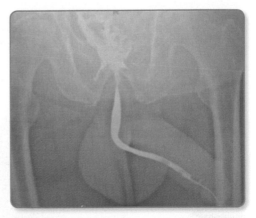

Figure 41 Retrograde urethrography demonstrating a complete urethral tear with contrast extravasation.

and extraperitoneal rupture (**Figure 42**). Urethral injury can be classified according to location: anterior urethra (penile lacerations, fractures or falls astride) or posterior urethra (pelvic fracture associated) or severity: partial or complete.

Scrotal injuries can range from skin lacerations to secondary haematoceles. Testicular injuries can be divided into contusions, haematomas and ruptures.

Treatment

Renal injury

Angiography and selective embolisation of bleeding vessels are indicated in patients with active bleeding from a renal injury but without other indications for renal exploration. The absolute indication for renal exploration is persistent life-threatening

Table 15 Renal trauma severity scale

Grade	Description
1	Contusion or nonexpanding subcapsular haematoma, no laceration
2	Nonexpanding perirenal haematoma, cortical laceration <1 cm deep without extravasation
3	Cortical laceration >1 cm without urinary extravasation
4	Laceration: through corticomedullary junction into collecting system (urinary extravasation) Vascular: segmented renal artery or vein injury with contained haematoma
5	Laceration: shattered kidney Vascular: renal pedicle injury or avulsion

Adapted from American Association for the Surgery of Trauma (AAST) renal trauma severity scale.

Table 16 Grading of ureteric injury

Grade	Description
1	Haematoma only
2	Laceration <50% circumference
3	Laceration >50% circumference
4	Complete tear <2 cm of devascularisation
5	Complete tear of >2 cm of devascularisation

Adapted from American Association for the Surgery of Trauma (AAST) for ureteric injury.

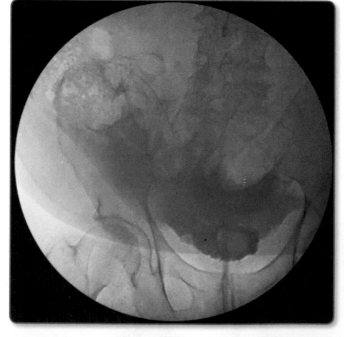

Figure 42 Cystogram showing intraperitoneal rupture following minimal bladder distension.

blood loss from a suspected renal injury resulting in haemodynamic instability.

Ureteric injury

Management of ureteric injury depends on the stage, location and timing of injury. Grade 1 injury is usually managed conservatively or with the insertion of a stent. Partial injury (Grades 2 and 3) requires insertion of a stent or urinary diversion by nephrostomy. In complete injuries (Grades 4 and 5), ureteric reconstruction is required and the type of repair is dependent on the site of injury. In general, proximal and midurethral injuries are managed by ureteroureterostomy, while distal injuries are treated with ureteric reimplantation.

Bladder and urethra injury

Intraperitoneal rupture of the bladder requires surgical repair. This involves a lower midline laparotomy and two-layer closure with absorbable sutures. Minimally invasive techniques have been described. Extraperitoneal ruptures are generally managed conservatively with a catheter for 10–14 days and antibiotics followed by a retrograde cystogram prior to removal of catheter.

Partial urethral injuries may heal with catheter placement alone. Follow-up is required to rule out subsequent strictures. Complete injuries associated with pelvic fracture are best treated with suprapubic diversion and delayed anastomotic urethroplasty. Anterior urethral injuries associated with penile fracture or lacerations should be repaired primarily.

Injuries to the external genitalia

Ruptured testes require early exploration and closure.

Complications

Early complications of renal trauma include secondary haemorrhage, infection and arteriovenous fistula or pseudoaneurysm formation. Late complications include hypertension and renal insufficiency. Ureteric injuries are often missed in an intraoperative setting. This can result in ureteric obstruction, urinoma, abscess formation, fistulation or stricture.

Intraperitoneal urinary extravasation following ureteric or bladder injury can result in urinary ascites, peritonitis, ileus and systemic sepsis. Injuries involving the bladder neck can result in incontinence or stricture. Urethral stricture, erectile dysfunction and incontinence may occur secondary to pelvic fractures. Hypogonadism can occur in bilateral external genitalia injuries or previously abnormal testes. Subfertility is a late complication. Sperm analysis and banking are recommended in bilateral injury.

Further reading

Moore EE, Cogbill TH, Malangoni M, Jurkovich GJ, Champion HR. Scaling system for organ specific injuries. Chicago: The American Association for the Surgery of Trauma, 2015.

Shergill IS, Arya M, Patel HR, Gill IS. Urological emergencies in hospital medicine. London: Quay Books, 2007.

Summerton DJ, Djakovic N, Kitrey ND, et al. Guidelines on urological trauma. Arnhem: European Association of Urology, 2014.

Related topics of interest

Gunshot injuries

Key points

- An appreciation of the physics involved when a bullet interacts with tissues is essential for understanding gunshot wounds and their management
- The consequences of a gunshot wound are related to both the anatomic structures involved and the amount of energy transferred into the tissue
- In all cases of torso, junctional or head/neck gunshot injury a contrast computed tomography is mandatory

Epidemiology

Internationally, firearms are involved in approximately 40% of civil homicides; however, there is wide variation between nations. In the Americas, two-thirds of homicides involve firearms whereas in Europe this figure is as low as 10–15%. The United Kingdom has strict legal controls on firearm ownership and consequently relatively low rates of gun crime as shown in **Table 17**.

In military conflicts, firearms are typically responsible for only a fifth of battlefield injuries, with explosive mechanisms such as improvised explosive devices predominating. Injuries caused by military firearms often involve higher-energy wounds than those seen in the civilian setting and wounds may be more complex.

Pathophysiology

Firearms convert the chemical energy in the propellant into the kinetic energy (KE) of the bullet. A bullet's kinetic energy is directly proportional to the mass of the bullet and the square of its velocity, thus:

$$KE = \frac{mV^2}{2}$$

Where KE is kinetic energy, m is mass of the projectile and V is velocity of the projectile.

As a consequence, increasing the velocity of a bullet will have a greater effect on its damaging power than increasing its mass.

The kinetic energy possessed by the bullet at the point it impacts the body is simply the maximum available to do work by damaging tissue. If the bullet lodges in the body, then all of the kinetic energy must have been transferred; if the bullet exits the body, then it still retains some kinetic energy and the amount deposited to cause tissue damage is equal to the difference between the kinetic energy on entry and that as the bullet leaves the body.

The bullet damages tissues in two ways:

1. By lacerating or crushing tissue directly in the path of the bullet, forming a permanent cavity approximately the width of the bullet. If the bullet fragments or strikes bone and accelerates a bony splinter, each of these new projectiles will also form their own permanent cavity

Weapon type	Firearm offences	Offences involving shots fired	Fatal injury	Serious injury	Minor injury
Shotguns	495	248 (50.1%)	16	56	36
Handguns	2651	332 (13%)	18	103	56
Imitation, BB/airsoft firearms	1377	1053 (76%)	0	8	624
Rifles/others	1478	597 (40%)	8	48	313
Air guns and rifles	3554	3160 (89%)	0	29	329
Total	9555	5388 (56%)	42	244	1358

Table 17 Firearm offences in England and Wales 2011/2012.

Data from Violent Crime and Sexual Offences, 2011/12. Statistical Bulletin London, Office of Nation Statistics, 2013. Serious injury is defined as requiring hospital admission. BB/airsoft guns are very low velocity air weapons

2. The temporary cavity or bubble that forms in the wake of the bullet expands radially from its path and then rapidly collapses back in on itself (**Figure 43**). The temporary cavity results from the shock wave imparted to the tissue by the bullet. Tissue that is elastic and will tolerate being stretched (e.g. lung and muscle) will be damaged less than tissue such as liver, which shears when placed under tension

Clinical features

The clinical effect of gunshot injuries depends on the anatomical region involved. A gunshot wound to the central nervous system, for example, will typically be rapidly fatal, whereas a superficial wound to the thigh may be tolerated fairly well. Haemorrhagic shock is likely to be the most significant initial clinical feature of a gunshot wound casualty, as damage to large vessels or very vascular organs such the liver and spleen will usually cause rapid blood loss.

Investigations

Initial investigations should be focused on assessing blood loss and planning surgical treatment. In the event of life-threatening haemorrhage, surgical treatment may be required prior to any investigations. As a minimum, serum lactate and haemoglobin analysis should be requested together with cross-matching blood products. However, in cases where haemorrhagic shock is suspected, dynamic thromboelastography (e.g. ROTEM) should be used to determine transfusion requirements and resuscitation must be with balanced blood components

In extremity injuries, plain X-rays may be sufficient to determine whether bones have been fractured and to look for retained projectiles. If there is a clinical suspicion of vascular injury, a CT angiogram will further define this. In all cases of torso, junctional or head/neck injury, a contrast CT is mandatory.

Diagnosis

The diagnosis of gunshot injury is usually clear from the history. Shotgun wounds are typically obvious clinically, with a characteristic appearance of wide but relatively shallow wounds with extensive tissue destruction. Differentiating between wounds caused by low energy handguns and higher energy rifles is often challenging

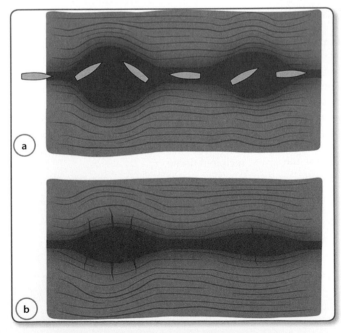

Figure 43 The temporary cavity formed when the cavitation bubble in the wake of the bullet expands radially from its path (a). This diagram shows that the cavitation is maximal at the point when the bullet is tumbling and flow of liquefied tissue around it is most turbulent. The cavity then collapses in on itself. Tissue that does not tolerate stretching will shear (b).

and patients will usually be able to offer little accurate information with regard to firearm type or even the range from which they were shot. Similarly, differentiation between high- and low-energy gunshot wounds based on the size of exit wounds is also unreliable. The path of bullets (and fragments) within the body may be wildly unpredictable and speculation and ill-founded assumptions about likely wound tracks are unhelpful.

The pattern of visible wounds together with radiographic data can give clues as to the amount of energy transfer. Bony fractures and bullet fragmentation are indicative of greater energy transfer and may suggest a more complex wound and greater tissue damage. However, forensic speculation is best left to specialists and is normally of forensic rather than clinical concern.

Treatment

Treatment of gunshot wounds is normally aimed at controlling haemorrhage and preventing infection, usually through surgery. Severe haemorrhage will require proximal control and then either primary repair, shunting or tying-off of vessels. Damage control surgery may be indicated with an abbreviated laparotomy allowing temporary treatment of haemorrhage and contamination by diversion of intestinal flow, packing of liver injuries and splenectomy.

In cases with penetrating abdominal injuries, even without evidence of on-going haemorrhage, laparotomy is normally mandated. However, it is not uncommon for low-energy projectiles to traverse the abdomen without causing organ damage.

With respect to the management of extremity injuries, surgical exploration is mandated if there is a suspicion of vascular injury. Otherwise, the objective of any surgery is the prevention of infection. The extent of surgical management of extremity gunshot wounds varies enormously. Simple injuries from low-energy hand gun bullets can be treated with superficial wound toilet, antibiotics and dressings. Gunshot wounds should never be closed primarily at the first surgical episode, either delayed primary closure or healing by secondary intention should be employed.

In more complex wounds produced by higher energy projectiles, or with features of greater energy transfer such bone fracture or bullet fragmentation, myofascial compartments should be released prophylactically and wounds irrigated with low-pressure saline. Cavitation is tolerated well by muscle tissue and significant necrosis is uncommon. Laying open the entire bullet tract is rarely indicated and instead, ribbon gauze soaked in saline can be passed along the tract using a Rampley's clip and the tract gently 'flossed' dislodging loose tissue or foreign material.

Fractures should be managed in accordance with normal orthopaedic principles albeit with the understanding that, at least initially, wounds are contaminated, and that bony union is often delayed in cases of fracture associated with bullet wounds. Gunshot wounds to the limbs should always be treated with several days of prophylactic antibiotics and the limb rested, e.g. in a plaster back-slab.

In neurovascular injury, there is likely to be both direct transection and subtotal damage to nerves or vessels. The zone of injury can extend away from the direct path of the bullet; in vascular or nerve grafting therefore, it is prudent to ensure that all of the damaged section of vessel or nerve is excised to ensure that the graft is attached to healthy recipient tissue.

Complications

The main complications of a gunshot wound are haemorrhage and infection. When wounds are closed immediately, infection is almost inevitable.

Further reading

Fackler ML. Wound ballistics. A review of common misconceptions. JAMA 1988; 259:2730–2736.

Midwinter MJ. Damage control surgery in the era of damage control resuscitation. J R Army Med Corps 2009; 155:323–326.

Brooks AJ, Clasper J, Midwinter M, Hodgetts TJ, Mahoney CPF. Ryan's ballistic trauma, 3rd edn. London: Springer, 2011.

Related topics of interest

- Blast trauma (p. 38)
- Blood product (1:1:1) resuscitation (p. 42)
- Selective nonoperative management of penetrating abdominal injuries (p. 254)

Hand injuries

Key points

- Hand injuries are common and mismanagement of apparently minor injuries may have a profound effect on the patient's quality of life
- Specialist follow-up by a hand surgeon is essential for all but the most trivial injuries
- A detailed knowledge of the nerve and muscle anatomy of the hand is essential for the optimal management of these injuries

Introduction

Hand injuries account for about 10% of emergency department attendances. These injuries can have profound effects on a patient's life with restriction of employment and other activities of daily living. Inadequate assessment and treatment can worsen morbidity from apparently minor hand injuries and early referral to a specialist hand team is often required for all but the most trivial of injuries.

Assessment and investigation

Bleeding is common after lacerations of the hand and upper limb. Most bleeding resolves with the application of mild pressure and elevation and clamping or ligation (which might damage associated structures) should be avoided. The neurovascular status of the digits or limb must be ascertained and recorded. In cases of vascular compromise, urgent referral to the hand specialist should be made. Tetanus vaccination status should be ascertained in open wounds. The vulnerability of the skeleton within the hand and the propensity for foreign body implantation means that radiographs are usually indicated. Ultrasonography may be useful when a foreign body is strongly suspected clinically but is not visible on radiographs. Ultrasonography is also of use when closed rupture of tendons or ligaments is suspected but clinical examination is inconclusive because of pain. CT or MRI for joint injuries may also be of help but is usually arranged by hand specialists. Despite the availability of these investigations, clinical examination remains the primary diagnostic modality for these injuries.

Lacerations

The anatomy of the hand means that with penetrating injuries, there is a high likelihood of deep structural injury. The assessing team should have a low threshold for surgical referral. Falling on to glass and knife wounds are common causes of injury to deep structures.

Tendon injuries

Substantial information can be inferred regarding injury to tendons by the attitude of the fingers and the position of the wound. A basic knowledge of anatomy is required to accurately identify these injuries. Complete disruption of a tendon usually results in absent flexion or extension of a joint distal to the injury. Partial injuries may still require repair and usually manifest as pain and weakness of the tendon when used against resistance. In penetrating wounds, the tendon injury may not lie under the laceration in a position of rest if the hand was in a different position (e.g. a fist) when the injury occurred.

Flexor tendons

The flexor tendons arise in the forearm. Flexor carpi ulnaris and radialis insert into the carpus; flexor digitorum profundus (FDP), flexor digitorum superficialis (FDS) and flexor pollicis longus (FPL) insert into the fingers and thumb. Disruption of FDS leads to inability to flex the proximal interphalangeal joints (PIPJs) of the digits. To test the FDS tendon in a single digit, it is necessary to neutralise the effect of the FDP tendon by holding the other fingers straight. The FDP tendons are deeper in the forearm and hand but become more superficial at the level of the PIPJ. The FDP tendons insert into the distal phalanx of each digit. The thumb has no FDS or FDP but has a separate flexor tendon known as FPL, which inserts into the base of the distal phalanx. The FDP to a digit can be assessed by immobilising the PIPJ and asking the patient to flex the distal interphalangeal joint (DIPJ). Similarly, the FPL can be assessed by flexing the thumb interphalangeal joint (IPJ), whilst immobilising the metacarpophalangeal joint (MCPJ).

Closed FDP rupture can occur in a so-called rugby-Jersey injury, when forced extension of a flexed fingertip occurs. There may be a fragment of bone attached to the tendon, which retracts down the digit and sometimes into the palm. Patients should be referred for urgent surgical repair.

Extensor tendons

Extensor tendons arise from the forearm and extend the MCPJs of the digits (except for the thumb where the IPJ is extended) or cause extension of the wrist. Two closed ruptures of extensor tendons are commonly seen.

Mallet deformity

Forced flexion to an extended DIPJ (e.g. by striking by a hard ball or catching in clothing) may result in rupture of the extensor tendon. The patient presents with a flexed DIPJ, with no active extension. There may be an associated fracture of the base of the distal phalanx. A mallet splint should be applied for 6 weeks to maintain the DIPJ in the extended position. It is important that the patient is told to support the fingertip when removing the splint. Early treatment and patient compliance is required to achieve a good outcome.

Closed central slip injury

The central slip or tendon is part of the extensor mechanism, which inserts into the base of the middle phalanx. When these injuries are neglected, a boutonniere deformity usually occurs with time. Tenderness at the insertion weak active extension of the IPJ and a history of a significant joint injury should cause suspicion of central slip injury.

Dislocations

Dislocations of interphalangeal injuries are common. Fortunately, most dislocations can be reduced by traction under digital 'ring block.' A check radiograph should be performed to confirm reduction. Follow-up is usually needed for these injuries in order to check the stability and integrity of vital ligaments. Imperfect reduction can lead to chronic pain and stiffness. Failure to reduce a dislocation is often due to interposition of soft tissues into the joint, when open reduction will be needed.

Volar plate injuries

Hyperextension injuries to the PIPJs are common. These injuries frequently damage the volar plate; a deep restraining ligament on the palmar side of the joint. There may be an associated small fracture at the base of the middle phalanx. Providing the joint is stable and there is no radiological evidence of subluxation, the majority of these injuries can be managed with neighbour strapping and mobilisation.

Nail bed injuries

Crush injuries to the tips of digits are very common. These injuries are particularly prevalent in children. There may a fracture through the distal phalanx tuft, but soft tissue repair is usually all that is required. When nail bed injury laceration occurs, a repair should be undertaken.

Fractures
Closed fractures

Assessment of a hand fracture relies on examination findings not just appearances on radiographs. It is important to assess whether there is loss of movement, e.g. extensor lag or deformity, particularly when the patient makes a fist. The presence of rotational deformity or crossing of fingers is an indication for surgery to reduce and hold the fracture.

The most commonly seen metacarpal fracture is the 'Boxer's fracture' or fracture through the 5th metacarpal neck. Provided there is no rotational deformity of the finger, these fractures are usually treated conservatively with neighbour strapping.

Fractures of the proximal and middle phalanges or metacarpal shaft with significant angulation with or without rotational deformity usually require surgery to achieve reduction and fixation. Displaced phalangeal fractures, in particular, are usually unstable and lead to angulation or rotational deformities of the digit.

'Fight-bites'

These injuries are sustained when punching somebody in the mouth with a clenched fist, resulting in an isolated laceration over an MCPJ. These patients may not give a reliable history and a high index of suspicion is essential. These injuries nearly always involve the joint and part of the extensor hood. Penetration into the joint predisposes the patient to septic arthritis from the organisms present in the human mouth. There may be cartilaginous fragments within the joint and on occasion, a piece of tooth may be found.

Treatment involves formal surgical washout and debridement. The position of the clenched fist should be recreated to identify the tract into the joint and the wound should be extended to allow access.

Nerve injuries

Nerve injuries may result in significant functional loss and pain from a neuroma, or even complex regional pain syndrome. To maximise recovery from such injuries, there must be a low threshold for making the diagnosis and referring for surgical exploration. Shortly after injury, patients may have difficulty appreciating sensory loss.

Assessment of both sensory and motor supply of nerves must be performed. Moving light touch is most commonly used to assess whether cutaneous nerve supply is intact. The absence of sweating may also be a helpful indicator that a nerve is injured.

The hand is supplied by the median, ulnar and radial nerves (**Figure 44**). The sensory territories for each nerve vary but largely follow the pattern of distribution below. The nerves

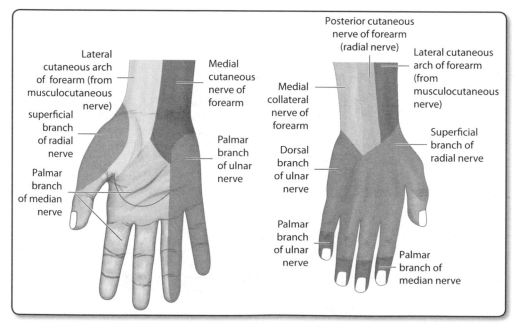

Figure 44 Cutaneous nerves in the hand. Reproduced from Chung K. Essentials of Hand Surgery. JP Medical Ltd, London.

then branch in the palm and give rise to digital nerves. There are two palmar and two dorsal nerves to each digit with the former being functionally most significant. At about the level of the DIPJ crease, the palmar digital nerves trifurcate making surgical repair more difficult.

Median nerve

The median nerve supplies the palmar sensation to the radial 3½ digits. It also supplies some small muscles of the hand [the radial two lumbricals, opponens pollicis, abductor pollicis brevis (APB) and flexor pollicis brevis]. The muscle most reliably supplied by the median nerve and easiest to examine is APB. This muscle can be assessed by asking the patient to hold their palm upwards and point the thumb vertically up towards the ceiling (palmar abduction). The patient is then instructed to hold the thumb in that position, whilst the examiner tries to push the thumb back into the palm. The APB can be palpated in the thenar eminence as it contracts. Much higher up in the forearm, the median nerve supplies other muscles including the FDP to the index and middle fingers, the FPL and the FDS tendons.

Ulnar nerve

The ulnar nerve supplies the sensation to the ulnar 1½ digits both on the palmar and dorsal surfaces of the hand. It also supplies the remaining small muscles of the hand not supplied by the median nerve. These muscles include the interossei muscles, abductor digiti minimi (ADM), ulnar two lumbricals and adductor pollicis brevis. Simple tests to check for ulnar nerve motor function include asking the patient to abduct the little finger (ADM),

spread the fingers apart against resistance and bring them together to hold a piece of paper or simply ask the patient to cross their fingers (interossei muscles). Further up the forearm, the ulnar nerve supplies other muscles including the FDP to little and ring fingers.

Radial nerve

The sensory area of the radial nerve is to the radial 3½ digits on the dorsum of the hand. There is overlap of this nerve territory and the most reliable area that can be tested is on the dorsum of the first webspace. Higher up the arm, the radial nerve supplies dorsal muscles such as the extensors to the digits and wrist.

Replantation of digits

Unfortunately, not all amputated digits are suitable for replantation and the decision should be made by a hand specialist in discussion with the patient. Although there are no absolute rules, attempted replantation is normally carried out in the following circumstances:

- When there is amputation of the thumb
- When multiple digits have been amputated
- When the injury is a clean cut ('guillotine')
- When the injury is in a child

The amputated digit should be wrapped in damp, saline-soaked gauze and placed in a polythene bag, labelled with the patient's details. The bag should then be placed in a bowl of ice. Ice should not come in to contact with the digit. Urgent referral to a hand specialist should be made to reduce ischaemia times.

Further reading

Lehfeldt M, Ray E, Sherman R. MOC-PS(SM) CME article: treatment of flexor tendon laceration. Plast Reconstr Surg 2008; 121:1–12.

Meals C, Meals R. Hand fractures: a review of current treatment strategies. J Hand Surg Am 2013; 38:1021–1031.

Wilhelmi BJ, Lee AWP, May JW. Hand amputations and replantation. New York: Medscape, 2014.

Related topics of interest

High-pressure injection injuries

Key points

- A high-pressure injection injury must be considered to be a true surgical emergency, since delays in surgical intervention substantially increase the risk of amputation
- The injected material must be identified at the outset, as solvent and solvent containing paint injections carry the worst prognosis
- Surgical intervention involves tracking of the injected substance by surgical exposure under a tourniquet, with copious lavage and meticulous removal under magnification. Early mobilisation significantly improves the chance of successful rehabilitation

Epidemiology

The industrial use of handheld high-pressure hoses or cylinders with fine nozzles, carrying potentially toxic fluids such as solvents or oils, has for decades posed a hazard to their users. Cases were reported as early as the 1920s. The very high pressures involved allow for easy inadvertent transcutaneous inoculation, forcibly dispersing the material through tissue compartments in fine droplets. Not surprisingly, the common site of injury is the nondominant hand, and more specifically the index finger. The early possible consequences are compartmental and vascular tamponade, and the local toxic effect of the injected substance on the tissues with inflammation and necrosis. In the longer term, the potential exists for persistent granulomata and superinfection. The result can be significant tissue loss including amputation, as well as later problems of fibrosis, scar contracture, loss of mobility and significant disablement.

Efforts have been made to promote awareness of these injuries by means of precautionary guidelines and safety regulations regarding hose integrity, hand protection with robust gloves, nozzle guards and careful nozzle handling. Despite this, injuries are still seen in an accident and emergency setting, with audited incidences documented at approximately 1 in 600 hand injuries, or 1–4 cases per year in large centres. The most commonly injected substance is grease (57% of cases, with pressures of 5000–10,000 psi), followed by paint (at 5000 psi), and then diesel fuel (14%, at 5000–6000 psi). A frequently reported reason is the unplugging of the nozzle of a paint gun by wiping it with the tip of the index finger. A wide range of other injected substances have been reported, including water, air, wax, cement and animal vaccines.

Pathophysiology

Tissue dispersal

The pressures and volumes involved are fundamental factors in determining the extent of dispersal and local pressure effects. Industrial high-pressure jets that reach the order of 5000–10,000 psi easily penetrate skin even without direct contact, indeed only 100 psi is needed to breach the skin. Wax injection studies into cadaver limbs have demonstrated that digital dispersal can be either outside the tendon sheath, in which case the passage of travel is alongside the neurovascular bundle, or within the tendon sheath. In the former case, the early consequence is more likely to be vascular compression, thrombosis and subsequent devitalisation. In the latter case, the material can travel significant distances along the limb, allowing greater longitudinal spread, with a tendency to cause tendon adhesions and long-term limitations in mobility. With more distal injections, the limited tissue spaces in the finger result in a greater likelihood of amputation, compared with, for instance, the greater capacity of the palm.

The nature of the fluid

Of the wide variety of pressurised fluids used in industry, the most damaging to tissues are solvents. These are frequently found in paints and are known chemical irritants. Solvents penetrate tissues widely due to their low viscosity and are capable of disrupting cell membranes, causing early tissue damage akin to that of a low-grade chemical burn. The effect of droplet dispersion of solvents in tissues is to cause early inflammation and oedema, local pressure, thrombosis and necrosis. Oils are less toxic, with more delayed consequences of widespread oleogranulomata and superinfection. Water- and oil-based paints are less damaging to tissues and essentially cause local volume effects. Water, saline and veterinary vaccines are more benign and have been treated nonoperatively.

Clinical features

The initial innocuous nature of the injury can mislead both patient and clinician, as the patient may present with little other than a puncture wound. However, the delay to surgical intervention is considered to be the principle factor influencing outcome. Clearly the injection pressure, and with that the volume likely to have been instilled, are further critical variables. The site of injury has a bearing on the tissue's capability to withstand the insult, the tight compartments of the finger fare worse that the greater capacity of the palm. Fingers that are poorly perfused at presentation have a high likelihood of being amputated. However, the nature of the injected fluid remains a key driver in the decision to operate: this applies to all solvents and solvent-based paints, greases, oils and fuels.

In the case of solvent injections, the typical clinical course after injury is one of increasing pain, swelling, redness, and lymphangitis, starting as early as 3–4 hours after the accident. Oil- or grease-based injuries may take some 3 days for symptoms to present. With further time, extending tissue necrosis may become apparent.

Even with expeditious surgery, potential longer term complications include decreased grip strength, a reduced range of motion, hypersensitivity, cold intolerance, and decreased two-point discrimination. Systemic consequences from the wider spread of the injected substance have been reported.

Investigations

In the initial patient workup attempts must be made to establish the specific circumstances of the injury including the probable pressure, approximate volume involved, the site of penetration and the time delay since the injury. This is in addition to standard recordings of handedness, the nature of employment and the presence of morbidities. A detailed examination of the injection site is performed for swelling, circulation, sensation and crepitus, with an attempt to gauge the extent of spread. The patient must also be assessed for possible generalised toxicity. An X-ray may reveal opacities, air, fractures and the presence of radiodense material such as paint or debris. An urgent MRI may help to demonstrate the extent of spread, but should not delay necessary surgical intervention.

Treatment

A high-pressure injection injury must be considered to be a true hand surgical emergency, unless the benign nature of the injected fluid, such as water or saline, proves it otherwise. Under a tourniquet, without forced exsanguination, the potentially involved compartments are released, and the tissues are then carefully explored to determine the extent of spread. Exposure in the digits is achieved with Brunner or midlateral incisions. Tendon sheath integrity should be checked, and if breached, will require washout and debridement. Copious saline lavage is used to achieve thorough washout and dilution with the meticulous removal of evident foreign material, aided by microscopy. Serial procedures may be considered, without initial full primary closure, and with a scheduled second look at 48 hours. The limb is placed in a resting splint in a safe position, with a view to early mobilisation. Antibiotic cover is recommended, and the use of steroids has been suggested in severe cases.

Complications

Outcomes have been audited with respect to the inoculated substance, the pressure and likely volume involved, the site of injury, and the time delay to presentation. The key outcome measure has been whether amputation has proved necessary. Digital amputation has been shown to be likely if the initial presentation is one of the vascular compromises. Delay to intervention is considered the most significant prognostic factor contributing to a poor outcome. The second is the nature of the injected substance, with solvent-based paints identified as the most toxic compound carrying the greatest morbidity. Overall, the amputation rates are of the order of 38–40% without treatment. This goes up to 50–80% when solvents, such as in oil-based paints, are involved.

Conclusion

A high-pressure injection injury represents one of the most urgent of hand surgical emergencies. This particularly applies when vascular compromise or compartment syndrome is evident, and when the injected material has been identified as being solvent based. Prompt compartmental release and exploration, with thorough lavage and meticulous debridement – serial if need be – followed by early mobilisation, is the necessary course of action. Antimicrobial prophylaxis is advised. Only with this will the consequences of significant disability be avoided or at least reduced.

Further reading

Burke F, Brady O. Veterinary and industrial high pressure injection injuries. Br Med J 1996; 312:1436.

Neal NC, Burke FD. High-pressure injection injuries. Injury 1991; 22:467–470.

Smith GD. High pressure injection injuries. Trauma 2005; 7:95–103.

Rees CE. Penetration of tissue by fuel oil under high pressure from a diesel engine. J Am Med Assoc 1937; 109:866–867.

Related topics of interest

Hip fractures and dislocations

Key points

- Impacted hip fracture should be considered in patients who have pain on walking after a fall
- Knee injury should be specifically excluded in patients with hip fracture or dislocation
- Multidisciplinary treatment and rehabilitation is essential for optimising outcome in hip fractures

Hip fractures

Epidemiology

Proximal femoral fractures involving the femoral neck are commonly referred to as hip fractures. In 2014 in England, Wales and Northern Ireland, 64,838 patients were admitted with neck of femur fractures according to the National Hip Fracture Database annual report for that year and the numbers are increasing year on year. The annual cost to the NHS of all hip fractures in the United Kingdom is estimated to be around £2 billion. These fractures form part of the fragility fractures group in elderly patients.

Aetiology

Apart from fragility fractures in elderly patients, in younger patients causes of hip fracture include high-velocity trauma sometimes associated with excessive alcohol consumption, as well as metabolic abnormalities including renal failure and vitamin D deficiency, and pathological fractures as a result of metastatic bone disease.

Classification

Neck of femur fractures can be divided into intracapsular or extracapsular fractures.

Intracapsular fractures

Fractures that are subcapital but proximal to the intertrochanteric line that forms the anterior attachment of the capsule are included in this group. They can either be displaced or undisplaced. Traditionally, these fractures were classified according to Garden's classification. This classification was based on the alignment of the trabeculae of the femoral neck and head of the femur. However, the functional ability of the patient preinjury and medical comorbidities dictate treatment options and as a consequence this classification is little used in current practice (**Table 18**).

Intracapsular fractures can lead to avascular necrosis of the femoral head due to disruption of blood supply to the femoral head if the fracture is displaced. The blood supply to the femoral head is predominantly by the ascending retinacular capsular vessels along the posterior capsule of the hip joint.

Extracapsular fractures

These are fractures at the level of the intertrochanteric line of the proximal femur.

Clinical presentation

In displaced fractures, the leg is externally rotated and shortened. Patients are unable to actively move the hip and cannot straight leg raise. However, in some cases, the fracture may be impacted and the leg in normal alignment, with active movements at the hip, including straight leg raising, being possible. Occasionally, impacted fractures may present late after a period of painful weight bearing following a fall.

Investigations

Plain X-ray of the pelvis and lateral X-ray of the affected hip will usually reveal the fracture. Pubic rami fractures are the most

Table 18 Garden classification	
Stage	Description
1	Undisplaced incomplete fracture including fractures with impaction in valgus
2	Complete but undisplaced fractures
3	Complete fractures, partially displaced but with contact between the two fragments
4	Complete fractures, displaced with no contact between the fracture fragments

likely differential diagnosis and should specifically and carefully sought when suspecting a neck of femur fracture on the plain X-ray. If pelvic X-rays do not reveal a fracture, an anteroposterior X-ray of the hip in 15° of internal rotation can be useful. MRI of the pelvis will reveal if there is an occult fracture. If there are contraindications to MRI, a CT scan of the pelvis is a useful alternative.

Management

The mainstay of management for those fit enough for surgery is operative treatment followed by early rehabilitation with mobilisation. Treatment of any associated medical problems will help in optimising patients for surgical treatment. This is most effectively achieved by combined care between orthopaedic surgeons, orthogeriatricians and a multidisciplinary rehabilitation team. Most hospitals now follow an admission care pathway for neck of femur fractures. Surgical treatment of intracapsular fractures includes internal fixation with cannulated screws if the fracture is undisplaced and hemiarthroplasty or total hip replacement if it is displaced.

Intertrochanteric fractures are treated with a dynamic hip screw or cephalomedullary nail depending on the fracture pattern. If the lateral cortex of the proximal femur is very thin or already involved in the fracture, a cephalomedullary nail is preferred. The treatment of pathological fractures must be carefully planned in consultation with a multidisciplinary team including oncologists and physicians as appropriate.

Complications

Specific complications of hip fracture and its management include nonunion and avascular necrosis in intracapsular fractures, failure of fixation and surgical site infection. More general complications include pulmonary embolism, deep venous thrombosis, chest and urinary infection and pressure sores.

Hip dislocations

Aetiology and pattern

Both the native hip joint and hip replacements can dislocate. Here we will concentrate on dislocations of the native hip joint. These dislocations result from high velocity injuries, most commonly from a road traffic collision or fall from a height. The mechanism of injury is typically due to the knee of the driver or front seat passenger hitting the dashboard of a car, the motorcyclist's knee hitting the tarmac or sporting injuries and these can be associated with either bony or ligamentous injuries to the knee. Most dislocations are posterior, but anterior dislocations are also encountered. Dislocations are commonly associated with either a posterior wall fracture of the acetabulum or a fracture of the femoral head. Complex acetabular fractures may result in medial displacement of the femoral head through the quadrilateral plate of the acetabulum and will need combined management with specialists in pelvic and acetabular fractures.

Clinical presentation

The leg is internally rotated, flexed and shortened in the case of posterior dislocation. In anterior dislocation, the leg will be externally rotated, flexed and shortened. There may be associated sciatic nerve injury with a foot drop in posterior dislocation of the hip. A careful examination of the distal vasculature is also important and knee examination is essential to exclude or confirm bony or ligamentous injury.

Investigations

X-ray of the pelvis or a trauma series CT scan is the investigation of choice. An X-ray of the knee is also important if there are signs of knee injury.

Classification

The Thompson and Epstein classification is used for posterior hip dislocations (**Table 19**).

Treatment

Closed reduction is carried out under general anaesthetic as soon as possible in order to prevent avascular necrosis of the femoral head and degeneration of the joint. Following reduction, skeletal traction should be applied with a distal femoral pin if the hip is unstable and there are no other associated injuries to the distal femur. A post reduction CT scan of

Table 19 The Thompson and Epstein classification for posterior hip dislocations	
Type	Description
I	Dislocation with a minor chip fracture
II	With a large single fracture off the posterior acetabular rim
III	With comminuted fractures of the acetabular rim (with or without a major fragment)
IV	With fracture of the acetabular rim and floor
V	With fracture of the femoral head

the hip is performed to look for any intra-articular fracture fragments. Open reduction may be required if there are associated femoral neck fractures or intra-articular fracture fragments blocking reduction of the hip.

Associated femoral head fractures will need internally fixing if they involve the weight-bearing portion superior to the fovea of the femoral head. Associated acetabular fractures may also need internal fixation. The approach depends on the fracture pattern of the acetabulum. As a consequence, these injuries are discussed with the pelvic and acetabular specialists.

Complications

Hip dislocation may be complicated by avascular necrosis of the femoral head or osteoarthritis of the hip as well as by the complications of prolonged immobility especially in the elderly.

Further reading

Alonso JE, Volgas DA, Giordano V, Stannard JP. A review of the treatment of hip dislocations associated with acetabular fractures. Clin Orthop Relat Res 2000; 377:32–43.

British Orthopaedic Association (BOA). Standards for Trauma, BOAST 1 Version 2, January 2012. London: BOA, 2012.

National Institute for Health and Care Excellence (NICE). The management of hip fracture in adults. Clinical Guidance CG124. London: NICE, 2011.

Related topics of interest

Human and animal bites

Key points

- A full history and examination is vital in order to assess the degree of infection risk associated with a bite
- Prophylactic antibiotics are only indicated for high-risk bites
- Most bite wounds should not be treated by primary closure

Epidemiology

Dog bites are the most common mammalian bite accounting for 60–90% of all bites presenting to emergency departments, cat bites for 5–20%; and human bites up to 23% of cases. In adults, most dog bites are to the extremities, whereas in children they are to the face. Human bites may be occlusal (inflicted by biting) or from a punch injury of the hand onto another person's teeth (the so-called 'fight bite' – characteristically over the knuckles).

Wound infection is the most common complication occurring in up to 20% of dog bites, 50% of human bites and 60% of cat bites.

Less frequent complications include fracture, most commonly of the bones of the hand, tenosynovitis, septic arthritis, septicaemia, teeth or teeth fragments as foreign bodies and tetanus infection. Dog and cat bite wounds most commonly become infected with *Pasteurella* spp., with other common bacteria including *Staphylococcus* spp., *Streptococcus* spp., *Moraxella* spp. and *Neisseria* spp. The most common organisms in human bites include *Staphylococcus* spp., *Streptococcus* spp., *Haemophilus* spp., or *Eikenella* spp.

Assessment

A thorough and detailed history is essential if complications are to be avoided. The wound must be examined carefully in order to ensure that no vital structures have been damaged. X-rays are indicated if there is a possibility of a retained tooth or tooth fragment in the wound (more common with smaller animals including cats) or if there is anything (such as bony tenderness) to suggest an underlying fracture. Assessment must include a careful assessment of the position of the hand at the moment of injury since different structures will lie under a wound with the fist clenched compared to one when the palm is open. The site and a description of the wound must be carefully recorded in the medical records along with careful measurements.

The history and examination should identify whether there are any risk factors for infection that require prophylactic antibiotics and must establish the patient's tetanus status.

For human bites, the risk of acquiring a blood-borne viral infection such as hepatitis B, hepatitis C or HIV must be assessed. Local and national guidance should be followed regarding relative risks in different demographic groups. When assessing bites in paediatric patients, it is important to consider whether there are child protection issues, and to refer to paediatrics if there are any concerns.

General management of bite wounds

If the bite has penetrated the skin, the wound should be encouraged to bleed and irrigated copiously with running water. Local anaesthetic infiltration may be required to facilitate adequate cleaning of the tissues. Tetanus prophylaxis (toxoid and immunoglobulin as appropriate) should be provided if it is indicated, according to standard guidelines.

Most bite wounds will not require closure and should be left open. Primary closure can be considered for large bite wounds that are <6 hours old with no risk factors for infection or in bites to the face or ear (which have a good blood supply and require the optimal cosmetic result). Primary closure should only be undertaken after extensive wound toilet and debridement, and will require cover by prophylactic antibiotics. Co-amoxiclav is recommended for the prophylaxis of high-risk wounds. Penicillin-allergic patients can be given metronidazole plus doxycycline (with the exception of children under 12 years of age, pregnant and breastfeeding women who will need to be discussed with the duty microbiologist).

Additional management of animal bites

Rabies is not endemic in the United Kingdom but may be at risk if the bite has been acquired whilst abroad. All people who suffer a bat bite in the United Kingdom should receive rabies vaccination. Cases should be discussed with the Health Protection Agency. Antibiotic prophylaxis is only indicated for high-risk wounds (see **Table 20**).

Additional management of human bites

The risk of acquiring hepatitis or HIV from a human bite is minimal, even when the assailant is known to be infected. The assailant is rarely available to provide a history or test for blood-borne viruses, although this is sometimes possible when the bite has occurred in a healthcare setting. Blood should be taken from the patient as a 'serum save' sample for baseline serology. An accelerated course of hepatitis B vaccine (0, 1 and 2 months apart) is generally administered, with the first dose being given in the emergency department. Patients who may be at risk of developing HIV should be discussed with the on-call infectious diseases consultant in order to decide if they require postexposure prophylaxis. Follow-up by the genitourinary or infectious disease team will be required at 6 weeks for repeat serology.

Antibiotic prophylaxis should be provided for all human bites that are <72 hours old. If the patient is being assessed after this time period and has no signs of infection, then antibiotics are unlikely to be of value. Patients should be advised to seek medical assistance in the event of the development of systemic symptoms such as rigors and if they notice proximal spread of the infection, pus formation, increased swelling or severe pain in the area of the bite.

Management of infection following a bite

Any discharge from the wound should be swabbed and sent to microbiology for culture before cleaning the wound. Infection is treated with the same oral antibiotics that would be used for prophylaxis. Patients presenting with severe cellulitis, or who are systemically unwell will require admission for intravenous antibiotics. Wound debridement or incision and drainage of any collection will require a surgical admission. Particular care must be taken when managing patients who are immunosuppressed, for example those with leukaemia or following organ transplantation.

Table 20 Risk factors for wound infection	
Patient factors	**Wound factors**
Age >50	All cat or human bites
Prosthetic valve or joint	More than 6 hours old
Postsplenectomy	Crush injury or devitalised
Diabetes mellitus	tissue
Immunosuppression	Deep puncture wounds
Postmastectomy	Involving joint, tendon,
Liver cirrhosis	ligament or fracture
	Hand or foot injury
	After primary closure

Further reading

Medeiros I, Saconato H. Antibiotic prophylaxis for mammalian bites. Cochrane Database Syst Rev 2001;(2):CD01738.

Morgan M. Hospital management of animal and human bites. J Hosp Infect 2005; 61:1–10.

National Institute for Health and Care Excellence (NICE). Bites – human and animal. London: NICE, 2013.

Related topics of interest

- Antibiotic therapy and infection control (p. 26)
- Hand injuries (p. 122)
- Microbiological considerations (p. 185)

Imaging in trauma – CT

Key points

- CT scanning is fundamental to major trauma management
- Whole-body CT (WBCT) is often indicated in major trauma, but should not replace clinical judgement
- A biphasic contrast protocol can eliminate the need for multiple scans, saving time and radiation dose

Introduction

CT scanning is now well established as a fundamental and indispensable part of the management of major trauma patients. No other imaging modality comes close to matching the combination of speed and diagnostic accuracy offered by a modern multislice CT scanner. CT is not, however, without its drawbacks, in particular time and availability, contrast dose and radiation dose. Nevertheless, a retrospective multicentre study from 2009 clearly showed an increased probability of survival in major trauma patients who had undergone WBCT (Huber-Wagner).

Practical considerations

Probably the most obvious concern when contemplating scanning an unstable trauma patient is the time taken, and sheer inconvenience involved, in getting the patient in and out of the scanner safely. Whilst a current multislice scanner can image a patient from head to toe in a matter of seconds, the process of moving the patient and all associated lines, tubes, ventilators and monitoring onto the scanner table invariably presents a logistical challenge. Whilst this problem is unlikely ever to be eliminated, it may be minimalised by intelligent design of the emergency department, and good teamwork. The first requirement is that the scanner needs to be as close as possible to the trauma bay, and available at short notice. When designing a trauma centre from scratch, this is easily achieved by siting a dedicated CT scanner within the emergency department. It is more difficult in a typical older hospital building without the necessary space. A CT room intended for trauma patients also needs to be bigger than many CT rooms, due to the amount of equipment and the large team that tends to accompany a polytrauma patient. Working in cramped conditions is not conducive to speed and efficiency. A well-trained trauma team with sufficient personnel to move the patient safely, while keeping track of lines and other equipment, is invaluable.

Indications for CT in trauma

CT is the investigation of choice for major trauma due to its unrivalled combination of sensitivity, specificity and speed. It is significantly more sensitive than plain film in the identification of spine or pelvic fractures (**Figure 45**), or pneumothorax or haemothorax – it is more sensitive and much more specific than that of ultrasound in the detection of intra-abdominal trauma (**Figure 46**). MRI is far too slow, with too many limitations, to be useful in the acute trauma situation.

In most clinical situations, CT is best used to answer a specific diagnostic question. For example, a noncontrast renal tract

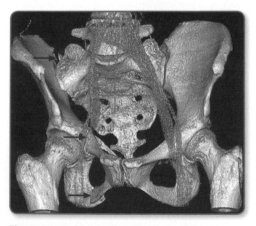

Figure 45 3D CT reconstruction image following pelvic trauma.

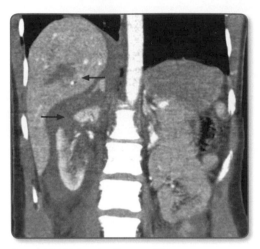

Figure 46 CT showing liver and kidney trauma.

Scanning and contrast protocols

Different parts of a trauma CT have different requirements in terms of intravenous contrast. Head CT in trauma should always be carried out without intravenous contrast, as one of the main aims is to detect intracranial haemorrhage, which appears white on plain CT. The presence of intravenous contrast, which also appears white, merely risks confusion.

The identification of fractures is not significantly affected by the presence or absence of contrast. The same applies to the identification of most lung trauma, such as pneumothorax or contusion.

Identification of soft tissue trauma, vascular trauma and, in particular, haemorrhage, requires good intravenous contrast opacification. Identification of vascular trauma requires that the contrast is within the arteries at the time of scanning, whereas optimal soft tissue enhancement of abdominal organs (such as is needed to identify subtle splenic lacerations) requires the contrast to have passed into the portal venous system. Originally, this was achieved by acquiring two scans, initially of the whole body in the arterial phase, then of the abdomen and pelvis in the portal venous phase. This would sometimes be preceded by a precontrast scan to identify any pre-existing densities that might be confused for contrast, and perhaps followed by a delayed scan, to look for pooling of contrast from haemorrhage, or leakage from the urinary tract. This system provides excellent diagnostic information, but multiple scans obviously significantly increase the radiation dose to the patient as well as the scanning time and the number of images for the radiologist to report, which increases the reporting time. Whilst there is no single, universal protocol, many trauma units have now moved to a split bolus contrast protocol that addresses these concerns. There are variations on this theme, but one protocol for an adult patient is a noncontrast CT of

CT is ideal for confirming a diagnosis of renal colic, but of limited usefulness for other causes of abdominal pain, for which a postcontrast scan is usually required. Similarly, in relatively minor trauma, a specific examination for a localised body area is likely to be appropriate. Examples include noncontrast scanning of the head and cervical spine in the case of an isolated head injury or postcontrast scanning of the abdomen and pelvis for a penetrating abdominal trauma. In the case of major trauma; however, a different approach is justified. Due to the high likelihood of multiple injuries across several anatomical sites, and the importance of speed, WBCT is often indicated. Depending on the clinical situation, this may include the lower limbs. The decision to proceed to WBCT is a clinical one based on the mechanism of the trauma and the clinical state of the patient. The advantages of speed and comprehensive coverage of possible injuries must be weighed against the downsides of radiation dose and reporting time. It should not be underestimated how long it takes even an experienced trauma radiologist to view and report the thousands of images involved in a WBCT, which can be a particular problem if there are multiple casualties.

the head, followed by 150 mL of contrast injected at 1.6 mL/s for the first 100 mL, then at 3.5 mL/s. The scan is triggered 70 seconds after the contrast injection starts, by which stage the initial contrast has reached the portal venous system, giving excellent opacification of abdominal organs, but there is still active filling of the arterial system, providing a good-quality angiogram. The scan is started at the circle of Willis and continues in a single acquisition through the torso and as far down the legs as is needed. In practice, the reduction in quality compared to separately acquired scans is minimal and more than outweighed by the savings in time and radiation dose.

Further reading

Beenen L, Sierink J, Kolkman S, et al. Split bolus technique in polytrauma: a prospective study on scan protocols for trauma analysis. Acta Radiol July 2015; 56:873–880.

Dreizin D, Munera F. Blunt polytrauma: evaluation with 64-section whole-body CT angiography. Radiographics 2012; 32:609–631.

Huber-Wagner S, Lefering R, Qvick LM, et al. Effect of whole-body CT during trauma resuscitation on survival: a retrospective, multicentre study. Lancet 2009; 373:1455–1461.

Royal College of Radiologists (RCR). Standards of practice and guidance for trauma radiology in severely injured patients. London: RCR, 2011.

Related topics of interest

Imaging in trauma – interventional radiology

Key points

- Interventional radiology (IR) plays an important role in trauma management, mainly in haemorrhage control
- Endovascular management of bleeding may reduce or eliminate the need for invasive surgery, particularly in blunt trauma

Introduction

IR is a subspecialty of radiology encompassing a wide range of procedures involving many different body systems that have in common minimally invasive access and imaging guidance. IR now plays a vital role in many areas of medicine, including haemorrhage control, notably in trauma.

Practical considerations

The availability of 24-hour IR cover is a requirement for level 1 trauma centre status. Given the relatively small number of IR consultants, this often presents a logistical challenge and is one that not all trauma centres have yet achieved. Where possible, the capability for IR should be considered in the layout of a trauma centre. A small IR room far from the emergency department and intensive care unit is not suitable for unstable trauma patients.

The optimal solution is a hybrid trauma theatre close to the emergency department and intensive care unit. This should be a fully equipped operating theatre with enough space to accommodate the radiological, surgical and anaesthetic teams that are likely to be involved with a polytrauma patient, and should ideally have a comprehensive built in X-ray system. Unfortunately, this is a very rare arrangement. The next best solution is an IR room in a suitable location with enough space and suitable anaesthetic infrastructure. A standard operating theatre with a portable X-ray machine is inadequate, as the imaging will be suboptimal, and the full range of equipment is often not to hand.

Indications for IR in trauma

The main role for IR in trauma is haemorrhage control (**Figure 47**). A closely related, but subtly different role is repair of vascular trauma. In the majority of cases, an IR referral will be the result of a CT showing active extravasation of contrast, indicating on-going haemorrhage. However in certain situations IR input may be indicated even in the absence of active extravasation: for example in an unstable patient with a significant pelvic fracture, with haematoma on CT and no other convincing cause for cardiovascular instability. In this situation, the haemorrhage may be venous in origin, hence the absence of an apparent arterial bleeding point, but may still benefit from embolisation.

In rare instances proceeding straight to angiography without CT may be appropriate although this carries the risk of missing other possible sources of bleeding and should really be considered to be a last resort. IR is most commonly useful in blunt visceral trauma, partly because the advantage of minimally invasive techniques is reduced if the patient will need open surgery anyway, for instance for a bowel injury. In isolated haemorrhage from a penetrating injury, particularly a solid visceral injury, embolisation may eliminate the need for open surgery, or reduce the extent of the surgery required. Haemorrhage control may be temporary, e.g. with intra-arterial balloons, or definitive with embolisation of bleeding vessels. Embolisation may be indicated in a delayed situation, for instance in development of hepatic artery pseudoaneurysms following trauma. Other applications for IR in trauma patients include the insertion of inferior vena cava (IVC) filters for pulmonary embolus (PE) prophylaxis.

Embolisation

Embolisation encompasses a range of techniques intended to occlude vessels via an endovascular approach. This can be divided into plugs and coils, Gelfoam, particles and liquid agents. Of these, plugs and coils with or without Gelfoam are most commonly used in trauma.

Coils are usually small lengths of platinum or stainless steel, often with fibres attached to encourage thrombosis, that are intended to coil up within a vessel in order to induce thrombosis and occlude the vessel. They are available in a wide range of shapes and sizes, and may be delivered via microcatheters (**Figure 48**) into very small vessels when required. Their main disadvantage is that multiple coils are usually required to produce a reliable occlusion that can be time consuming and expensive. In addition, if coil selection is misjudged, or the delivering catheter moves during deployment, part or all of the coil may end up somewhere other than the target area, which can lead to occlusion of the wrong vessels. Typically coil embolisation is indicated where a specific arterial bleeding point has been established from a vessel that can be safely sacrificed, e.g. renal haemorrhage where microcoil embolisation of a small-end artery can stop

haemorrhage whilst sacrificing a minimal amount of renal tissue, thereby avoiding nephrectomy (**Figure 49**).

Amplatzer plugs are expanding metal mesh plugs that can be deployed through a sheath or large catheter and aim to occlude an artery by producing a solid framework

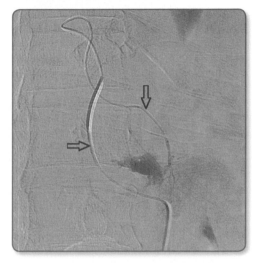

Figure 48 A selective angiogram with the right facing arrow showing the main catheter still in the common hepatic, and the downwards arrow showing a microcatheter going into the bleeding branch of the left hepatic artery.

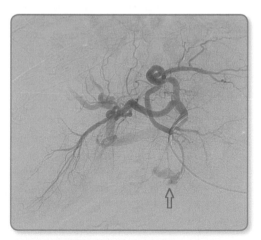

Figure 47 Liver embolisation: a catheter is visible in the common hepatic artery with the arrow showing clear extravasation of contrast.

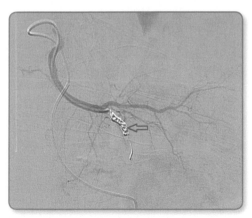

Figure 49 Postcoil embolisation of the bleeding vessel showing no further bleeding, but continued flow in other branches. The arrow indicates the embolisation coils.

for thrombus. They have the advantage of being a single device (instead of multiple coils), and are suitable for permanent occlusion of relatively large arteries. The main disadvantage is that they are relatively bulky and inflexible, and so may be difficult or impossible to place in small or tortuous arteries. A typical example of use of an Amplatzer plug would be proximal occlusion of the splenic artery in splenic trauma.

Gelfoam is a collagen-based product that can be mixed with contrast to make a thick paste that is injected via a suitably positioned arterial catheter. This can be used to occlude fairly large vessels. The main advantages of Gelfoam are that it is relatively quick, cheap and temporary, so that the vessels are likely to recanalise in a few weeks after the risk of rebleeding has passed. Gelfoam can be used, for example, to occlude one or both divisions of one or both internal iliac arteries in order to establish rapid haemorrhage control in an unstable patient with pelvic fractures.

Vascular injury: stent grafts

A stent graft is a springy metal tube with artificial graft material (e.g.

polytetrafluoroethylene) attached that is intended to reline a vessel from the inside. If an injured artery cannot be safely embolised, endovascular repair with a stent graft may be appropriate. The prime example is in thoracic aortic injury, which is relatively common, although often fatal at the scene following high-velocity road traffic collisions. For the patient to survive to reach hospital, the aortic tear must either be incomplete (a pseudoaneurysm) or contained (tamponaded). Endovascular placement of a stent graft avoids the risk of catastrophic haemorrhage due to losing the tamponade effect and has a much lower morbidity and mortality than open repair.

Stent grafting may also be used for injuries to other arteries that would otherwise require significant open-surgical procedures for repair (such as the iliac or subclavian arteries), particularly in patients who may be poor surgical candidates. Stent grafting is relatively contraindicated in areas with significant movement, such as the common femoral or popliteal arteries, due to the risk of stent failure after repeated flexing.

Further reading

Medsinge A, Zajko A, Orons P, Amesur N, Santos E. A case-based approach to common embolization agents used in vascular interventional radiology. AJR Am J Roentgenol 2014; 203:699–708.

Rousseau H, Elaassar O, Marcheix B, et al. The role of stent-grafts in the management of aortic trauma. Cardiovasc Intervent Radiol 2012; 35:2–14.

Related topics of interest

Imaging in trauma – MRI

Key points

- Patient safety during MRI is paramount
- MRI is the primary modality for investigating internal derangement of joints
- MRI has a complimentary role to CT in the management of the seriously injured patient

Introduction

MRI provides outstanding soft tissue contrast. It does not use ionising radiation and has a myriad of applications in imaging patients with traumatic injury.

How the image is produced?

Humans are predominantly composed of water molecules that contain hydrogen atoms each with a single positively charged proton. The MRI scanner contains a magnet that generates a magnetic field, causing the protons to align. A radiofrequency wave is briefly applied that flips the nuclei, altering the magnetisation vector from longitudinal to transverse. Once the pulse is switched off, the nuclei relax, returning to their original state and producing a signal, identifying their location, which is detected by a receiver coil and converted into an image.

MRI safety

The radiographer and patient complete a safety questionnaire before any MRI. A list of absolute and relative contraindications to MRI is set locally, and may include pacemakers, implantable cardiac defibrillators, otic implants, ferromagnetic implants, and, of potential relevance in trauma, metal foreign bodies. Use in the first trimester of pregnancy is currently absolutely contraindicated. In addition, all anaesthetic and monitoring equipment used must be MRI compatible. Open scanners may be useful when clinicians require easier access to the patient, e.g. those with pulmonary or cardiovascular disease or requiring sedation, or in patients with a very high body mass index or size and who would not fit into a conventional scanner.

Which sequences are used?

A pulse sequence is the set of parameters used to generate an image. Each has its uses and limitations. Sequences may be performed in any plane (usually axial, coronal or sagittal). The common sequences are T1, proton density (PD), T2 and short tau inversion recovery (STIR). The first three can be performed with fat saturation (FS) to remove the high signal from fat (e.g. PDFS), whilst the latter is a different method of achieving the same aim. Many acute pathological conditions manifest at least partly as oedema and are more conspicuous when fat signal is removed. Areas are described in terms of their signal characteristics with respect to muscle, e.g. oedema is high on T2-weighted imaging. Numerous other sequences are available. For example, a volume gradient echo sequence can be obtained and reconstructed in any plane, and is excellent for imaging very small structures, e.g. to analyse the ligaments of the wrist.

Each institution has a 'routine' protocol for every body part with a number of complimentary sequences designed to answer the common clinical questions. There are usually between three and five sequences per part scanned, taking approximately 4 minutes each. A radiologist decides if further sequences are necessary, based on clinical information or the images acquired. Contrast is rarely used.

There is a balance between performing many sequences, which would theoretically give more information, and the need to keep scanning times short, both for reasons related to the patient factors (e.g. long scan times may contribute to movement artefact due to patient discomfort) and external factors (the desire for high-patient throughput).

Up to 15% of patients experience claustrophobia. There are a number of methods of countering this problem, including keeping the scan time to a minimum (and acquiring the most important sequences first), music via headphones, sedation, hypnosis and changes in scanner design. 'Open' magnets are less commonly available, but designed to reduce claustrophobia. However, there is a trade-off with image quality.

The major trauma patient

The primary imaging modality for the severely injured patient is CT. The latest trauma radiology guidelines from the Royal College of Radiologists states that MRI should be available at all times in major trauma centres, but that MRI is not indicated in immediate trauma care, for a variety of reasons, including image acquisition time. It takes much longer to perform MRI than CT. For example, a whole spine MRI examination may take 1 hour, whereas the image acquisition time for whole-body CT is seconds. MRI is better used as part of targeted approach. Imaging may need to be performed before treatment can take place, e.g. MRI of the spine for clarification of potential injury before application of an external fixation device (a contra-indication to MRI) for limb trauma in a patient with multiple injuries.

Imaging the central nervous system

MRI has a complimentary role to CT. MRI gives a clearer guide to spinal stability, as it is possible to have significant, unstable, ligamentous injury that does not appear on a CT image. Conversely, CT identifies subtle fractures that might be overlooked on MRI. It is not generally current practice to perform whole spine MRI on unconscious trauma patients following normal CT. MRI depicts soft tissue injury, including the spinal cord, manifesting as oedema with or without haemorrhage, and intraspinal haematoma, as well as identifying osseous and disc and ligament injury. MRI may also evaluate brachial plexus injury, differentiating root avulsion (preganglionic) from lesions distal to the dorsal root ganglion (post ganglionic), which is a key determinant in treatment pathways. Brain MRI is more sensitive to diffuse axonal injury than CT, and should be considered in patients with neurological deficit not explained by CT findings.

Musculoskeletal imaging

MRI is often used to identify fractures when the initial plain film is normal and there is persistent clinical suspicion of bony injury. In these cases, bone marrow oedema on fluid sensitive sequences will alert the reporter to the abnormal area, which can then be scrutinised to identify the fracture. In contrast, undisplaced fractures can be difficult to confidently diagnose on CT. Common anatomical sites for this scenario are the hip (to confirm or exclude neck of femur fracture) and the wrist (to confirm or exclude scaphoid fracture). MRI can help determine whether a fracture is pathological, particularly if there is a reason to suspect bony metastases.

The pattern of bone marrow oedema may indicate the mechanism of injury and hence the intra-articular structures likely to be involved. For example, contusion at the posterolateral tibial plateau and midlateral femoral condyle is classical for the pivot shift injury, and the anterior cruciate ligament is likely to be torn. MRI accurately demonstrates internal derangement within joints such as the knee and wrist. It provides excellent demonstration and grading of cartilage, ligament, muscle and tendon injuries. Therefore, it can be used both as a diagnostic and prognostic tool.

Further reading

Helms CA, Major NM, Anderson MW, et al. Musculoskeletal MRI, 2nd edn. London: Saunders, 2008.

McRobbie DW, Moore EA, Graves MJ, et al. MRI from picture to proton, 2nd edn. Cambridge: Cambridge University Press, 2007.

The Royal College of Radiologists. Standards of practice and guidance for trauma radiology in severely injured patients. London: The Royal College of Radiologists, 2011.

Related topics of interest

- Imaging in trauma – CT (p. 135)
- Injuries of the thoracic, lumbar and sacral spine (p. 150)
- Mild traumatic brain injury (p. 188)

Imaging in trauma – ultrasound

Key points

- Ultrasound is effective for rapidly identifying free intraperitoneal fluid but is operator dependant
- Modern CT scanning reduces the value of the focussed abdominal/assessment sonography in trauma (FAST) scan in individual patients
- FAST is useful in triage, and may be useful in prehospital settings

Introduction

Ultrasound is an extremely useful imaging modality with numerous applications. Compared to other imaging modalities, ultrasound machines tend to be far cheaper and more portable and there is no known health risk from diagnostic ultrasound frequencies. One of the major disadvantages of ultrasound is that it is entirely user dependent. An ultrasound machine in the wrong hands can be the source of diagnostic errors, often due to missing significant findings, or confusing normal anatomy with pathology.

Principles of ultrasound

An ultrasound probe contains a piezoelectric plate that creates ultrahigh frequency (usually between 2 and 15 MHz) soundwaves that can be transmitted into the body. Different body tissues have slightly different acoustic impedance (AI), which is dependent on the density and the stiffness of the material. Whenever the ultrasound wave passes into a tissue with different AI, a proportion of the energy is reflected back and detected by the probe. The speed of sound in different body tissues is relatively constant, so the time taken for the echo to return indicates the depth of the tissue interface. Gas and bone have very different AI compared to body tissues, so an interface with either causes reflection of most of the sound energy. This causes one of the drawbacks of diagnostic ultrasound: it cannot

see effectively through gas or bone. Simple fluid contains no interfaces, so appears completely black and is easily identified. As there is a limit to how much energy can safely be transmitted to the tissues, and a proportion of the energy is reflected at each tiny tissue interface, the useful depth that can be effectively imaged by ultrasound is limited.

Focussed abdominal/ assessment sonography in trauma

The FAST scan has been in use for decades, and is part of ATLS protocols. The original FAST scan involves the examination of four areas, the perihepatic/hepatorenal space, perisplenic space, pericardium and pelvis, for free fluid. These are the areas where free intraperitoneal fluid will tend to accumulate in a prone patient, and in the context of trauma, free intraperitoneal fluid is likely to be blood.

Pericardial fluid can be reliably detected by ultrasound, and in penetrating trauma, it is a strong indicator of cardiac injury. Early detection gives the opportunity for drainage before tamponade develops.

FAST should be carried out as a concurrent activity with the primary survey and initial resuscitation. The lack of space around a trauma patient means that a small handheld machine is an advantage, as is dexterity in the sonographer.

In the early days of FAST, its detection of free intraperitoneal fluid made it extremely valuable. A trauma patient with free intraperitoneal fluid required a laparotomy, and the competing diagnostic techniques were diagnostic peritoneal lavage which is slow, invasive and oversensitive, and CT which, at the time, was slow and inefficient. Over the last few decades, ultrasound technology has improved significantly, such that small handheld machines are now available that are comparatively inexpensive, whilst providing most of the capability of full-size machines. However other technology has also improved greatly, meaning that the role of FAST is no longer so clear cut. The latest generation of CT scanners is extremely fast and, when suitably sited within or very close to the emergency department and manned by well-trained staff with suitable trauma protocols, it can produce whole-body imaging with which ultrasound cannot compete. In skilled hands, FAST is very sensitive in detecting free fluid in a slim patient. However, imaging in obese patients (a significant proportion of Western populations) is limited by the useful range of sound waves in adipose tissue, potentially significantly decreasing diagnostic accuracy. FAST is intended to detect free blood, not the source of the bleeding. This may be apparent to a skilled sonographer, for instance a large splenic laceration may be seen, but more subtle injuries are unlikely to be identified without a much more detailed, and slower, examination. Ultrasound is also unreliable for identifying free intraperitoneal gas, which is a vital indicator of bowel damage, especially in penetrating abdominal trauma. CT, however, will almost always identify the source of the bleeding, thereby allowing better planning of management, as well as being sensitive to tiny quantities of free intraperitoneal gas. This is particularly relevant as trauma management is also changing: free intraperitoneal blood no longer automatically indicates laparotomy, as visceral injuries are now often ideally managed nonoperatively, or via interventional radiology, depending on their severity. Changes in resuscitation practices, such as large volume blood transfusion via rapid transfusion devices and large-bore central lines, as well as novel techniques such as resuscitative endovascular balloon occlusion of the aorta (REBOA), mean that there are very few patients who are too unstable to stand the short delay of a CT scan.

The combined effect of these changes is that the vast majority of major trauma patients will have an early CT, markedly reducing the value of the FAST scan.

Arguably the most useful role for standard FAST now is in triage. In a multiple casualty situation, FAST is helpful in prioritising the more severely injured patients to go to CT first. The portability of ultrasound machines means that this triage role can increasingly be carried into the prehospital setting, where it may help to decide the order in which patients are transported to hospital, and the choice of hospital (e.g. deciding between a smaller local hospital and a more distant major trauma centre).

Extended FAST

FAST may be extended to look at the chest, aiming to identify pneumothorax or haemothorax. Small anterior pneumothoraces can be detected with greater sensitivity than by chest radiograph. This application is again potentially useful in a prehospital setting, informing judgements on requirement for chest decompression prior to transfer to hospital.

Other applications of ultrasound in trauma

Ultrasound is routinely used in obtaining vascular access in most settings, and may be useful in trauma patients. In skilled hands and slim patients, however, the landmark technique is often quicker in a trauma situation. Ultrasound may also be useful in deciding when to stop an unsuccessful resuscitation. In a critically injured patient with no cardiac output for some time, the lack of any visible myocardial movement on ultrasound scanning indicates that further attempts at resuscitation are likely to be futile.

Further reading

American College of Emergency Physicians. Policy Statement: emergency ultrasound guidelines. Ann Emerg Med 2009; 53:550–570.

Royal College of Radiologists (RCR). Ultrasound training recommendations for medical and surgical specialties, 2nd edn. London: RCR, 2012.

Walcher F, Weinlich M, Conrad G, et al. Prehospital ultrasound imaging improves management of abdominal trauma. Br J Surg 2006; 93:238–242.

Related topics of interest

Immediate trauma care in sport

Key topics

- Organisers of high risk sports should always ensure that they have protocols and action plans in place for dealing with the full range of potential injuries that might arise from playing the sport, even if these injuries are rare
- Sporting national bodies should ensure that, within the spirit of the game, all steps are taken to avoid or modify elements of play that are associated with the highest risks of injury
- Management of sports injuries must be tailored to the injured player and reflect the level of participation of the player in the activity

Introduction

Though sports-related trauma injuries are relatively rare, they still occur frequently enough that is a well-defined need for doctors, physiotherapists and other professionals looking after athletes and teams to be personally equipped with the skills and equipment required to deliver immediate care in the sporting setting. It is the practitioner's duty to be trained and to ensure that their skills are reviewed and refreshed regularly.

Emergency action planning

The development of an 'Emergency Action Plan' through a risk assessment considering the sporting environment, available communications, skill retention and team working in emergency situations is an essential part of immediate care preparedness in sport. Such plans should consider potential situations that might result in injury at both training and match venues and include standard operating procedures for particular scenarios. Minimum standards of equipment and responsibilities with regard to equipment checking and skill maintenance of practitioners should be in place.

Initial assessment and management

The treatment of seriously injured athletes requires rapid initial assessment and initiation of appropriate care in a safe environment following a systematic approach to ensure injuries are identified and treated in the correct order. This process constitutes the S<C>ABCDE of immediate care, where S represents SAFE (Shout for help, Assess the scene, Free from danger, Evaluate the player).

Catastrophic haemorrhage control

In the very rare circumstance of an athlete presenting with catastrophic haemorrhage, the application of a pressure dressing and the use an arterial tourniquet or haemostatic agents should be considered in an attempt to arrest the bleeding.

Airway maintenance with C-spine protection

If there is any possibility of a cervical spine injury the neck must be controlled by manual in-line immobilisation as part of the initial approach. The airway assessment begins by checking if the athlete is able to respond with a clear verbal response to voice commands. Listening to the quality of the voice may give information about the airway status and clues to any impending problems. Most episodes of airway obstruction can be easily managed with simple airway manoeuvres. Situations necessitating more advanced interventions are rare in sport, but practitioners must be skilled and equipped to provide appropriate management.

Breathing with adequate ventilation

It is important to determine the respiratory rate and check for equal expansion of the chest wall. A rapid palpation of the chest wall at this time may reveal areas of crepitus or tenderness. The more detailed assessment of breathing will normally take place in the medical room or ambulance where inspection of the thorax, assessment of the respiratory rate and expansion as well as percussion, auscultation, and examination for tracheal deviation and cyanosis are undertaken.

Circulation with haemorrhage control

It is essential through the systematic approach to recognise early signs of shock and if necessary attempt to stop or stem any visible bleeding, while transferring the athlete to the appropriate emergency department for more definitive care.

Assessment of the circulation includes the radial pulse for rate and volume, the colour of the player, noting pallor, the patient's mental status including their conscious level and agitation and the presence of any external or internal bleeding. The presence of the radial pulse usually indicates the blood pressure is adequate for end-organ perfusion, acting as a guide to whether intravenous fluids are required, administered in 250 mL aliquots of crystalloid, in blunt trauma. When shock is evident the major areas of occult bleeding are assessed: namely the chest, abdomen, retroperitoneum, pelvis and long bones.

Disability: neurological status

The on pitch baseline observation of neurological status employs the AVPU system (A: Alert, V: Responding to voice, P: Responding to painful stimulus, U: Unresponsive). Once in the medical room a more detailed neurological examination should be undertaken using the Glasgow Coma Scale. This should be repeated frequently and recorded along with all observations in the primary survey to identify improvement or deterioration.

A significant head injury requires meticulous cervical spine immobilisation at all times, early application of high flow oxygen, attention to airway, breathing and circulation, safe extrication and urgent transfer to the nearest emergency department if there is no improvement.

An athlete suspected of having concussion should be removed from play and assessed by a licensed healthcare provider trained in the evaluation and management of concussion. Diagnosis involves the clinical assessment of a range of domains including symptoms, cognition and balance. There is no same day return to play for an athlete diagnosed with concussion and most sports have their own mandatory guidelines.

Exposure and environment control

There should be limited exposure in the field of play with the athlete protected from the environment. Once in a more protected environment, the athlete may be exposed allowing a thorough examination and assessment, time allowing which must not delay transfer to definitive care.

Resuscitation

The management of life-threatening injuries as identified is essential to optimise the athlete's condition. All athletes suffering any significant injury should receive oxygen administered at 10–15 L/min via a well-fitting nonrebreathe mask. Continuous monitoring of vital signs and neurological status are essential. Athletes with significant injuries must be re-evaluated constantly and particularly after intervention.

Secondary survey

The secondary survey includes a SAMPLE history (S: Signs and symptoms, A: Allergies, M: Medications, P: Past medical history, L: Last meal and drink, E: Events and environment of the injury/illness) and a systematic head-to-toe examination. Preprepared documentation with the athlete's personal details, contact details including a next of kin and the AMP parts of SAMPLE already completed, speeds up this process.

Definitive care

The transport of critically injured athletes should be undertaken by qualified ambulance crews with appropriate equipment immediately available in case of deterioration in the athlete's condition. The mnemonic ATMIST is now widely adopted by prehospital medical teams for the handover of trauma patients.

- A: Age of the athlete (sex of athlete often also included)
- T: Time of the injury and expected time of arrival
- M: Mechanism of injury
- I: Injuries present and suspected
- S: Signs including physiological parameters
- T: Treatment given and needed

Spinal injury in sport

Although spinal injuries are rare in sport, it is important practitioners providing pitch side care are able to recognise and manage spinal injuries appropriately. A high index of suspicion for a spinal injury should be considered. Removal from the field of play should be undertaken by an experienced and well-trained team that has undertaken pre-event rehearsal of extrication procedures.

Factors suggesting spinal injury include:

- A suspicious mechanism of injury
- A reduction in conscious level

- Neurological signs or symptoms
- Distracting injury
- Midline cervical spine tenderness
- Intoxication with alcohol or drugs
- Inability voluntarily rotate neck >45° to the right and left

Musculoskeletal trauma

Limb injuries are common in sport and early appropriate management is essential. Field of play management should include rest, ice elevation and effective analgesia, wound management and splinting of the injured limb.

Medical equipment

To deliver immediate trauma care the appropriate equipment maintained and stored in accordance with the manufacturer's guidelines should be immediately available next to the field of play. Medical equipment should be maintained in accordance with the manufacturer's guidelines.

Further reading

Greaves I, Porter K, Smith J. The Principles and Practice of Immediate Care. Edinburgh: Royal College of Surgeons, 2004.

Steggles B. Faculty of Pre-hospital Care Manual of Core Material: Level 1 and Level 2. Edinburgh: Royal College of Surgeons, 2004.

Related topics of interest

Injuries of the thoracic, lumbar and sacral spine

Key points

- A high index of clinical suspicion for spinal injury is essential in the polytrauma patient
- The spine must be protected until a diagnosis and plan can be made regarding mobilisation or surgery
- Early surgical spinal fixation should be considered in the trauma patient

Epidemiology

Trauma to the vertebral column may be associated with significant mortality and morbidity if injuries are not diagnosed and treated in an appropriate manner. Concomitant injury to the spinal cord and cauda equina can result in devastating consequences for the patient with significant impact on physiological, psychological and socioeconomic status.

It has been estimated that the incidence of spinal injuries ranges from 19 to 88 per 100,000 population with the overall mortality having remained relatively unchanged at 17% over the past 20 years. The incidence of spinal cord injury is thought to range from 15 to 50 per 1,000,000 people with an estimated 10,000 new cases per year in the United States and 1000 new cases per year in the United Kingdom and Ireland. Analysis of data from the Trauma Audit and Research Network (TARN) suggests that the prevalence of significant spinal injury without neurological compromise is in the region of 10% and the majority of injuries sustained are located in the thoracolumbar spine. Approximately 2% of patients on the registry had sustained a spinal cord injury.

When any patient with multisystem trauma is being managed, it is important to recognise the importance of early spinal immobilisation whilst investigations are being undertaken to assess the severity of the injuries. Approximately 45% of major trauma patients will have a spinal injury and it can often be a challenge to fully assess the patient in the acute setting. It may be difficult or impossible to get a history and derive meaningful clinical examination findings from a patient with a head injury or a haemodynamically unstable patient who has a low Glasgow Coma Scale Score. Immobilisation of the spinal column will help to reduce secondary insults to the spinal cord in an unstable spinal fracture or dislocation. If this is likely to be prolonged, consideration should be given to the use of blocks and tape or similar and the removal of the cervical collar, the presence of which may increase intracranial pressure.

Pathophysiology

The parts of the spinal column most likely to fracture can be predicted from a knowledge of its anatomy. The most commonly injured area is the thoracolumbar region that comprises the eleventh and twelfth thoracic, and first and second lumbar vertebrae (T11 to L2). The functions of the spine are to protect the spinal cord, to provide stability, to provide mobility and to control the transmittance of movement of the upper and lower extremities. Injury to the spine can result in loss of spinal function leading to long-term morbidity.

A knowledge of normal spinal biomechanics will aid understanding of the pathology and adverse mechanics that will in turn guide decisions regarding subsequent management for the spinal fracture or dislocation. At each level in the thoracolumbar spine, there are six degrees of freedom, meaning that at each vertebral level, motion can occur in six independent ways of which three are translational and three are rotational. A normal functioning spinal segment contributes to a prescribed motion or retains a given position therefore remaining stable after a force has been applied to the spinal column. If the spinal segment is subjected to a force and is unable to maintain its anatomical relationship to its surrounding structures, then it can be said that there is mechanical instability. The point of application and energy imparted by an excessive force to the spine will dictate the pattern of failure and hence the fracture and/or dislocation seen clinically.

Soft-tissue injury to muscles, ligament and intervertebral discs should not be underestimated. The posterior ligamentous complex (PLC) of the spine (ligamentum flavum, intertransverse ligament, facet capsular ligament, interspinous ligament and supraspinous ligament) is an essential component of the posterior tension band allowing the vertebral column to remain upright when standing. An injury to the PLC can result in post-traumatic deformity and add to morbidity if it is not recognised promptly.

Clinical features

Any patient who is suspected to have a spinal injured will be examined with full precautions in-situ including a collar, cervical blocks or restraints and in-line immobilisation on a spinal board or scoop stretcher. The spinal column should be assessed as soon as practically possible in order to transfer the patient onto a pressure relieving surface and hence avoid the sequelae of skin breakdown at pressure points on the scalp, back, pelvis and heels. In-line immobilisation and log-rolling is used to examine the back and complete the neurological assessment of the perineal and perianal region including sphincter function. The principles of minimal patient handling should be followed.

In a fully alert co-operative trauma patient, pain will usually be the main presenting feature of a fractured vertebra in the thoracic, lumbar or sacral spine. There is often protective muscular spasm following spinal trauma and palpable muscle tenderness as well as midline bony tenderness may be present. However, the absence of pain does not mean that a spinal injury is excluded as patients with cervical and thoracic cord injuries may be insensate from the level of injury. Clinical suspicion should remain and careful detailed neurological examination will help define the level of injury.

In an obtunded patient, a high level of clinical suspicion and precautions must remain until all appropriate investigations are complete. Palpable midline posterior spinal bony deformity may be the only external examination finding to suggest spinal trauma. Absent reflexes and flaccid limbs are also a sign of spinal cord injury. Signs of neurogenic shock (hypotension, bradycardia) should alert the treating team and supportive measures must be instituted to prevent secondary neurological injury caused by hypoperfusion to the spinal cord.

Investigations

Imaging of the spine should be carried out if the mechanism of injury is significant and the treating teams are suspicious of a spinal injury. Plain X-rays in a trauma patient are no longer adequate for assessing the thoracic, lumbar and sacral spine, given the difficulties in interpretation of these films due to overlying ribs, soft tissue, pelvis and resuscitation equipment. Reconstructed images of the spine can be taken from a standard CT of the chest, abdomen and pelvis, providing two- and three-dimensional images from which to make an accurate diagnosis of the spinal injury.

An MRI of the spine should be completed once a vertebral injury has been identified. A decision about mechanical and clinical stability can only really be made once both CT and MRI are reviewed in conjunction. When appropriate, a standing X-ray can be requested looking for preservation of the normal spinal alignment. If there is increased post-traumatic deformity on axial loading of the spinal column, surgical fixation of the fracture may need to be considered.

Diagnosis

The current concepts in vertebral fractures were first described by Holdsworth in 1964, who recognised that the mechanism of injury was an important factor in the resultant fracture pattern. He described a two-column concept in which the spine was divided into anterior and posterior columns. Denis in 1983 introduced the concept of a middle or third column that was composed of the posterior half of the vertebral body, the posterior longitudinal ligament and the posterior annulus fibrosus. The failure of the middle column was believed to correlate with the fracture type and neurological injury as well as creating acute instability. Magerl in 1994 described a classification system that allowed identification of a spinal injury using radiographic and clinical characteristics and which provided a description of the severity of the fracture. However, significant inter- and intra-observer variation has been noted using both Denis' and Magerl's classifications.

The thoracolumbar injury classification system (TLICS) described by Vaccaro in 2006 is thought to provide the best method for therapeutic decision making in injuries to the thoracolumbar spine. This system uses injury morphology, integrity of the PLC and neurological status as the three main determining categories in the management of fractures and dislocations. Point values are assigned to subgroups within the three categories and a score is derived from the summation of the subgroup scores. A TLICS score of ≤3 suggests that the fracture can be managed nonoperatively; a score of 4 suggests that the injury can be managed nonoperatively or operatively depending on other patient or injury factors, surgeon preferences and patient wishes; a score ≥5 suggests that surgical treatment will be required (**Table 21**).

Treatment

Any treatment for injuries to the thoracic, lumbar and sacral spine should aim to restore normal function. Clinical management strategies depend on the severity of the fracture but can be stratified broadly into:

- Conservative therapy
- Isolated posterior stabilisation with or without decompression
- Isolated anterior decompression and stabilisation
- Combined anterior and posterior stabilisation

Conservative therapy can be applied to all age groups and includes bed rest and postural

Table 21 Thoracolumbar injury classification system	
Morphology	• Compression fracture – 1 point • Burst fracture – 2 points • Translational rotational injury – 3 points • Distraction injury – 4 points
Posterior ligamentous complex integrity	• Intact – 0 points • Suspected injury or indeterminate – 2 points • Injured – 3 points
Neurological involvement	• Intact – 0 points • Nerve root – 2 points • Cord/conus medullaris (incomplete) – 3 points • Cord/conus medullaris (complete) – 2 points • Cauda equina – 3 points

reduction followed by casting or bracing. Traditionally, patients with unstable fractures were kept on strict bed rest for 6–8 weeks followed by orthotic support and gradual mobilisation, but this was found to have high morbidity and as a result treatment objectives have shifted toward earlier mobilisation.

Surgical approaches to the spine can be either anterior or posterior and aim to decompress the spinal canal, reduce the fracture, restore vertebral height and provide stability. Posterior instrumented fixation involves pedicle screw systems and can be performed either open or through percutaneous minimally invasive techniques. The long-term outcomes for percutaneous pedicle screw stabilisation without fusion in the context of spinal trauma remain to be seen.

Indications for anterior surgery include anterior canal compromise with neurological deficits, deformity >20° kyphosis and 50% loss of anterior vertebral height, progressive kyphosis and late pain secondary to fracture malunion.

There is evidence to suggest that in the context of a multiply injured patient, early spinal stabilisation leads to shorter intensive care unit stays, reduced time spent on mechanical ventilatory support, fewer pulmonary complications and hence shorter hospital stays. The benefit of early surgery is seen in both spinal cord injured and noninjured patients although cord hypoperfusion needs to be avoided in the perioperative period for cord-injured patients.

Complications

Early recognition of a thoracic, lumbar or sacral injury with application of protective measures should minimise secondary injury in the form of further vertebral injury, neurological injury and vessel injury. Prolonged periods of bed rest can be avoided with modern fixation techniques and instrumentation and hence the morbidity associated with extended spinal immobilisation can be avoided. Surgical fixation of spinal injuries is not without risk and the surgeon will need to have detailed discussions with the patient and relatives in order to gain informed consent.

Further reading

Hasler RM, Exadaktylos AK, Bouamra O, et al. Epidemiology and predictors of spinal injury in adult major trauma patients: European cohort study. Eur Spine J 2011; 20:2174–2180.

Rihn JA, Anderson DT, Harris E, et al. A review of the TLICS system: a novel, user-friendly thoracolumbar trauma classification system. Acta Orthop 2001; 79:461–466.

Velez DA, Newell DW. Spine injuries. In: Moore AJ, Newell DW (eds), Neurosurgery principles and practice. London: Springer, 2005:379–406.

Related topics of interest

Intraosseous access

Key points

- Intraosseous access is an effective and underused technique in the trauma victim
- Intraosseous access insertion is no more painful than insertion of a wide bore cannula
- All drugs, fluids and blood products can be given via an intraosseous needle, and cross-match, haemoglobin, electrolytes and venous pH samples taken from it

Introduction

Rapid circulatory access is a prerequisite for fluid resuscitation as well as the administration of critical care drugs in trauma and periarrest patients. Peripheral cannulation is often challenging in the shocked and peripherally shut down patient, and the difficulty of insertion is often proportional to the degree of need. Intraosseous infusion was first described in 1922 and proposed as a possible site for transfusion following investigation of the circulation in the sternum. It was first used in children in the 1940s for blood transfusion and delivery of antibiotics, but its use declined in the 1950s following the introduction of plastic intravenous cannulae, and the use of alternative vascular access techniques. Over the last few years intraosseous devices have become more widely accepted in adult practice, especially in the military during the recent conflicts in Iraq and Afghanistan where the injury patterns sustained made peripheral intravenous access particularly challenging.

The most commonly used devices are the First Access in Shock and Trauma (FAST) system (FDA approved 1997) that uses a spring to fire a trochar into the sternum and the EZ-IO (FDA approved 2004) that uses a battery powered driver, similar to a handheld drill, to place a specially designed needle into bone. Simple handheld screw or push in needles are now rarely used.

Intraosseous devices are simple to use, can be used in a variety of situations, in and out of hospital, and have been frequently used in the military during tactical helicopter evacuation. Both EZ-IO and FAST access can be established in under 1 minute. First time success rates for EZ-IO range from 84% to 98% and for FAST1 are 72% to 74%. Ultimate success rates are 92–100% and 72–100%, respectively.

The pain of inserting an intraosseous needle is similar to that of placing a wide-bore venous cannula, although unlike peripheral cannulation, pain may also result from the infusion of fluids into the bone marrow space mediated by pressure sensors within the bone structure. This pain can be mitigated, if there is time, by instilling 3 mL of 1% lidocaine through the needle before starting the infusion.

Anatomy and physiology

Diffusion occurs from the red marrow into venous sinusoids in the medullary cavity. These sinusoids drain into venous channels that leave the bone via emissary veins before entering the circulation. Circulation times for drug administration have been shown to be similar to peripheral intravenous access in terms of pharmacokinetics and pharmacodynamics. Rates of volume infusion have been shown to be acceptable; up to 250 mL/min in some studies; however fluid infusion will require pressure rather than gravity drainage.

Indications

The main indications for use of an intraosseous access route are:

- Failure of two attempts to gain peripheral access in a situation in which it is required
- Cardiac arrest – when loss of pulses makes location of a vessel challenging
- Hypovolaemic shock – when rapid access is needed and peripheral intravenous access is difficult

In many cases, intravenous access can be substituted for intraosseous access once a degree of venous filling has been achieved. Absolute contraindications to intraosseous access include suspected or confirmed fracture in the bone (not the limb) intended as the insertion site (insertion in these circumstances may lead to extravasation and subsequent compartment syndrome), attempted placement in the same site in the past 48 hours (e.g. the sternum) because of consequent extravasation into soft tissue compartments through the previous puncture site, and joint replacement at the site of insertion. Abnormalities of bone strength such as osteogenesis imperfecta, or osteoporosis, and infection at the site of insertion (which risks osteomyelitis) are relative contraindications.

Uses

Fluid and drugs

All drugs, fluids and blood products can be infused through intraosseous access and times of onset of action have been shown to be similar in terms of pharmacodynamics and pharmacokinetics. There is some evidence from animal models that the infusion of hypertonic saline can be harmful to bone marrow, and therefore should be used with some degree of caution; however, this is not supported by papers describing its use in humans.

Laboratory investigations

All routine investigations needed including cross-match, haemoglobin, electrolytes and venous pH can be done using bone marrow aspirated from the needle. However the laboratory must be informed prior to sending the sample because most laboratory batch processing systems are not calibrated for bone marrow aspirates.

Insertion sites

EZ-IO

- Anteriomedial aspect of tibia, 2–3 cm (2 finger breadths) below and medial to tibial tuberosity
- Proximal humerus – most prominent aspect of greater tuberosity
- Anterior superior iliac spine

FAST1

- Sternum, 1.6 cm below angle of Louis (sternal angle)

Procedure

FAST1

The chest is exposed and the template patch aligned with the patient's sternal notch. Having removed the cap from the device, the cluster of needles is placed in the 15 mm 'Target Zone,' holding the device perpendicular to the manubrium (**Figure 50**). Downwards pressure with the hand and elbow in line will result in a distinctly palpable click. Pulling straight back on the device after the release is felt will release it, exposing the infusion tubing to which the connector tube can be attached. This is then connected to the infusion tube luer lock and to the intravenous line. The protective plastic dome can then be placed over the template patch to prevent dislodgement.

EZ-IO

The EZ–IO (**Figure 51**) needle is available in a number of sizes, each of which is colour coded: pink (paediatric) 15 mm; blue (adult) 25 mm; yellow (obese or muscular patients or humeral head access) 45 mm; and; 15-gauge.

The driver is positioned at the insertion site with the needle at 90° to the bone surface and the skin gently pierced with the needle until the needle tip touches the bone. The bone cortex is penetrated by squeezing the driver's trigger and applying steady,

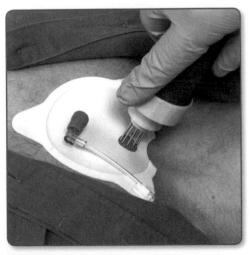

Figure 50 Inserting a FAST IO. Reproduced with permission from MedTree.

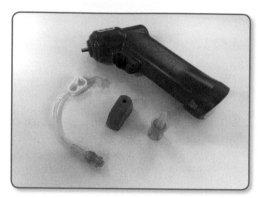

Figure 51 The EZ-IO device.

downward pressure. The trigger is released and the insertion stopped when the hub is almost flush with the skin. The catheter hub can then be stabilised and the power driver removed from the needle set. The stylet is then removed from the catheter by turning counter-clockwise.

Complications

The risk of introducing infection into a long bone leading to osteomyelitis is assessed in some series as being in the region of 0.6% that is why sterile technique must be used and inserting intraosseous devices through areas of obvious infection, such as cellulitis, is not recommended. Damage to a growth plate is a common concern in paediatrics, but no study to date has demonstrated any long-term effects on long-bone growth in children who have had intraosseous devices used on them. Compartment syndrome is a recognised complication with 16 cases recorded in the literature to date, 5 of which resulted in amputation. Extravasation of fluid is the most common complication of intraosseous placement; this may occur from a misplaced needle, from multiple attempts in the same bone, or from movement of the needle enlarging the penetration site. Good practice dictates that the area where the intraosseous is inserted be monitored for signs of extravasation. More common minor complications are seen that relate to failure of the device; placement failure, failure to infuse and misplaced/dislodged needles. Rarely the FAST1 needle can be difficult to remove leaving a retained metallic foreign body within the sternum requiring surgical removal under anaesthetic.

Further reading

Paxton JH. Intraosseous vascular access: a review. Trauma 2012; 14:195–232.

Santos D, Carron PN, Yersin B, et al. EZ-IO intraosseous device implementation in pre-hospital emergency service: a prospective study and review of the literature. Resuscitation 2013; 84:440–445.

Spivey WH, Lathers CM, Malone DR, et al. Comparison of intraosseous, central, and peripheral routes of sodium bicarbonate administration during CPR in pigs. Ann Emerg Med 1985; 14:1135–1140.

Related topics of interest

Intravenous fluids – colloids

Key points

- Colloids and crystalloids have been superseded by blood products as the fluids of choice in the initial management of severe trauma
- There is no evidence to suggest a survival benefit associated with the use of colloids rather than crystalloids in trauma
- Postulated advantages in terms of reduced resuscitation fluid volume requirements for colloids compared to crystalloids have been proven to be false

Introduction

Colloids are defined as suspensions of molecules within a carrier solution that are relatively incapable of crossing the healthy semipermeable membrane between the intravascular and interstitial spaces, because of the size of the molecules. Colloids for clinical use are broadly divided into two categories, natural and semisynthetic. The natural colloid in use for human therapy is human albumin, and a 4–5% solution is viewed as the reference colloid. The semisynthetic fluids in current clinical use fall mainly into one of three groups:

1. Hydroxyethyl starch
2. Succinylated gelatin and urea-linked gelatin–polygeline preparations
3. Dextran solutions

Current position of colloids in resuscitation

In recent years, colloids have been pushed into 'third place' as fluids of choice for the initial treatment of trauma casualties behind crystalloids and blood products (packed red cells, platelets and plasma). Emerging evidence suggests that blood products are the fluids of choice for severely injured casualties, although a degree of caution must be attached to this statement, as the evidence is currently limited because of a lack of prospective randomised clinical trials and detailed scientific studies comparing blood products to other resuscitation fluids. By contrast, a crystalloid versus colloid debate has lasted several decades, with many clinical trials of varying degrees of power. The comparison between crystalloids and colloids has been complicated by the wide range of colloids available. However, a recent Cochrane systematic review concluded that there was no evidence of a survival benefit associated with using colloids (compared to crystalloids, for further detail see 'Intravenous fluids – crystalloids', p. 161) and that because of the higher financial cost of using colloids, it was difficult to justify the continued use of colloids in resuscitation. The current UK guideline for prehospital management of hypovolaemic trauma casualties states that crystalloids are the fluid of choice when prehospital fluids are indicated although blood products are increasingly available in the prehospital environment.

Several points are noteworthy. In broad terms (but there are exceptions to this) colloids are not inferior to crystalloids, they are simply more expensive. Initial concern regarding the safety of using albumin as a resuscitation fluid in trauma was allayed by the SAFE (Saline versus Albumin Fluid Evaluation) trial. However, a subgroup analysis did reveal an increased mortality amongst albumin-treated patients who had suffered traumatic brain injury. Furthermore, a range of other trials has raised concerns regarding the safety of various hydroxyethyl starch solutions, which has led to several authors calling for a ban on their use for resuscitation, although this opinion is not universal (see Topic 'Intravenous fluids – starches'). The end result is that colloids have fallen behind crystalloids as a choice for resuscitation, and blood products are overtaking crystalloids as the choice for the more severely injured casualty. The remainder of this chapter considers the rationale for the early promise held by colloids, and why they have so far not lived up to this promise.

The ideal resuscitation fluid

Amongst a range of considerations, the ideal resuscitation fluid should expand intravascular volume with a minimum of infused volume to reduce the dilution of, for example, clotting factors in plasma. The infused fluid should also be retained in the intravascular space rather than migrating into the interstitial space where it will cause oedema that will lead to secondary problems.

Theoretical promise of colloids

Movement of fluids between the intravascular and interstitial spaces is governed by Starling forces. The theoretical promise of colloids was based on Starling forces as they were understood at the time, as it was anticipated that a large colloid molecule that could not cross the barrier between the intravascular and interstitial spaces, was likely to be retained in the vascular space until it was eventually metabolised or removed by a secondary process. Confined to the intravascular space, therefore, colloids would exert an oncotic pressure, which would retain water and hence the infused volume within the vascular space. By contrast, crystalloids are principally composed of electrolytes in water that are able to cross the barrier. Therefore, over a period of tens of minutes the crystalloid solution could be assumed to extravasate so that only a proportion of the original infusion remained in the vascular space and as a result a larger volume of crystalloid solution would be needed to produce a sustained expansion of the intravascular space, as a significant proportion of the infusion migrated into the interstitium, contributing to tissue oedema. Based on the relative permeability of the barrier and the original volumes of the intravascular and interstitial compartments, a ratio of 1:3–5 (colloid to crystalloid) was expected to produce equivalent expansions of the intravascular space, giving a clear benefit for colloid therapy. Unfortunately, this expected benefit has not been realised in practice.

Real world disappointment with colloids

In clinical practice, the ratio of colloid to crystalloid needed for resuscitation has been of the order of 1:1.2–1.4, which is substantially worse than the 1:3–5 ratio that was predicted. There are several reasons for this. First, the expected permeability for the barrier between the intravascular and interstitial spaces was based on healthy individuals. However, an inflammatory response develops quickly after severe trauma, tissue hypoperfusion/ischaemia and resuscitation/reperfusion. This inflammation increases the permeability of the barrier to larger molecules, thereby diminishing the oncotic effect of the colloid. Second, the initial premise underpinning how the barrier functioned was based on an oversimplified model. Our understanding of the nature of the barrier between the interstitium and the intravascular spaces, which is central to the operation of Starling's forces, has developed considerably over recent years and has had a significant impact on the realistic expectations of a colloid used for resuscitation.

Key developments in our understanding of Starling forces

The barrier between the intravascular and interstitial spaces is made up of the glycocalyx, endothelium and basement layer of the exchange vessels in the microcirculation, and is much more complex than previously thought (**Figure 52**). In the classical version of Starling's forces, filtration out of the intravascular space occurred at the arteriolar end of the capillaries, driven by the high hydrostatic pressure in this region of the vessel. By the venular end, the hydrostatic pressure had fallen sufficiently for the plasma oncotic pressure to dominate and draw fluid back onto the vascular space. In the revised glycocalyx model and Starling equation, there is no sustained reabsorption in most capillaries,

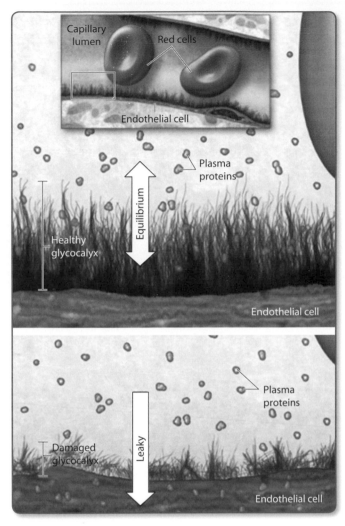

Figure 52 Endothelium and fluid permeability. From Myburgh JA, Mythen MG. Resuscitation fluids. N Engl J Med 2013; 369:1243–1251. Reprinted with permission from Massachusetts Medical Society.

which limits any attempt to prevent or treat tissue oedema by transfusing colloids. In addition, the rate and extent of extravasation of isotonic crystalloid solutions is lower than anticipated by the classical Starling equation, particularly in hypovolaemia. These revisions narrow the theoretical gap in efficacy between crystalloids and colloids, as has been observed in clinical practice. To further complicate matters, the glycocalyx itself can become damaged by the secondary consequences of trauma and fluid resuscitation (**Figure 52**). Since the glycocalyx plays a pivotal role in the movement of fluid into tissue, fluids such as plasma that are thought to protect the glycocalyx may yet be identified as the ultimate colloid resuscitation fluid.

Conclusion

Colloids are not the resuscitation fluid of choice in trauma. This is because the early expectations for this class of fluid were built in part on a premise that has subsequently been shown to be incomplete, particularly in trauma patients. The distinction between crystalloids and colloids in terms of efficacy is consequently less than anticipated, which, in addition to the financial cost and in some cases safety concerns associated with colloids has limited their potential use in trauma.

Further reading

Bunn F, Trivedi D. Colloid solutions for fluid resuscitation. Cochrane Database Syst Rev 2012; 7:CD001319.

Finfer S, Bellomo R, Boyce N, et al. A comparison of albumin and saline for fluid resuscitation in the intensive care unit. N Engl J Med 2004; 350:2247–2256.

Myburgh J, Cooper DJ, Finfer S, et al. Saline or albumin for fluid resuscitation in patients with traumatic brain injury. N Engl J Med 2007; 357:874–884.

Myburgh JA, Mythen MG. Resuscitation fluids. N Engl J Med 2013; 369:1243–1251.

Perel P, Roberts I, Ker K. Colloids versus crystalloids for fluid resuscitation in critically ill patients (Review). Cochrane Database Syst Rev 2013; 2:CD000567.

Woodcock TE, Woodcock TM. Revised Starling equation and the glycocalyx model of transvascular fluid exchange: an improved paradigm for prescribing intravenous fluid therapy. Br J Anaesth 2012; 108:384–394.

Related topics of interest

Intravenous fluids – crystalloids

Key points

- Crystalloids have no primary role in the resuscitation of the shocked trauma victim in specialist centres
- Outcomes with crystalloids are no worse than with colloids, crystalloids are cheaper than colloids and therefore preferred when immediate access to blood products is not available
- Hypertonic solutions can no longer be recommended for use in trauma

Introduction

Much has changed in recent years with the development of new trauma resuscitation strategies influenced at least in part by military research and battlefield practice. Patients with life-threatening trauma are now resuscitated using the principles of damage control resuscitation (DCR). One important principle of DCR is blood and blood product based resuscitation. In major trauma, crystalloid-based resuscitation has been shown to be inferior to resuscitation using blood products, and is associated with worse outcomes. However, if blood or blood products are unavailable, or the casualty's injuries or physiological state are not life threatening, then crystalloid resuscitation still has utility.

Crystalloids versus colloids

A recent Cochrane review concluded that there was no evidence from randomised controlled trials that resuscitation with colloids reduced the risk of death compared to crystalloids in a range of critically ill patients, including trauma casualties. The authors of this review went on to recommend that as a consequence of this finding and the greater expense associated with colloid use, it was difficult to justify the continued use of colloids. The recommendation to use crystalloids in preference to colloids for prehospital resuscitation accords with UK national guidelines for initial management of trauma casualties and recent guidelines from other countries.

Isotonic crystalloids

Crystalloid solutions fall into two main groups: balanced and unbalanced. In unbalanced solutions, the concentrations of certain ions (principally chloride) do not match the physiological levels seen in plasma. By contrast, balanced solutions incorporate buffers and alternative ions to allow more physiological concentrations of key ions. In the United Kingdom, only three crystalloid solutions are recommended for trauma resuscitation. These are 0.9% or normal saline (NS, unbalanced) lactated Ringer's solution (more commonly known in the United Kingdom as Hartman's solution, LR, balanced) and the newer Plasma-Lyte solution (PL, balanced). The ionic compositions of these fluids are given in **Table 22**.

The principal aim of using balanced versus unbalanced solutions is to avoid clinically significant elevations in plasma chloride. If excessive, hyperchloraemia can lead to hyperchloraemic acidosis and be associated with, for example, microvascular dysfunction and disturbances in renal blood flow and kidney function. Hyperchloraemic acidosis has received significant attention in intensive care medicine, but opinion as to its clinical significance in the early management of trauma is divided.

A recent small randomised, double-blind, parallel-group clinical trial demonstrated that resuscitation of trauma patients with Plasma-Lyte (compared to 0.9% saline) resulted in

Table 22 Ionic composition of common resuscitation crystalloids	
0.9% (normal) saline	Na$^+$ 150 mM, Cl$^-$ 150 mM, 300 mOsm, pH 5.5
Hartman's solution	Na$^+$ 130 mM, K$^+$ 4 mM, Ca^{2+} 1.5 mM, Cl$^-$ 109 mM, lactate- 28 mM, 300 mOsm, pH 5–6.5
Plasma-lyte	Na$^+$ 140 mM, K$^+$ 5 mM, Mg 1.5 mM, Cl$^-$ 98 mM, acetate- 27 mM, gluconate- 23 mM, 295 mOsm, pH 7.4

improved acid–base status over the first 24 hours after injury, although there was no difference in mortality in the two groups. In animal trials, balanced solutions have shown some benefit over unbalanced solutions in relation to acid base status (depending on how this is assessed) and global organ blood flow, but little overall advantage compared to unbalanced solutions in terms of effects on the inflammatory state or damage to the endothelium and glycocalyx. In comparison to the effects of prolonged profound shock, the effects of the additional chloride may be the lesser evil when 0.9% saline is the only resuscitation fluid available.

Initial resuscitation for severely injured patients is based on a strategy of permissive hypotension, aiming for cerebration in the awake patient, or 70–80 mmHg in penetrating trauma and 90 mmHg in blunt trauma. The National Institute for Health and Clinical Excellence (NICE) has recommended that in older children and adults with blunt trauma, no fluid be administered in the prehospital resuscitation phase if a radial pulse can be felt, or for penetrating trauma if a central pulse is palpable. This is beneficial as this avoids over-resuscitation with crystalloid, haemodilution and the dangers of disrupting nascent clots and iatrogenic rebleeding in the casualty. All fluids should be warmed. In a prehospital environment, this seldom occurs that predisposes to hypothermia and overall worsening of the lethal triad of trauma (**Figure 53**).

It should be noted that the evidence base underpinning the benefits of hypotensive resuscitation (or permissive hypotension) relate to short periods (1–2 hours) before full resuscitation. Beyond this time, the penalties of the inherent shock state may start to dominate, and alternative (hybrid) strategies of resuscitation may need to be considered, especially if there is concomitant lung injury and hypoxaemia. The period of hypotension should therefore be kept to a minimum, with rapid transfer to the operating theatre for definitive care. Once haemostasis has been achieved, resuscitation targeted to measures of cardiac output or oxygen delivery improves outcome.

Hypertonic saline

Hypertonic solutions include 5% hypertonic saline (Na$^+$ 856, Cl$^-$ 856, 1711 mOsm, pH 5) and RescueFlow (7.5% sodium chloride and 6% dextran). These solutions expand the intravascular volume by far more than the volume of fluid infused as they mobilize interstitial fluid into the vascular space. Care must be taken when administering hypertonic solutions, as there is often a delay before blood pressure starts to rise in response to the fluid, and pressure may continue to rise after the infusion is stopped, risking an 'overshoot' of an intended pressure target. A number of clinical studies have examined the efficacy of hypertonic solutions in trauma but overall they have not shown a difference in mortality or other clinically important outcomes associated with the use of hypertonic saline, although most of these studies were not adequately powered to show significant differences. Furthermore, a recent randomised controlled trial of prehospital use of hypertonic solutions was terminated by the data and safety monitoring board after randomisation of 1331 patients, having met prespecified futility criteria. A study based on an in vivo model of blast and nonblast injury found that although hypertonic saline-dextran performed well in the absence of blast injury, it was significantly inferior to normal saline in the presence of blast injury. Finally, a number of studies have shown that hypertonic saline solutions are associated with an attenuated inflammatory response after trauma/shock and resuscitation and hypertonic solutions have been proposed to improve cerebral perfusion and reduce cerebral oedema in patients with traumatic

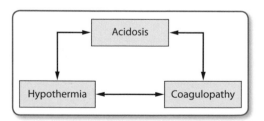

Figure 53 Schematic representation of the 'lethal triad of trauma' and the interaction between the components.

brain injury. One of the main concerns with the use of hypertonic saline is its potential to cause central pontine myelinolysis due to a rapid increase in serum sodium levels.

Summary

In severe trauma, blood products are the best choice of fluid for early resuscitation of casualties. However, in less severe trauma or when blood products are not available then crystalloids are the fluids of choice. Current debate is focusing on the issue of balanced versus unbalanced crystalloid preparations, although at present there is more opinion than hard evidence in either direction.

Further reading

Harris T, Thomas GOR, Brohi K. Early fluid resuscitation in severe trauma. BMJ 2012; 345:e5752.

Kirkman E, Watts S, Cooper G. Blast injury research models. Philos Trans R Soc Lond B Biol Sci 2011; 366:144–159.

Myburgh JA, Mythen MG. Resuscitation fluids. N Engl J Med 2013; 369:1243–1251.

Patanwala AE, Amini A, Erstad BL. Use of hypertonic saline injection in trauma. Am J Health Syst Pharm 2010; 67:1920–1928.

Perel P, Roberts I, Ker K. Colloids versus crystalloids for fluid resuscitation in critically ill patients (Review). Cochrane Database Syst Rev 2013; 2:CD000567.

Woodcock TE, Woodcock TM. Revised Starling equation and the glycocalyx model of transvascular fluid exchange: an improved paradigm for prescribing intravenous fluid therapy. Br J Anaesth 2012; 108:384–394.

Related topics of interest

Intravenous fluids – starches

Key points

- Hydroxyethyl starch (HES) may be associated with increased coagulopathy, which may be a particular problem in trauma patients
- HES administration appears to be an independent risk factor for acute kidney injury and death after blunt, but not penetrating, trauma
- HES cannot currently be recommended for use in trauma

Introduction

HESs are a heterogeneous family of semisynthetic compounds used to make colloid-based plasma volume expanding solutions. HESs were initially hailed as potentially safer, cheaper, alternatives to colloid solutions based on human and animal-based material such as albumin. However, in recent years there has been considerable controversy around HES solutions and several key trials and publications have been retracted. The end result is a deep division between experts with some groups expressing deep concern regarding any use of HES for resuscitation, while others are keen to see it remaining on the list of options for clinical use and further evaluation.

Chemistry

There is marked heterogeneity between various HES molecules resulting in a range of pharmaceutical products with significantly different pharmacokinetic and pharmacodynamics properties. These differences in pharmacological properties derive from differences in the chemistry of various HES molecules.

Starch molecules are made up of glucose units that are either joined by linking carbon atom 1 (C1) of one glucose unit to carbon atom 4 (C4) of the next (α 1:4 linkage), or C1 of one glucose unit to C6 of the next (α 1:6 linkage) (**Figure 54**).

To increase the water solubility and reduce breakdown by plasma α-amylase the starch molecule is chemically hydroxyethylated to give HES. The hydroxyethyl groups can be added to C2, C3 or C6 of the glucose units within the starch molecule, although in practice this occurs mainly at C2 and C6. It is hydroxyethylation at C2 that is most important with respect to protection against amylase. The end result is a range of HES molecules, each one of which is typically characterised by:

- The average in vitro molecular weight (450–700 kDa (high), 100–200 kDa (medium), or 70 kDa (low)
- The degree of substitution by hydroxyethyl groups, quantified as molar substitution (MS, ratio of hydroxyethyl groups to glucose units)
- The ratio of hydroxyethyl substitution at C2 versus C6 (high ratios, >8, significantly reduce degradation by serum α-amylase)
- The source of the original plant starch (waxy corn or potato)

To make a preparation for clinical use, pharmaceutical companies dissolve a specific HES in a solvent that is usually either normal saline or a balanced Ringer-type crystalloid solution, although less commonly HES can be dissolved in hypertonic (7.5% saline) crystalloid solutions. The most common concentrations of HES solutions are either 6% (6 g HES per 100 mL crystalloid solution, which is iso-oncotic with plasma) or 10% (which is hyperoncotic compared to plasma). The initial effect of a 6% HES solution will be to expand the plasma volume by the amount of HES solution given, while a 10% HES solution will initially expand the plasma volume by 1.45 times the volume infused (since it is hyperoncotic, it will mobilise interstitial fluid into the vascular space to give additional volume expansion).

The standard short-hand for HES is HES MW/MS, for example HES 130/0.4 is a medium molecular weight (130 kDa) tetrastarch.

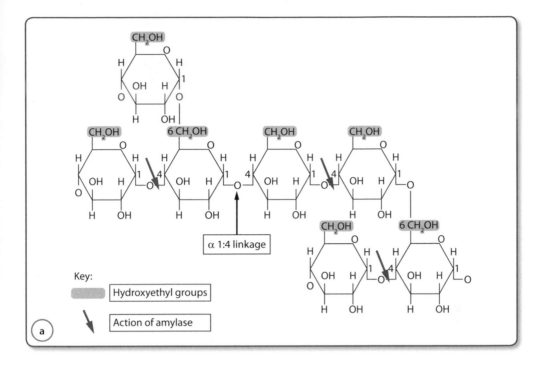

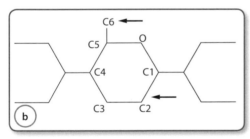

Figure 54 (a) Hydroxyethyl starch (HES) molecule and (b) carbon positions in a glucose unit of a HES molecule.

Use of HES for resuscitation: animal models of trauma and haemorrhagic shock

Animal trials show that although HES has significant advantages over crystalloid with respect to volumes of fluid required for resuscitation after haemorrhagic shock, the evidence of any additional haemodynamic benefit is mixed. Some studies have shown HES to attenuate secondary inflammation after haemorrhagic shock and resuscitation; however, others studies have shown no effect. There seems to be little benefit or even detriment associated with HES in respect of the microcirculation, the endothelium and intestinal barrier function. HES was found to be inferior to blood products with regard to clotting in models of traumatic shock. There may be important differences between various HES molecules, but currently the body of literature is too small to form any firm conclusions.

Use of HES as a trauma resuscitation fluid: human studies

There are relatively few reports of the use of HES in early resuscitation after trauma. HES, in limited volumes, has been used as a plasma volume expander in US civilian trauma practice. In US military battlefield resuscitation, a 500 mL bolus of HES is recommended for patients who are hypotensive or obtunded if blood products are not immediately available. In the United Kingdom, HES (tetrastarch only since this is the only one found in the British National Formulary) is not recommended as fluid for resuscitation by the NICE guidelines.

Data from two unblinded and one blinded randomised controlled trial suggested that there may be an important difference in the response to HES in penetrating versus blunt trauma. These studies examined several HES preparations covering high and medium molecular weights and ranging from hetrastarch to tetrastarch. The overall conclusion was summarised by one study which stated 'HES is an independent risk factor for acute kidney injury and death after blunt, but not penetrating, trauma, which underscores a fundamental difference between these two injury types.' These observations highlight the importance of clinicians considering the mechanism of injury when selecting treatment. Finally, there are concerns that HES may be associated with increased coagulopathy, which would be a particular problem in trauma patients.

Other uses of HES as resuscitation fluid

HES was been a popular resuscitation fluid in critically ill patients in Europe. A Cochrane review examined the use of HES for resuscitation in a range of critically ill patients and concluded that 'the current evidence suggests that all HES products increase the risk in AKI (acute kidney injury) and RRT (renal replacement therapy) in all patient populations and a safe volume of any HES

solution has yet to be determined. In most clinical situations, it is likely that these risks outweigh any benefits, and alternate volume replacement therapies should be used in place of HES products.' Although this review based its conclusions on 42 studies, only one of these represented a trauma population. Clearly, the situation is complex and caution needs to be employed when applying generalised conclusions to trauma groups.

HES products are now contraindicated in critically ill patients or patients with sepsis or burns; however, HES could be used in patients with acute blood loss, where treatment with crystalloids alone is not sufficient. If HES is used, the maximum dose is currently 30 mL/kg and it should only to be used in the first 24 hours of fluid resuscitation treatment. Renal function must be monitored for at least 90 days in patients receiving HES. Clinicians are advised to give careful consideration to the expected benefits versus the potential and uncertain harm of HES prior to using it in trauma and surgery.

Conclusion

In summary, the use of HES as a resuscitation fluid is a complex and contentious area. The early promise suggested by preclinical trials has not translated to widespread use, and there is significant concern that the risks associated with using starch solutions may outweigh the possible benefits. Part of the problem may be the heterogenous nature of various starch molecules and their widely differing pharmacological properties, which makes it difficult to make comparisons between various trials and reports. Until more evidence becomes available, perhaps the safest advice to follow is that issued in the United Kingdom in NICE guideline 174, which states that tetrastarch should not be used for fluid resuscitation.

Further reading

Allen CJ, Valle EJ, Jouria JM, et al. Differences between blunt and penetrating trauma after resuscitation with hydroxyethyl starch. J Trauma Acute Care Surg 2014; 77:859–864.

Bellomo R, Bion J, Finfer S, et al. Open letter to the executive director of the European Medicines Agency concerning the licensing of hydroxyethyl starch solutions for fluid resuscitation. Br J Anaesth 2014; 112:595–600.

Coriat P, Guidet B, de Hert S, et al. Counter statement to open letter to the Executive Director of the European Medicines Agency concerning the licensing of hydroxyethyl starch solutions for fluid resuscitation. Br J Anaesth 2014; 113:194–195.

Datta R, Nair R, Pandey A, Kumar N, Sahoo T. Hydroxyethyl starch: controversies revisited. J Anaesthesiol Clin Pharmacol 2014;30:472.

Mutter TC, Ruth CA, Dart AB. Hydroxyethyl starch (HES) versus other fluid therapies: effects on kidney function. London: The Cochrane Library, 2013.

Related topics of interest

Lethal triad

Key points

- The 'lethal triad' in trauma is hypothermia, acidosis and coagulopathy
- Management of these should be anticipatory and preventative or if the triad is established, aimed at rapid identification and correction
- A 'damage control' approach is essential if the lethal triad is to be effectively managed

Epidemiology

The lethal triad of acidosis, coagulopathy and hypothermia is driven in trauma patients by haemorrhage, decreased tissue perfusion and shock together with dilution and consumption of clotting factors (**Figure 55**). Hypothermia (<35°C) is present in up to 43% of seriously injured patients, an incidence that increases if the patient is entrapped in a wet or exposed, cold environment. Hypothermia is directly correlated to the injury severity score and is an independent risk factor for the development of multiple organ dysfunction syndrome and mortality.

Acidosis may be endogenous (due to poor tissue perfusion) or exogenous (due to administered fluids such as 0.9% saline). In major trauma patients with shock, approximately 50% will have an elevated blood lactate level (>2 mmol/L) and 14%

will have a base excess >6 mEq/L. Lactate clearance is an independent predictor of mortality in this patient population.

Approximately, 25% of trauma patients present to the Emergency Department with hypocoagulopathy defined as a prothrombin time >1.5 times normal and this too is an independent risk factor for mortality. Hypothermia and acidosis have synergistic effects on the function of the coagulation system.

Pathophysiology

Hypothermia leads to α-adrenergic stimulation with vasoconstriction, exacerbating any organ hypoperfusion that may be already present secondary to hypotension from the injury. This leads to worsening acidosis. Both hypothermia and acidosis may be further exacerbated by aggressive fluid resuscitation, especially with normal saline. Hypothermia and acidosis combined with consumption, dilution and failure to replace clotting factors leads to a coagulopathy.

Trauma-induced coagulopathy (TIC) has two components: (i) acute traumatic coagulopathy (ATC) that is associated with tissue hypoperfusion and with more severe injury and (ii) systemic acquired coagulopathy (SAC) resulting from consumption and dilution of clotting factors.

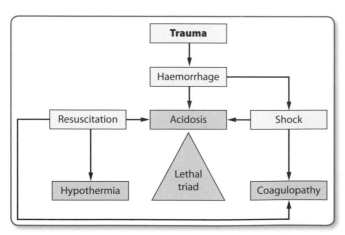

Figure 55 Drivers of the lethal triad.

Tissue hypoperfusion per se is believed to induce ATC through activation of protein C via endothelial protein C receptor thrombin and thrombomodulin, inhibiting the clotting cascade and promoting fibrinolysis (through inhibition of plasminogen inhibitor activator 1). Even if major surgical bleeding is controlled at this stage, the patient will continue to bleed from all cut surfaces prolonging the cycle of hypothermia, acidosis and coagulopathy.

Hypothermia impairs the coagulation pathways. Protease activity falls as the temperature decreases. Factor VII activity declines linearly with temperature, retaining only 80% of its activity at 33°C. Platelet activation is decreased secondary to diminished interaction between von Willebrand's factor (vWF) and collagen glycoproteins Ib and X (GPIb/X). A core temperature of 34°C is a critical point at which significant changes in platelet physiology occur and enzyme activity decreases. Hypothermia is directly correlated to injury severity and is an independent risk factor for mortality.

Acidosis also significantly affects haemostasis. At a pH <7.4, a normal platelet will change internal structure and lose its ability to change shape. At pH 7.1, thrombin production in clot propagation is decreased by 50%, fibrinogen by 35% and platelet activity by 50%.

Clinical features

The most severely injured trauma patients represent only approximately 10% of trauma cases but the majority of in-hospital trauma deaths. Ninety per cent of trauma patients are not in shock and are hypercoagulable rather than hypocoagulable following injury. The 10% of patients most severely injured are in shock, and at risk of ATC and TIC. Identification of these patients is initially based on information gained from the history of the mechanism of injury, injury patterns discernible clinically, initial physiological parameters at the scene and their response to prehospital treatment and on arrival at the emergency department.

Investigations and diagnosis

In addition to clinical assessment and identification of the patients at risk of developing the lethal triad, routine serial measurement of core temperature, blood gases with lactate and clotting function should be performed. The later may be either point of care or laboratory based. There has increasingly been a move towards whole blood thromboelastography (viscoelastic assessment) in assessing coagulation status due to the recognition that traditional factor based assays do not reflect the true coagulation status of trauma patients. However, ATC is still defined by a prothrombin time ratio (PTr) >1.2, and while functional thromboelastographic definitions have been suggested (clot amplitude at 5 minutes <35 mm), this has not been universally adopted. Any test must be readily and rapidly available as it is a dynamically changing condition. Monitoring of all the parameters of the lethal triad during resuscitation and surgery is important in order to ensure that the patient's physiology is not deteriorating.

Treatment

The key to treatment of the lethal triad is recognition, as well as the avoidance of interventions that may exacerbate the condition (such as prolonged exposure, cool fluids or crystalloid-based resuscitation). Active temperature management including warming mattresses, air-warming blankets and warmed fluids is essential. The resuscitation protocol must be based on blood products with individualised management guided by near patient testing.

Acidosis is corrected by re-establishing adequate tissue perfusion during resuscitation. While hypotensive resuscitation is the recommended initial resuscitation strategy, this should be time limited and bleeding should be controlled and adequate tissue perfusion established in a timely fashion (within an hour).

Best practice now limits or effectively eliminates the use of crystalloid in the early stages of trauma resuscitation by using a massive haemorrhage protocol based on infusion of blood components. Coagulopathy is corrected by resuscitation using blood products and tranexamic acid within 3 hours of injury.

A damage control (DC) approach is based on the premise that the physiological derangements of acidosis, coagulopathy, and hypothermia occurring as a result of haemorrhagic shock are exacerbated by surgery, which should be limited to control of haemorrhage and removal of contamination until the patient's physiology is restored and the lethal triad corrected or improving before more definitive surgical repair is considered.

The decision to perform a damage control surgery (DCS) procedure is an active decision that should be made early in the patient assessment (immediately preoperatively or with a few minutes of starting the procedure) in order to avoid promoting the changes in the parameters of the lethal triad with further blood loss, hypotension, hypoperfusion,

acidosis and coagulopathy. Attempts to define physiological measures mandating a DCS approach have been suggested. An estimated ISS of >25, systolic blood pressure <70 mmHg, core temperature <34°C and pH <7.1 have been suggested as indicators for DCS. Other authorities have suggested lactate or base deficit, blood transfusion requirement or injury mechanism and patterns as possible indicators of the need for DC rather than conventional surgery. However, by the time these changes have become established the patient is already compromised. Proactive measures to limit the lethal triad by active counter hypothermia measures, maintaining adequate tissue perfusion and correction of coagulopathy are desirable and must be instituted as early as possible, including in the prehospital phase. This 'bundle' of measures is included in the concept of Damage Control Resuscitation. Active monitoring is required to establish the direction of trends in temperature, acid–base (including lactate clearance) and coagulation.

Further reading

Davenport R, Manson J, De'ath H, et al. Functional definition and characterization of acute traumatic coagulopathy. Crit Care Med 2011; 39:2652–2658.
Duchesne JC, Kimonis K, Marr AB, et al. Damage control resuscitation in combination with damage control laparotomy: a survival advantage. J Trauma 2010; 69:46–52.
Spahn DR, Bouillon B, Cerny V, et al. Management of bleeding and coagulopathy following major trauma: an updated European guideline. Crit Care 2013; 17:R76.

Related topics of interest

Long-bone fractures

Key points

- Careful clinical assessment including a detailed history and neurovascular examination is essential
- The possibility of a pathological fracture should be considered in unusual cases
- The complications of long-bone fractures may be life threatening

Fracture types

Long-bone fractures may be classified according to cause (aetiological classification):

- Traumatic fractures occurring in normal bones as a result of trauma
- Pathological fractures occurring in abnormal bone (e.g. osteoporosis or neoplasm)
- Stress fractures occurring in normal bone that has been subjected to repeated stresses (e.g. metatarsal fractures in soldiers) or by the configuration of the fracture
- Transverse fractures with or without a wedge (butterfly) fragment caused by a bending force
- Spiral fractures caused by a rotational force
- Compression (buckle) fractures caused by an axial force
- Oblique fractures caused by a combination of the above

In addition, fractures may be undisplaced or displaced. Traditionally, the displacement of the distal fragment is described in relation to the proximal fragment. This does not necessarily represent how the displacement occurred. In each plane, the displacement has a direction and a magnitude, e.g. valgus displacement of 30°. In addition, displacement in the coronal and sagittal planes may be translation or angulation (**Table 23**).

Fractures may also be open or closed. Most fractures are *closed*, that is to say the broken bone is covered by an intact soft tissue envelope. When the soft tissue envelope has been disrupted, so that the

Table 23 Configurations and directions of fracture fragments
Configurations of displacement
a. Translation
b. Angulation
c. Combination of a and b
Directions of displacement
a. In the coronal plane
i. Varus (towards the midline)
ii. Valgus (away from the midline)
b. In the sagittal plane
i. Apex anterior or anterior translation
ii. Apex posterior or posterior translation
c. In the axial plane (judged by clinical examination)
i. External rotation
ii. Internal rotation

broken bone is in communication with the exterior, the fracture is open. Contrary to common belief, open fractures can result from either low- or high-energy trauma. Open fractures have a significant incidence of infection and nonunion if they are not managed in a timely and appropriate manner. The British Orthopaedic Association (BOA) and the British Association of Plastic, Reconstructive and Aesthetic Surgeons (BAPRAS) have provided standards of care for the management of open lower limb fractures (BOAST 4), which call for a combined orthopaedic and plastic approach to both the initial management and subsequent definitive fixation and soft tissue cover of open fractures.

Initial management

Careful management of any fracture in the emergency department is essential. The neurovascular status of the limb should be examined carefully and documented and the limb restored to its normal alignment and splinted under appropriate analgesia. Following reduction, the neurovascular status should be re-examined. X-rays of the bone including the joints above and below the fracture should be taken in two planes at 90° to each other.

Open fractures should be managed in the same way, and the wound covered with a clean, moist, nonadhesive dressing. Antibiotics should be administered at the earliest opportunity in line with local policy. Photographs of the wound, should obviate the need to repeatedly remove the dressing prior to surgery.

Principles of fracture management

Reduction

The aim of the management of any fracture is to restore the normal anatomy of the bone and soft tissues by reduction of the fracture. Some fractures will not require anatomic reduction, for example rib fractures. Reduction may be achieved by closed or open means. In closed reduction traction on the limb may be all that is necessary to reduce a long-bone fracture by the principle of ligamentotaxis – applying tension to the ligaments and other soft tissues that pulls the bony fragments to which they are attached back into alignment. More often, manipulation – using a combination of traction and other forces (usually the reverse of those which caused the original displacement) will be required. Analgesia or anaesthesia will be required depending on the type of fracture and the age of the patient. Open reduction is achieved by surgical intervention and direct reduction of the fracture fragments.

Maintenance of reduction

Once the anatomical position has been restored, this should be maintained until bony union has occurred. This can also be achieved by closed or open means. Closed maintenance of reduction can be achieved with plaster of Paris or fibreglass casts (the joints above and below the fracture are normally immobilised), splints, traction or external fixation. Open maintenance of reduction by internal fixation usually uses intramedullary (nails) or extramedullary (plates and screws, K-wires) methods.

Rehabilitation

After fracture union, it is important to restore function by encouraging movement of joints and muscle groups as soon as it is safe to do so. If fractures are treated by stable fixation (internal or external), early mobilisation is possible.

Fracture healing

Indirect fracture healing occurs if the fracture has been treated by closed means, or if the method of fixation used provides relative stability (it maintains length and alignment but does not rigidly immobilise the bone), for example an intramedullary nail.

This type of healing passes through the following stages:

- Haematoma formation between the fractured ends of bone
- An inflammatory stage, characterised by invasion of the haematoma by inflammatory cells
- Formation of callus, which is an amorphous tissue composed of cartilage and fibrous tissue
- Consolidation of the callus into woven bone
- Remodelling of woven bone into lamellar bone, with reconstitution of the medullary canal

Direct fracture healing occurs when the bone ends have been anatomically reduced and rigidly immobilised, such as by internal fixation with plates and screws. Movement between fracture fragments usually induces the formation of callus in order to limit this movement. In direct fracture healing, this movement is eliminated by the rigidity provided, so the stages of callus formation are bypassed and healing occurs directly across the fracture. Callus is not seen on radiographs, so fracture union can be difficult to determine. This process takes longer than indirect healing.

Regional injuries

Humeral shaft fractures

These are commonly treated nonoperatively in casts followed by functional splints. Indications for operative management and internal fixation include:

- Open fractures

- Pathological fractures
- Bilateral fractures
- Multiple injuries
- Failure to maintain alignment nonoperatively

Humeral shaft fractures (**Figure 56**) may be associated with radial nerve injury and careful clinical examination is mandatory. The Holstein-Lewis fracture pattern (spiral fracture of the distal third of the humerus) is said to be associated with radial nerve involvement. The majority of these are neuropraxias and are treated expectantly. Radial nerve palsy following surgery requires exploration of the nerve.

Forearm fractures

The radius and ulna articulate at each end to form the proximal and distal radioulnar joints. Fractures of the shaft of a single forearm bone may result in disruption of these joints. Fracture of the radius (**Figure 57**) with dislocation of the distal radioulnar joint is a Galeazzi fracture, while fracture of the proximal ulna with dislocation of the radial head is a Monteggia fracture. In adults, displaced forearm fractures are usually treated by operative reduction and internal fixation, as they together form a 'joint,' and malunion, rotational deformity and functional deficit are common with nonoperative treatment.

Femoral fractures

Femoral shaft fracture is a significant injury, commonly resulting from high energy trauma. Life-threatening complications may result, including blood loss leading to shock (up to 1.5 L of blood may be lost into the thigh in a closed femoral shaft fracture, and immediate restoration of alignment and splintage can reduce blood loss), as well as the incidence of fat embolism and thromboembolism (both deep vein thrombosis and pulmonary embolism).

Adult femoral shaft fractures are usually treated by internal fixation with intramedullary nails (**Figure 58**); in situations where this is contraindicated, such as where

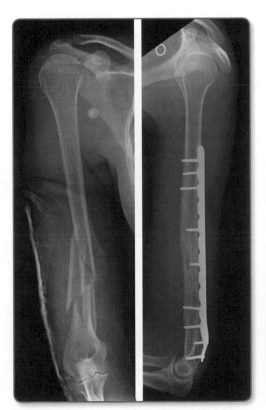

Figure 56 A humeral shaft fracture treated by plate fixation.

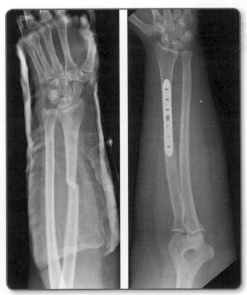

Figure 57 A radial shaft fracture treated by plate fixation.

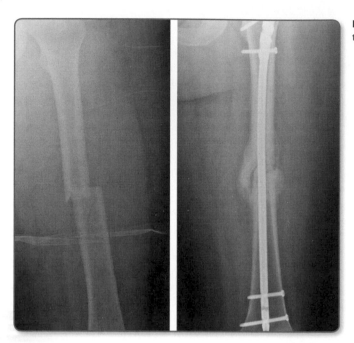

Figure 58 A femoral shaft fracture treated with an intramedullary nail.

there is a narrow medullary canal or there are significant chest injuries, plating or external fixation may be used.

Tibial fractures

Tibial shaft fractures may occur after either high- or low-energy trauma. Internal fixation is favoured in most cases, although undisplaced or mildly displaced fracture patterns with inherent stability may be managed in a cast followed by functional bracing. Fractures of the middle third can be treated by intramedullary nailing (**Figure 59**), but this should be performed with caution in fractures of the proximal or distal third, as the introduction of the nail itself will not reduce the fracture in these locations and other fixation methods such as plating or external fixation may need to be considered.

Long-bone fractures in children

Long-bone fractures in children are commonly treated nonoperatively by immobilisation in a cast or splint, with

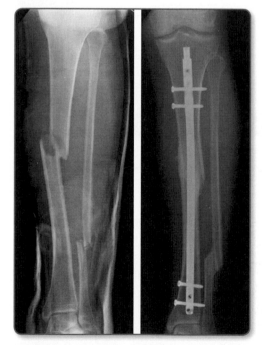

Figure 59 A tibial shaft fracture treated by an intramedullary nail.

some exceptions. Displaced fractures of the forearm bones are internally fixed with plates or flexible intramedullary nails in order to prevent rotational deformity. Femoral shaft fractures in adolescents are also treated by flexible intramedullary nails in order to prevent malunion and facilitate early mobilisation.

Complications of long-bone fractures

The early complications of long-bone fractures include:

- Blood loss

- Neurovascular compromise
- Compartment syndrome
- Fat embolism (commonly after femoral fractures)
- Thromboembolism (deep vein thrombosis, pulmonary embolism)

Late complications include:

- Infection (osteomyelitis)
- Nonunion
- Malunion
- Ischaemic (Volkmann's) contracture after vascular injury or missed compartment syndrome

Further reading

British Orthopaedic Association (BOA) and British Association of Plastic, Reconstructive and Aesthetic Surgeons (BAPRAS). BOAST 4: The management of severe open lower limb fractures. London: BOA, BAPRAS, 2009.
Dandy DJ, Edwards DJ. Essential orthopaedics and trauma, 5th edn. Edinburgh: Churchill Livingston, 2009.

McRae R, Esser M. Practical fracture treatment, 5th edn. Edinburgh: Churchill Livingston, 2008.
Solomon L, Warwick DJ, Nayagam S. Apley and Solomon's concise system of orthopaedics and trauma, 4th edn. Florida: CRC Press, 2014.

Related topics of interest

Lyophilised plasma in trauma resuscitation

Key points

- Resuscitation with high ratios of plasma to packed red blood cells is now standard practice for resuscitation in major trauma
- Observational evidence suggests that prehospital resuscitation with red blood cell concentrate and plasma is beneficial
- Freeze-dried (lyophilised) plasma is an alternative to thawed fresh frozen plasma (FFP), whose shelf-life and storage conditions limit its suitability for prehospital emergency care, for austere environments and for low-volume trauma centres

Epidemiology

Trauma-induced coagulopathy (TIC) (part of the lethal triad) is found in between one-quarter and one-third of major trauma casualties and, when present, increases mortality fourfold.

Pathophysiology

TIC occurs early after injury is related to the magnitude of injury burden and is driven by a combination of tissue hypoperfusion and severe tissue damage. TIC is multifactorial, contributing factors include clotting factor dysfunction and consumption, platelet dysfunction, hyperfibrinolysis and, possibly, autoheparinisation from shedding of the endothelial glycocalyx. To these may be added hypothermia, acidosis and dilution from inappropriate resuscitation fluids.

Clinical features

TIC causes prolonged bleeding from wounds (both traumatic and surgical), from arterial and venous cannulation sites and from mucosa and serosa. Haematomas form in the absence of local injury, although they may not be apparent in the acute trauma patient.

Investigations

Haematological investigations should include standard laboratory tests (full blood count, prothrombin time, activated partial thromboplastin time), fibrinogen tests and near-patient viscoelastic tests [rotational thromboelastometery (ROTEM) or thromboelastography]. Routine electrolytes, acid–base balance and serum calcium concentrations should be also monitored.

Diagnosis

No formal definition of trauma-induced coagulopathy has been agreed. Standard laboratory tests [prothrombin time ratio (PTr) and activated partial thromboplastin time] are prolonged and a PTr > 1.2 has been suggested as diagnostic. Such tests are rarely available in <45 minutes – a timeframe that may represent complete blood volume replacement in massive haemorrhage.

Where available, viscoelastic tests showing reduced clot strength within 5 minutes of test initiation may be diagnostic (e.g. ROTEM EXTEM Clot Amplitude <35 mm); these are not yet widespread in civilian practice. None of these investigations are suitable for diagnosing TIC in the prehospital environment.

Treatment

Principles of haemostatic resuscitation should be adopted from the point of first contact with the patient. TIC is treated presumptively with blood-product-based resuscitation including FFP. This has been widely adopted for in-hospital treatment of major haemorrhage and is associated with improved survival. Military and civilian air ambulances are increasingly carrying red blood cell concentrate with or without thawed plasma in order to deliver this resuscitation strategy in the prehospital environment. Observational studies have demonstrated an association between prehospital blood product resuscitation and improved survival after battlefield trauma and, to a lesser extent, in the civilian context. Individualised resuscitation is possible in-hospital if viscoelastic testing is available.

Plasma-rich resuscitation strategies are limited by logistical constraints. In a military or civilian acute medical response setting, transport and storage of frozen components may compromise agility. FFP may take up to 40 minutes to thaw and is therefore poorly suited to situations where rapid availability is required. Current UK guidelines limit the shelf-life of thawed FFP to only 24 hours (other countries permit shelf-lives of up to 14 days, accepting a rapid reduction in Factor VIII activity beyond 24 hours). The universal plasma donor group (group AB) is rare, with only 4% of the UK donor pool having this ABO group. Consequently wastage of this scare resource must be avoided. However, group A plasma shown to have low titres of anti-A and anti-B may be substituted to meet demand. Where frequent use is anticipated (e.g. in high-intensity military conflict or high-volume civilian trauma centres), maintaining a constant supply of thawed universal plasma is viable without unacceptable wastage.

Freeze-dried (lyophilised) plasma has been used as an alternative in settings where rapid plasma availability is desired but the requirement is infrequent or where the supply chain is vulnerable to disruption (including civilian prehospital care, trauma centres receiving lower case volumes or smaller-scale military operations with extended supply chains or delayed evacuation).

The German Red Cross and French military are established producers of lyophilised plasma that can be stored at 2–25°C for up to 15 months. The German product is group specific, whereas the French one is based on a minipool to provide a 'universal plasma.' Both products are issued as powder in glass bottles. These can be reconstituted within 5 minutes with 100–200 mL of water for injection and administered from either bottle or fluid bag. An administration set with air vent and standard filter (170–230 μm) is required for transfusion from the bottle, whereas administration from the fluid bag can use a standard blood giving set. Haemostatic profiles are similar to conventional FFP. The product should be administered within 4–6 hours of reconstitution.

Clinical considerations

Clotting factor concentrations

Clotting factor concentrations in reconstituted lyophilised plasma are lower than in the FFP from which they are manufactured but remain above the minimums specified in British and European quality standards for FFP. In vitro clot formation is preserved, as is the ability to correct coagulopathy in animal models.

Hypocalcaemia

As with other plasma components, lyophilised plasma contains citrate, which may lead to hypocalcaemia. Monitoring and correction of serum calcium concentration (preferably with intravenous calcium chloride) should feature in major haemorrhage protocols.

Disease transmission

Like the plasma from which it is derived, transfusion of lyophilised plasma carries risks of transmission of viral or prion disease. Blood safety measures include quarantine or pathogen-inactivation processes prior to lyophilisation to reduce the risk of blood-borne viruses. Plasma is leucodepleted and sourced from countries with a low risk of vCJD to minimise the risk of prion disease.

Immunity

The risk of transfusion-related acute lung injury (TRALI) is minimised through the use of male only plasma. Although lyophilised plasma carries the same theoretical risks of TRALI as FFP, no such complications have been reported in the literature despite transfusion of over 500,000 units. Plasma should be either universal or ABO compatible to minimise the risk of immune haemolysis.

Further reading

Glassberg E, Nadler R, Gendler S, et al. Freeze-dried plasma at the point of injury: from concept to doctrine. Shock 2013; 40:444–450.

O'Reilly DJ, Morrison JJ, Jansen JO, et al. Prehospital blood transfusion in the en route management of severe combat trauma: a matched cohort study. J Trauma Acute Care Surg 2014; 77:S114–120.

Sailliol A, Martinaud C, Cap AP, et al. The evolving role of lyophilized plasma in remote damage control resuscitation in the French Armed Forces Health Service. Transfusion 2013; 53:65S–71S.

Related topics of interest

- Blood product (1:1:1) resuscitation (p. 42)
- Lethal triad (p. 168)
- Viscoelastic assessment of coagulation in trauma (p. 318)

Maxillofacial and dental injuries

Key points

- Maxillofacial injuries are common in both major and minor trauma
- Maxillofacial injuries are important due to their involvement with and proximity to the airway
- Maxillofacial injuries can be divided into life-threatening injuries requiring immediate attention (within the primary survey) and those requiring less urgent attention (identified during the secondary survey)

Primary survey issues

Some maxillofacial injuries will present during the primary survey as a result of airway obstruction due to a foreign body (e.g. teeth, dentures or vomit), bleeding into the airway, deformity (e.g. from displaced midface or mandibular fractures) or direct laryngeal/tracheal trauma. Haemorrhage from facial injuries may also be severe and require immediate management. The airway must be cleared of all debris, using a finger sweep or appropriate suction (Yankauer) and when practical, imaging of the airway should confirm that dental fragments teeth or foreign bodies have not been aspirated into the airway. Inability to intubate may require surgical airway (cricothyroidotomy) to secure the airway.

Grossly displaced facial fractures can be manually reduced to alleviate airway obstruction; this may also tamponade and reduce haemorrhage. In cases of gross mandibular mobility, a traction tongue suture can help to pull the tongue forward and prevent further obstruction. The suture can be secured to the patient's chest or clothing. Maxillary disimpaction or repositioning anteriorly can also relieve airway obstruction. Midface or nasal packing may be required in order to establish haemorrhage control. Anterior nasal packing can be achieved with the use of bismuth/iodoform paraffin paste impregnated ribbon gauze, proprietary nasal tampons (e.g. Merocel or Nasopore) or inflation tamponade devices (Rapid Rhino). Posterior nasal packing can be achieved by the insertion of a Foley catheter into each side of the pharynx via the nose. The balloon is inflated with sterile saline, and the catheter retracted so that the balloon occludes the posterior nasal space. Continued bleeding following these manoeuvres may mean that interventional radiology or formal surgical intervention is required to arrest haemorrhage.

Secondary survey issues

In the case of the polytrauma patient these injuries may only be identified on a trauma series CT study. In less severely injured patients, they are diagnosed using a combination of clinical examination and plain radiological investigations.

Regional injuries – bony injuries

Mandible and maxilla

Signs of fracture of the mandible or maxilla include disturbed occlusion, mobility of fractures, swelling, tenderness or bruising. Sublingual ecchymosis is virtually pathognomonic of mandibular fracture. The patient may complain of pain, paraesthesia of the lower lip or chin (mandibular fracture) or cheeks and midface (maxillary fracture), as well as altered occlusion. Initial investigation is usually by plain radiography: dental panoramic tomogram and PA films for suspected mandibular fracture, facial views including occipitomental 10° and 30° films for maxillary fractures. However, many facial injuries are best evaluated on high-resolution CT imaging, usually best requested after discussion with a maxillofacial surgeon.

No immediate treatment is required unless the fracture is grossly mobile and at risk of obstructing the airway. Bridle wires around the teeth can be used to stabilise fractures. The usual method of treatment is open reduction and internal fixation alone, or in combination with mandibulomaxillary fixation.

Zygoma and orbits

These fractures may present with bony deformity including depression of the malar body, arch or infraorbital rim, swelling and bruising. Lateral subconjunctival haemorrhage with no posterior limit is often described as pathognomonic of zygomatic fracture. Orbital fractures may be complicated by restriction of eye movements or altered position of the globe, which is usually difficult to see initially due to swelling. The patient may complain of pain, swelling, tenderness, paraesthesia of the cheeks or midface and diplopia. Increasing pain behind the eye, proptosis or decreased visual acuity may signify acute intraorbital (retrobulbar) haemorrhage that is a surgical emergency. Where orbital involvement or globe injury is suspected, ophthalmological review is mandatory, and orthoptic examination should be arranged.

Initial investigation is usually with plain X-rays (occipitomental facial views at 10° and 30°) but CT scanning is the only reliable way of confirming orbital fractures and should always be requested where clinical suspicion is high.

No urgent treatment is required unless there is ophthalmic injury or retrobulbar haemorrhage is suspected. This requires urgent orbital decompression via lateral canthotomy with cantholysis, and urgent ophthalmological review.

Frontal bone and base of skull

The usual presentation is with facial bony deformity, swelling and bruising. Bilateral periorbital ecchymoses (Panda or Raccoon eyes) can be suggestive of a base of skull fracture, as can mastoid bruising (Battle's sign). Checks should be made for cerebrospinal fluid rhinorrhoea and otorrhoea, and if present, specimens sent for testing for β-2 transferrin. Pain and paraesthesia of the forehead may occasionally be present. The investigation of choice is usually CT scanning – which is generally performed due to the associated high clinical suspicion of head injury.

No urgent treatment is required unless there is overlying soft tissue injury or evidence of significant neurological deficit, particularly signs of orbital apex compression (including decreased visual acuity and ophthalmoplegia). Monitoring for signs of evolving head injury is the priority.

Frontal bone fractures involving the sinus are still an area of controversy. Outer table only fractures may require intervention for cosmetic reasons, while those involving displacement of the inner or both tables are likely to require surgery to render the sinus 'safe,' thereby reducing the lifetime risk of meningitis.

Cervical spine injury

Cervical spine injury occurs in a significant proportion (1–6%) of patients with facial trauma, and must therefore be excluded. Immobilisation should be maintained during maxillofacial examination, until clearance of the C-spine is complete.

Soft tissue injuries

In general, injuries should be closed as soon as is practical. Infection is rarely an issue, although all wound closure should be accompanied by thorough wound debridement, and wounds are usually covered with antibiotics, especially in the case of bite injuries. In anatomically sensitive areas (e.g. overlying the distribution of facial nerve branches or the parotid duct), thought should be given to the possibility of damage to underlying structures. If there should be any suspicion of injury, wounds will require formal exploration by an experienced surgeon, when any necessary repairs may be undertaken.

Penetrating neck wounds should be managed with care: angiographic examination may be required to establish the presence of large vessel damage. Pressure should be applied to control haemorrhage, and exploration should only be performed in an operating theatre environment.

Areas of tissue loss may be reconstructed by means of skin grafts or local flaps; however when extensive (as in the case of shotgun injuries for example), free tissue transfer may be required. Specialist opinion should be sought for any significant soft tissue injury.

Dental injuries

Avulsion

Avulsed teeth (teeth that are completely displaced from their socket) are treated by reimplantation and splinting to an intact tooth as soon as possible following injury or the tooth should be stored in an appropriate storage medium (milk, saline or saliva) until reimplantation can be attempted. Success is dependent on the degree of damage to the tooth, the extra-alveolar time and the stage of development of the tooth at the time of avulsion. Primary teeth should not be reimplanted.

Luxation

Luxation is displacement of a tooth in a direction other than axial. Such teeth require repositioning and splinting. If repositioning is impossible, or the patient presents some time after injury, the teeth may be orthodontically realigned. Primary teeth should not be repositioned.

Intrusion

Intrusion is axial displacement into the socket. Intruded teeth may be left to re-erupt over time, or re-positioning can be performed. Intruded primary teeth are probably best extracted to prevent further damage to their permanent successors. With the exception of avulsion injuries, where time is of the essence and outcome is directly related to the speed of treatment, expert opinion for dental injuries should be sought prior to treatment.

Further reading

Newlands C, Kerawala C. Trauma in oral and maxillofacial surgery. Oxford specialist handbooks in surgery. Oxford: Oxford University Press, 2010.

McPherson DW, Webb RM. Immediate care in the emergency room. In: Maxillofacial trauma and esthetic facial reconstruction, 2nd edn. Missouri: Elsevier Saunders, 2011.

Related topics of interest

Metabolic response to trauma

Key points

- Trauma triggers a hormonal and metabolic response that aims to allow the patient to survive the insult, repair damage and restore the body's normal homeostasis and function
- Changes in fluid balance and energy stores are seen. The more significant the trauma the greater the response
- Understanding these changes is important in helping to predict where dysfunction may occur and in optimally managing these critically ill patients to improve morbidity and mortality

Introduction

It has been said that people do not die from trauma, but from the effects of trauma. It is essential, therefore, that clinicians have an awareness of how trauma effects body systems. The metabolic response to trauma is usually divided into the ebb and the flow phases (**Table 24**). The ebb phase is defined as a period of reduced metabolism, fall in body temperature and oxygen consumption in order to conserve energy stores. This starts immediately after a significant traumatic insult and may last for several hours. Psychological fear and stress as well as loss of circulating volume cause an increase in circulating levels of catecholamines. This aims to maintain blood flow to vital organs and manifests as alertness and agitation, tachycardia and peripheral vasoconstriction. Cortisol and glucagon levels rise and insulin levels fall. Hyperglycaemia occurs as a result of high catecholamine levels triggering release from the liver and low insulin levels causing failure in uptake and utilisation. This does, however, provide a continued supply of substrate for the brain that may be important early in the disease process. Catecholamines are the driving force in this acute phase as the body tries to achieve haemodynamic stability.

The flow phase follows the ebb phase and is thought to last anywhere from a few days to 3 weeks or more. The maximum response is often seen by 5–10 days, although metabolic changes may be seen still many months later. The flow phase is defined as a period of hypermetabolism and catabolism that is typically hormone driven (catecholamines and cortisol) and promotes repair and supplies energy to the injured body. The body's oxygen requirements and basal metabolic rate rise, which can lead to a rise in body temperature. Protein and fat are consumed (proteolysis and lipolysis), glucose production is stimulated and salt and water retained. This highly catabolic phase leads to substrate consumption and falls in protein levels and can lead to an increased risk of infection and weakness. Early hypercalorific nutritional replacements enterally delivered are recommended and may help prevent metabolic depletion and its complications.

A third phase may then follow known which is referred to as the convalescent or anabolic phase during which recovery continues and a positive nitrogen balance is achieved.

Specific metabolic responses
Hormones and glucose

Traumatic stress triggers the release of:

- ACTH that stimulates glucocorticoid and mineralocorticoid production

Table 24 The ebb and flow phases (summary)	
The ebb phase	Metabolic rate is reduced
	Body temperature falls
	Oxygen consumption falls to conserve energy stores
	Circulating levels of catecholamines increase to maintain blood flow to vital organs
	Cortisol and glucagon levels rise
	Insulin levels fall
The flow phase	Metabolic rate increases
	Oxygen requirement rises
	Catecholamines and cortisol promote repair and supply energy
	Body temperature rises
	Protein and fat are consumed (proteolysis and lipolysis)
	Glucose production is stimulated
	Salt and water are retained
	Protein levels fall (consumption)

- Cortisol which is catabolic, triggering lipolysis, proteolysis and glucose production. It also has anti-inflammatory effects
- Glucagon that triggers gluconeogenesis and glycogenolysis
- Catecholamines that are catabolic, sympathomimetic and inhibit insulin
- Growth hormone that has anti-insulin effects and stimulates protein synthesis and lipolysis
- ADH, especially triggered by hypovolaemia, which stimulates water retention
- Aldosterone that promotes salt and water retention

Hyperglycaemia is commonly seen as a result of a number of pathways driven by high cortisol and catecholamine levels. Gluconeogenesis and glycogenolysis in the liver are stimulated, insulin levels fall and the body develops a peripheral insulin resistance, thus circulating levels remain high. Poorly controlled glucose levels in diabetics are associated with increased morbidity, especially due to infections. It is less clear whether the same is true in the trauma patient, although control within normal ranges avoiding hypoglycaemia is recommended.

Lipolysis

Cortisol, growth hormone and catecholamines stimulate fat breakdown to provide further substrate for liver gluconeogenesis. In blunt trauma patients, fat stores are only utilised when calorific intake does not meet expenditure needs and thus with adequate intake fat stores may be maintained. Lipolysis appears to be relatively impaired in the obese trauma patient, leading to greater utilisation of other energy substrates.

Proteolysis

Cortisol-induced proteolysis in muscle leads to tissue loss and negative nitrogen balance. The amino acids can then be used for energy or acute phase protein production in the liver. The protein consumed is typically skeletal muscle leading to loss of muscle mass. This in part accounts for the muscle weakness seen post-trauma that leads to difficulties in

weaning from ventilation and mobilisation. Research into amino acid replacement (e.g. glutamine) in feeding regimes has shown promising results, although further work is needed. Post-traumatic protein loss currently appears to be independent of early additional protein administration and feeding.

Fluid and electrolytes

Triggered by intravascular losses, the body releases ADH and aldosterone that work to prevent fluid excretion by the kidneys via salt and water retention. Once haemodynamic stability is achieved this fluid is typically maintained in the extracellular fluid (having moved from the intravascular compartment because of increased vascular permeability) until it is cleared by redistribution and the lymphatic system. Measured sodium levels often fall, especially in shocked patients. This change is complex and dependant initially on resuscitation fluid type and volume used, and then hormonal changes and failure of the cellular sodium–potassium pump. Measured levels of potassium often remain within normal limits, although they will change with muscle damage and renal dysfunction.

Cellular metabolism and systemic inflammatory response syndrome

Hypovolaemia and shock post-trauma and increased oxygen requirements lead to reduced oxygen supply to cellular mitochondria and switching from aerobic to anaerobic metabolism. This leads to the production of acid and lactate that accumulates and causes a metabolic acidosis. Bicarbonate is consumed and where possible ventilation stimulated to excrete carbon dioxide in order to try and maintain a normal pH.

In response to tissue damage the systemic inflammatory response is triggered leading to cytokine and acute phase protein production, along with neutrophil, platelet and clotting cascade activation. This aims to aid healing, protect tissue and limit blood loss. However, severe damage may lead to an out of control response causing disordered coagulation with an increased thrombotic risk, as well as bleeding and multiorgan damage.

Response modification

There have been a number of attempts to attenuate and prevent the body's response to stress, implying that the response is detrimental. Overall the results have been limited. In certain types of surgery, high-dose opiates may modify or inhibit the body's stress response; however, large doses are needed that carry significant side effects. Clonidine and benzodiazepines have also been shown to have some effect in inhibiting the stress response; however, the outcomes of this are currently unclear. Epidural anaesthesia has been shown to supress the stress response to surgery in the lower limbs, but only when placed before an insult and thus of little assistance in acute trauma.

Further reading

Desborough JP. The stress response to trauma and surgery. Br J Anaesth 2000; 85:109–117.

Gosling P. The cellular, immune, and metabolic response to trauma. Crit Rev Clin Lab Sci 1998; 35:59–112.

Sritharan K, Thompson H. Understanding the metabolic response to trauma. Br J Hosp Med 2009; 70:M156–158.

Related topics of interest

- Acute respiratory distress syndrome (p. 9)
- Nutrition in trauma and burns (p. 208)
- Systemic inflammatory response syndrome (SIRS) (p. 279)

Microbiological considerations

Key points

- Following trauma, patients are at high risk of early and late infective complications and infection remains a significant cause of mortality and morbidity
- For certain traumatic injuries, a short course of antimicrobial prophylaxis is recommended. Additionally, vaccination should be offered in some trauma situations
- Specimens should be collected for microbiological investigation when infection is suspected. Where possible, they should be taken prior to initiation of antimicrobial therapy
- The most important treatment for many early trauma-related infections is surgical debridement. In such patients, prompt wound cleansing with debridement of necrotic and devitalised tissue and removal of environmental debris is essential

Background

Infection remains a prevalent complication of trauma with significant morbidity and mortality. Infective complications can be divided into early (acquired at the time of injury and manifesting promptly) and late (acquired at the time of injury with late presentation or acquired as a complication of subsequent healthcare).

Trauma is a risk factor for infection for many reasons:

- Breach of skin and mucosal surfaces may occur, with contamination of sterile sites. To cause infection, micro-organisms can reach the site of infection through an inoculating injury (e.g. a bowel penetrating stab wound leading to bacterial peritonitis) or contiguous spread of normal flora from an adjacent site (such as a base of skull fracture leading to bacterial meningitis)
- Severe trauma associated with blood transfusion or organ failure may lead to suppression of immunity

- The monitoring and treatment of such patients predisposes them to healthcare acquired infection. Patients with devices such as intracranial pressure bolts and intra-vascular lines are at particularly high risk

Initial risk assessment

During initial evaluation of the trauma patient, a brief infection risk assessment should be undertaken. This ensures that prompt prophylaxis (antimicrobials, immunoglobulins and vaccinations) can be administered when necessary. Additionally, if infective complications develop later then appropriate empirical antimicrobials can be administered.

There are specific indications for short, prophylactic antimicrobial courses in specific trauma situations, including severe open lower limb fractures (see further reading). Such prophylaxis cannot prevent all infective complications and is no substitute for surgical management. Where prophylaxis is recommended, broad-spectrum agents that cover well-adapted community pathogens (such as *Staphylococcus aureus*, β-haemolytic *Streptococci* and *Clostridia* spp.) are used. Conversely, there are many situations with a lack of clinical evidence for antimicrobial prophylaxis, e.g. cerebrospinal fluid (CSF) leak.

There are trauma-related indications for vaccination, such as pneumococcal vaccine following base of skull fracture with CSF leak or splenectomy. Additionally, tetanus and blood-borne virus risk assessments may be indicated and should be made in accordance with national/local guidelines.

When assessing a trauma admission clinicians should consider:

- Mechanism of injury – injuries involving heavy environmental contamination or inoculation of a foreign body pose a very high infection risk
- Extent of injury – consideration should be given to any devitalised or necrotic tissue, perforated viscus, base of skull fracture or compound bony fracture

- Geographical location of trauma – the epidemiology of pathogens varies by country and environment (e.g. sea or freshwater, farmyard or road surface)
- Healthcare abroad – a patient who has received healthcare abroad may have become colonised or infected with multidrug resistant micro-organisms. This can have an impact on infection prevention precautions and antimicrobial therapy (prophylaxis or treatment)
- Patient factors – age, comorbidities, medications or other factors that may render the patient immunosuppressed. The threshold for commencing antimicrobial treatment may be lower in such patients. Low virulence micro-organisms that can colonise otherwise healthy trauma patients may cause invasive infection in the immunosuppressed

If the mechanism of trauma is unusual, out of context or unknown then it is important to consider infection as a potential precipitant for trauma. For example, a young person could injure themselves during a seizure secondary to viral encephalitis. To manage the traumatic injuries without addressing the underlying pathology in such patients could be disastrous.

Management principles

Infection can be difficult to diagnose in the context of severe trauma. Patients often have a systemic inflammatory response syndrome and therefore raised inflammatory markers. Furthermore, postoperative patients or those with burns raised intracranial pressure or organising haematomas may be pyrexial. This can make the clinical picture difficult to interpret.

The basic principles of diagnosing and managing an infected patient apply to early and late trauma-associated infection. Where possible, antimicrobials should be withheld until appropriate microbiology specimens have been taken. However, antimicrobials should never be withheld in patients with severe sepsis (with or without septic shock). Delays in administering appropriate antimicrobials to this patient group lead to increased mortality.

Following sampling, empirical antimicrobial therapy should be commenced. Empirical antimicrobials are usually broad-spectrum agents that cover well-adapted community pathogens (e.g. co-amoxiclav). In patients failing to respond, a well-documented history and examination can direct microbiologists and clinicians to likely pathogens and therefore appropriate second line agents. For example, an infected open wound sustained in fresh water would be exposed to different micro-organisms (e.g. *Aeromonas* spp.) and may require the addition of Ciprofloxacin compared to one sustained in an urban road traffic collision (see p. 26).

Where microbiology samples have been collected, it is possible to rationalise the empiric antimicrobials with the results of culture and sensitivities using a narrow spectrum agent where possible.

It is important to note that the mainstay of treatment for many early trauma-related infections is timely and thorough surgical debridement. The importance of prompt wound cleansing with debridement of necrotic and devitalised tissue and removal of environmental debris cannot be overestimated. This also allows for sampling of deep tissues for microbiological and histological investigation. Antimicrobials alone will not successfully treat an infection without adequate source control.

Where traumatic wounds present ≥6 hours after injury or are inoculated with debris, surgeons often opt for a delayed primary closure. Although there is a lack of systematic evidence to advocate delayed primary closure, it is generally thought to reduce the risk of on-going infection (see further reading). Additionally, this method allows for daily wound inspection prior to wound closure.

Further reading

British orthopaedic association (BOA) and British association of plastic, reconstructive and aesthetic surgeons (BAPRAS) BOAST 4: The management of severe open lower limb fractures. London: BOA and BAPRAS, 2009.

Eliya-Masamba MC, Banda GW. Immediate closure or delayed closure for treating traumatic wounds in the first 24 hours following injury. London: The Cochrane Library, 2013.

Public Health England. Immunisation against infectious disease. London: Public Health England, 2013.

Related topics of interest

Mild traumatic brain injury

Key points

- Traumatic brain injury (TBI) is a leading cause of death and disability in young adults and children
- The severity of TBI is graded according to the conscious level [Glasgow Coma Scale (GCS) score] at presentation, the duration of post-traumatic amnesia (PTA) and the radiological findings
- The prognosis of mild TBI is usually, but not invariably, good. About 15% of people will develop persistent postconcussional features and 2–4% will suffer permanent symptoms. Mortality is low compared to severe TBI but age and comorbidity are risk factors for a poor outcome

Epidemiology

TBI is a leading and rising cause of disability worldwide. The incidence of TBI is estimated to be between 200 and 790 per 100,000 population per year, with significant variations between countries and urban or rural settings. Young males are most at risk, but increasing life expectancy is linked to a rising incidence in the elderly due to falls and frailty. The vast majority of TBI cases, between 85% and 95%, are classed as mild. Road traffic collisions (RTCs) are the leading cause of mild TBI (mTBI) followed by falls, assaults and sports. mTBI is also common in military conflict and has been dubbed the signature injury of the recent wars in Iraq and Afghanistan.

TBI is defined as a nondegenerative, noncongenital insult to the brain from an external mechanical force, possibly leading to:

- A period of loss of consciousness (LOC)
- Loss of memory for events immediately before or after the accident
- Alteration in mental state at time of accident
- Focal neurologic deficits, which may or may not be transient

For TBI to be classed as mild the following criteria must be met:

- The LOC must be approximately 30 minutes or less
- The GCS at presentation must be 14–15
- There must be no abnormalities on computed tomography (CT) scan
- The period of post-traumatic amnesia (PTA) must not be longer than 24 hours
- The length of hospital stay must be < 48 hours
- There must be no operable intracranial lesion

Pathophysiology

The pathophysiology of mTBI is complex. Mild traumatic brain injury is caused by acceleration and/or deceleration of the brain inside the skull, which can be linear, rotational or a combination of the two. The energy transfer to the brain is sufficient to distort and strain axons causing depolarization, impaired neurotransmission, loss of transmembrane ionic balance and calcium influx into cells. Cerebral blood flow may also be transiently reduced. The immediate effect is a brief period of altered consciousness and sometimes (rarely) seizures. Once ionic balance and neurotransmission are restored, normal consciousness returns, but this is often followed by a long phase of altered brain metabolism, mitochondrial impairment and neuroinflammation. Impaired brain metabolism may persist for days, weeks or even months, and neuroinflammation can be detected for years after mTBI. The significance of these persistent abnormalities is unclear but the brain may remain particularly vulnerable to further insults during the recovery phase, for example to a second concussion in contact sports.

Clinical features

mTBI presents with a wide variety of cognitive, physical, emotive and behavioural symptoms (postconcussional symptoms) including:

- Fatigue

- Headaches/migraines
- Vertigo
- Impaired coordination/balance
- Visual disturbances
- Impaired attention, concentration and memory
- Sleep disturbances
- Irritability and behavioural changes
- Anxiety
- Low mood
- Failure to cope
- Slow thinking processes

Loss of sense of smell and seizures may also, rarely, complicate mTBI.

Investigations

Initial assessment and resuscitation follows conventional <C>ABCDE principles. CT scanning of the head is the gold standard for acute phase TBI investigation. The NICE guidelines for CT head scanning are as follows:

An immediate CT should be performed if:
- The GCS is <13 (any point)
- The GCS is 13 or 14 within 2 hours of injury
- There is a suspected skull fracture (depressed, compound, skull-base)
- There is focal neurological deficit
- There are post-traumatic seizures
- There has been >1 episode vomiting in adult (>2 in child)
- There is a dangerous mechanism of injury (e.g. ejection or a pedestrian versus vehicle RTC)

A CT within 8 hours is indicated if:
- There is retrograde amnesia of >30 minutes before event
- If there is amnesia or LOC after event with the presence of high-risk criteria
  - Age >65 years
  - Alcohol use
  - Coagulopathy

Some centres pursue a policy of immediate scanning in the elderly on warfarin. To be considered minor, the CT scan must be normal. Additional vascular imaging (CT-angiography) may be indicated in selected situations (e.g. suspicion of carotid injury following skull-base fracture). There is no role for emergency MRI in the acute-phase of TBI of any severity. Advanced MRI investigations (MR spectroscopy, functional MRI and diffusion tensor imaging) can detect abnormalities after mTBI, but these are not in routine clinical use.

Treatment

No specific pharmacological treatment is currently available for mTBI. Individual symptoms are treated in a targeted fashion (e.g. headaches, vertigo, depression or anxiety). Neuropsychological assessment is recommended for patients with persistent neurocognitive symptoms.

Educational support has been shown to be beneficial, for example using consultation with a head injury expert to monitor recovery, managing expectations and addressing issues around returning to work or education. The mainstay of the management of mTBI is physical and cognitive rest until symptoms subside. Return to play requires particular attention in contact sports in view of the heightened vulnerability of the brain after injury, which varies between individuals. Most sporting bodies such as the Rugby Football Union have official codes covering return to play which are clear, strict and enforceable. Complete symptomatic recovery is required before return to contact sports, with children and adolescents requiring longer periods of rest than adults.

Complications

Sequelae following TBI include:
- mTBI slightly increases the risk of epilepsy in the first few years after injury but after 5 years the risk is the same as the general population
- Cognitive impairment (memory loss, concentration and attention deficits, slow processing speed)
- Vertigo
- Chronic headache or migraines
- Mental health problems (depression, anxiety, substance abuse)
- Loss of sense of smell and impaired taste

Further reading

Ellenbogen R, Abdulrauf S, Sekhar L. Principles of Neurological Surgery, 3rd edn. Elsevier: Saunders, 2013:325–347.

Samandouras G. The Neurosurgeon's Handbook. Oxford: Oxford University Press, 2010:208–216.

Valadka A, Andrews B. Neurotrauma: Evidence-Based Answers to Common Questions. Thieme: New York, 2004.

Related topics of interest

- <C>ABCDE resuscitation (p. 63)
- Imaging in trauma – CT (p. 135)
- Moderate-to-severe brain injury (p. 191)

Moderate-to-severe brain injury

Key points

- Mortality from severe traumatic brain injury (TBI) has steadily decreased over the past few decades but whether this equates with improved quality of life for survivors is debateable
- The brain trauma foundation (BTF) provides evidence-based guidance and recommendations for the management of severe TBI
- Achieving good outcomes following severe TBI is a truly multidisciplinary process requiring input from neurosurgeons, trauma teams, intensive care physicians and, following the acute phase of injury, rehabilitation physicians and psychologists

Epidemiology

Moderate-to-severe TBI is classified according to the presenting Glasgow Coma Scale (GCS) score (9–13 and 3–8, respectively). Intracranial haemorrhages complicate 25–45% of severe TBI cases and 3–12% of moderate TBI cases.

Trauma Audit and Research Network (TARN) data has demonstrated that the general mortality following TBI and the mortality of severe TBI were significantly increased in patients treated in non-neurosurgical compared to specialist neurosurgical centres (61% vs 34% and 34% vs 26%, respectively). NICE guidelines recommend that patients with isolated severe TBI should ideally be transferred to and managed at a specialist neurosurgical unit regardless of the need for neurosurgical intervention.

Pathophysiology
Primary brain injury

Primary brain injury is injury sustained by the brain immediately at the time of impact. Extra-axial primary brain injuries include:

- Extradural haemorrhage: It occurs between the skull vault and dura, classically due to a ruptured middle meningeal artery (rarely due to venous sinus rupture) following skull fracture
- Acute subdural haemorrhage: It occurs between the brain pial surface and the dura due to rupture of bridging veins traversing from the cortical surface to the dural sinuses, or rupture/laceration of cortical vessels or pia. Subdural haematoma usually indicates major intracranial trauma or high-velocity impact
- Chronic subdural haemorrhage: It follows rupture of bridging veins in patients with atrophic brains (e.g. the elderly, those with high levels of alcohol use or patients with coagulopathy). The subdural bleeding presents in delayed fashion due to pre-existing cortical atrophy allowing degradation of acute blood into chronic blood
- Traumatic subarachnoid haemorrhage: Trauma is the commonest cause of subarachnoid haemorrhage

Intra-axial primary brain injuries include:

- Contusions: Small discrete areas of ruptured parenchymal vessels surrounded by oedematous necrotic brain
- Intracerebral haemorrhage: Larger contusions (> 2 cm) containing more blood
- Diffuse axonal injury: In these patients, severe acceleration–deceleration or rotational forces result in shearing injury to neurons and axons. Radiologically, the stereotypical appearance is petechial haemorrhages in typical locations (corpus callosum, basal ganglia, thalamus, white matter tracts, grey–white matter junction and brainstem)

Secondary brain injury

Secondary brain injury is pathological insult suffered by the brain immediately following primary injury and evolves over days. It occurs either adjacent to the injury site or away from it (or both). The pathological process involves a combination of cerebral vascular dysfunction with ischaemia (impaired autoregulation, cerebral blood flow (CBF) and cerebral oxygenation), cerebral oedema and oxygen free-radical mediated neurotoxicity and neuronal destruction.

Risk factors worsening secondary brain injury include:

- Increased intracranial pressure (ICP)
- Hypotension (a single episode at any stage of patient's care can double mortality)
- Hypoxia
- Hypercarbia
- Hyperthermia/pyrexia
- Seizures
- Infection (systemic, intracranial)
- Hydrocephalus
- Metabolic dysfunction (e.g. electrolytes and glucose)

ICP is the pressure within the fixed volume of the cranial vault derived from four components: (mainly) intracranial volume (ICV) [$ICV_{total} = V_{brain}(85\%) + V_{CSF}(10\%) + V_{blood}(5\%) + V_{additional\,mass}(0\%)$], brain compliance/elastance and gravitational vector relative to craniospinal axis. $V_{additional\,mass}$ is nonexistent contributing 0% in the normal physiological state. It represents additional volume in a pathological state (e.g. haemorrhage or oedema following TBI or a tumour). Compliance is the change in volume per unit pressure. Elastance is the reciprocal of compliance (or the change in pressure per unit volume). Cerebral perfusion pressure (CPP) is the pressure gradient maintaining brain perfusion and CBF. CPP = Mean Arterial Pressure (MAP) – ICP. In normal physiology, cerebral autoregulation describes mechanisms that maintain a constant CBF (750 mL/min) over a wide range of CPPs (50 – 150 mmHg).

The Monroe-Kellie doctrine states that the skull has a fixed volume with brain, cerebrospinal fluid (CSF), blood and additional mass each contributing to total intracranial volume (and thus ICP). An increase in one component must be offset by a decrease in other components to prevent an increase in ICP.

Compensatory mechanisms accommodate pathological increases in volume from additional masses and prevent ICP elevation.

CSF is the most amenable to manipulation with efflux into dural sinuses or lumbar subarachnoid cisterns. Venous blood follows with efflux into systemic veins.

Initially, there is high compliance and low elastance as additional volumes are accommodated with little change in ICP. Compensatory mechanisms are, however, limited and beyond a critical threshold when they are saturated, ICP begins to rise exponentially with additional volume as brain compliance decreases and elastance increases.

The brain is the least amenable to manipulation and when compensatory measures are saturated, the exponential rise in ICP leads to two deleterious effects: impaired CPP (decoupling of flow-metabolism as flow is insufficient to meet metabolic demand, precipitating ischaemia, infarction and cytotoxic oedema; a vicious circle ensues with further rise in ICP) and brain shift and herniation (transtentorial/uncal, tonsillar). This can lead to catastrophic neurological injury and eventually death.

Management in the acute phase of TBI aims to limit neurological dysfunction from secondary brain injury via optimisation of CPP, to normalise ICP and other physiological parameters and to achieve as much neurological recovery as possible.

Clinical features

The symptoms and signs of TBI depend on the initial severity and injury morphology, the neurological structures compromised and pre-existing neurological function. Patients require careful observation and assessment for their baseline neurological dysfunction and for any deterioration or improvement. Monitoring should not only evaluate conscious level and baseline neurological examination (cranial and peripheral nerves) but also seek the stereotypical signs or symptoms suggestive of cerebral herniation.

Uncal herniation

The uncus of the medial temporal lobe passes through the tentorial incisure compressing the ipsilateral rostral midbrain structures and resulting in ipsilateral oculomotor (CN 3) nerve palsy and impaired parasympathetic innervation to the pupil (leading to an ipsilateral fixed, dilated pupil unresponsive to light). Compression of the ipsilateral cerebral peduncle may also occur, leading to contralateral hemiparesis. Involvement of periaqueductal grey matter may lead to confusion of the ascending reticular activating formation to drowsiness and of the posterior cerebral artery to unilateral or bilateral occipital lobe infarction with blindness.

Tonsillar herniation

The cerebellar tonsils pass through the foramen magnum with compression of the cardiorespiratory centre in the medulla resulting in Cushing's reflex (the triad of hypertension, bradycardia and altered respiration) and ultimately cardiorespiratory arrest.

Investigations

CT head scan is the gold standard in acute TBI. CT reliably demonstrates haemorrhages and fractures and allows assessment of ICP within the cranial cavity. Features of raised ICP on CT-head include:

- Ventricular collapse and effacement
- Midline shift (MLS)
- Effacement or loss of cortical sulcal CSF spaces
- Collapse of basal cisterns
- Loss of grey–white differentiation

Assessment follows <C>ABCDE protocols. There should be a low threshold for repeating a CT-head scan if there is any deterioration in neurological function or conscious level.

Diagnosis

Moderate-to-severe TBIs are classified based on presenting GCS scores of 9–13 and 3–8, respectively).

Treatment

Initial resuscitation and stabilisation are as per <C>ABCDE protocols. Treatment protocols, guidance and care recommendations formulated from best available evidence for TBI management were initially published in 1995 by the BTF. These were updated in 2007.

Decision-making for surgical evacuation of intracranial haemorrhage takes into consideration the severity of injury, the degree of neurological compromise, the patient's conscious level and the probability of achieving a satisfactory neurological outcome. BTF guidelines should be used for guidance. For example, with acute extradural haematoma (AEDH), recommendations for craniotomy and evacuation include:

- Volume > 30 cm³ regardless of GCS
- MLS > 5 mm
- Clot thickness > 15 mm
- GCS < 9 with pupillary changes
- Low temporal AEDH
- Deteriorating clinical examination

In acute subdural haematoma, recommendations for craniotomy and evacuation include:

- Clot thickness >10 mm (regardless of GCS)
- MLS > 5 mm (regardless of GCS)
- GCS < 9 and either ICP > 20 mmHg or fixed dilated pupil

Society of British Neurological Surgeons (SBNS) guidelines recommend that craniotomy for acute subdural haematoma should be performed within 4 hours of injury and for AEDH within 2 hours of deterioration.

The Medical Research Council Study 'Corticosteroid randomisation after significant head injury' trial demonstrated that corticosteroid use provided no benefit in terms of death and disability following TBI and that outcomes at 6 months were worse with steroid use. Prophylactic antiepileptic drugs have an impact on the incidence of early post-traumatic seizures (< 7 days) but do not affect the incidence of late post-traumatic seizures (> 7 days).

There is evidence that ICP and CPP serve as outcome predictors. Higher mean ICPs are associated with a higher mean mortality. Very high CPPs are associated with less favourable outcomes. Most goal-directed therapeutic protocols are based on both ICP (< 20 mmHg) and CPP control (≥ 65 mmHg). The indications for ICP monitoring include:

- GCS < 9 with ANY abnormality on scan
- GCS < 9 with NORMAL scan and two risk factors (Age > 40 years, systolic BP < 90 mmHg, decorticate/decerebrate posturing)

- Patients with altered conscious level where neurological examination to evaluate for deterioration is not reliable or possible, e.g. those under sedation required for multiple injuries

An example of a modern goal-directed approach for intensive care management of moderate-to-severe TBI is given in **Table 25**.

Complications

Uncontrolled intracranial following TBI precipitates a vicious circle of impairment of CPP, decoupling of flow-metabolism, ischaemia, infarction with brain shift, herniation, catastrophic neurological injury and eventually death.

Table 25 A goal directed approach to head injury

Maintenance of systemic parameters	
Airway + breathing	$Pao_2 > 11$ kPa, $Sao_2 > 97\%$, $PaCo_2$ 4.5–5.3 kPa
Circulation	Central venous pressure 6–10 cmH$_2$O, normotension and normovolaemia
Disability + exposure	Normal temperature and glucose < 7 mmol/L
Maintenance of brain parameters	
Target pressure	ICP < 20 mmHg, CPP > 65 mmHg
Specific measures for ICP control (first stage - early)	
Conservative	Head up, loosen or remove cervical collars (to allow drainage via jugular veins), control sepsis, control seizures
Medical	Sedation and paralysis (decreased cerebral metabolic and neuronal activity with decreased metabolic demand). Burst hyperventilation for hypocarbia (vasoconstriction with decreased cerebral blood volume and ICP, short lasting only). Osmotic diuresis (mannitol, hypertonic saline)
Surgical	Craniotomy and evacuation of surgical target (e.g. haemorrhage) CSF diversion (e.g. external ventricular drain)
Specific measures for ICP control (second stage - late)	
Medical	osmotic diuresis (hypertonic saline), hypothermia (decreases cerebral metabolic activity), barbiturate coma (thiopentone) (aim to achieve burst suppression on electroencephalography for decreasing metabolic activity)
Surgical	Decompressive craniectomy

CPP, cerebral perfusion pressure; CSF, cerebrospinal fluid; ICP, increased intracranial pressure.

Further reading

Bullock MR, Povlishock JT (for Brain Trauma Foundation). Guidelines for the management of severe traumatic brain injury. J Neurotrauma 2007; 24:S1–106.

Edwards P, Arango M, Balica L, et al. Final results of MRC CRASH, a randomised placebo-controlled trial of intravenous corticosteroid in adults with head injury: outcomes at 6 months. Lancet 2005; 365:1957–1959.

Patel HC, Bouamra O, Woodford M, et al. Trends in head injury outcome from 1989 to 2003 and the effect of neurosurgical care: an observational study. Lancet 2005; 366:1538–1544.

Related topics of interest

- Brain stem death and organ donation (p. 53)
- Cervical spine injuries (p. 66)
- Mild traumatic brain injury (p. 188)

Mortality patterns

Key points

- Globally, 5.8 million people of all ages and economic groups die from trauma each year
- Of these 5.8 million deaths, the top three leading causes are road traffic collisions (1.3 million per year), suicides (844,000 per year) and homicide (600,000 per year)
- Current consensus suggests that the trimodal distribution model is flawed

Introduction

Mortality and morbidity due to trauma are worldwide problems, with varying consequences for individuals, healthcare systems and society as a whole. According to the latest figures published by the World Health Organisation, injuries account for 10% of all deaths worldwide. Globally, 5.8 million people of all ages and economic groups die from trauma each year, this equates to approximately 662 deaths per hour or 11 deaths per minute worldwide. Of these 5.8 million deaths, the top three leading causes are road traffic collisions (1.3 million per year), suicides (844,000 per year) and homicide (600,000 per year). In addition to this, many millions seek medical treatment as a result of trauma and a proportion of these people are left with life changing or life limiting injuries.

In the western world, death secondary to trauma is the leading cause of death in the first four decades of life. In England and Wales, 10,000 people a year die as a result of trauma. In addition to this, many thousands are left disabled, leading to increased healthcare costs and loss of contributions to the nation's economy.

In the United Kingdom, 98% of trauma is caused by blunt forces. The vast majority of these cases are individuals involved in road traffic collisions and falls. Assaults, deliberate self-harm, explosions, crushing injuries and burns are amongst the other common causes. The proportion of trauma resulting from gunshot and knife wounds is 2% in the United Kingdom, the majority of this 2% being injuries sustained from a sharp object rather than gunshot wounds. The proportions of penetrating to blunt trauma cases differ according to the country being studied. As a comparison, in the United States, penetrating trauma accounts for 20% of trauma cases, with the majority of these cases being due to gunshot wounds. The most common preventable cause of death in all trauma cases is uncontrolled haemorrhage.

The trimodal distribution of deaths

There have been many attempts to identify the mortality patterns in trauma. One of the first people to describe a trend was R. Adams Cowley in the 1950s. From his personal observations in Baltimore USA and his study of deaths in the US Army during World War II, he concluded that the vast majority of deaths occurred in the first 60 minutes after injury. He identified the top cause of death in this initial period as exsanguination, mainly from chest, abdominal, pelvic or vascular limb injuries. From this, he concluded that early intervention in this initial phase postinjury would provide the patient with the best outcome. He termed this period 'The Golden Hour.'

> "There is a golden hour between life and death. If you are critically injured you have less than 60 minutes to survive. You might not die right then, it may be three days or two weeks later – but something has happened in your body that is irreparable."

Soon after this, with a grant from the US Army, Cowley started the first clinical shock trauma unit in the United States in Baltimore. In the late 1960s, he pioneered the first trauma helicopter service in a further attempt to decrease the time from trauma to specialised treatment, rather than waiting for the patient to arrive at the trauma centre.

In 1983, Donald Trunkey further added to our understanding of mortality trends in trauma. He studied trauma deaths in San Francisco over a 2-year period and noted a particular distribution that he described as the trimodal distribution of trauma deaths (**Figure 60**). This model describes three main peaks of deaths after trauma; immediate, early and late. The following diagram summarises the mortality trends in the trimodal distribution.

Immediate deaths occurred within the first hour, accounted for 45% of deaths and were because of nonsurvivable central nervous system injuries or exsanguination. These patients usually died on scene or soon after arriving at the receiving hospital. Early deaths occurred 1–4 hours after injury, accounted for 34% of deaths and were again largely because of exsanguination or brain injury. The last peak was the late deaths, accounting for 20% of deaths and occurring within a few weeks after injury. The causes of death in these individuals were predominantly multiorgan failure and sepsis.

Recent developments

After being widely accepted by the medical profession, the trimodal distribution fuelled the development of more efficient, organised prehospital care and the establishment of major trauma centres and networks, first in the United States and then more widely. It has now been over three decades since Trunkey first described this distribution. Recently, there have been many civilian and military population-based studies, which have

attempted to confirm or refute the existence of the trimodal distribution.

The results of these studies have showed great variability in the distribution of deaths. The vast majority of data sets concluded that the trimodal distribution was not valid. Some studies stated that the majority of deaths did occur in the first hour after injury, followed by a rapid decline in mortality rates (unimodal). A larger number of studies showed a bimodal distribution of death, with fewer late deaths than expected according to the trimodal distribution. A very small number of studies concluded that the trauma deaths in their population actually followed a tetramodal distribution; they termed this: death at 2 minutes, 2 hours, 2 days and 2 weeks.

A logical and commonly accepted explanation in the skew of deaths towards the first 4 hours after injury and the general decrease in the mortality rate due to preventable causes is the maturation of trauma systems in developed countries. The development of such systems has led to the establishment of systems offering rapid access to pre-hospital care interventions and to the continuing improvement of these systems in the light of clinical advances. Examples of significant improvements include the use of tranexamic acid, rapid diagnosis due to technological advancements, resuscitation with blood components and advanced surgical intervention in haemorrhaging patients. A number of these changes have been introduced and validated on the battlefield and transferred to civilian

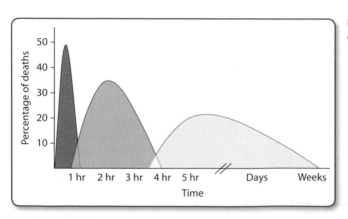

Figure 60 The trimodal distribution of death in trauma.

use. One of the explanations for the demise of the late peak in the trimodal distribution is the improvement and advancement in critical care medicine that we have seen in the last three decades.

Conclusion

Although we have come a very long way in our management of trauma cases since the latter half of the last century, many millions of people still die due to preventable causes. We are therefore in need of further research to broaden our understanding of how major trauma might be prevented and of the treatment of patients who have been its victim. There is evidence to suggest that the trimodal distribution of death is now evolving into a bimodal distribution of death due to improved survival in the early in-hospital death.

Further reading

Baker CC, Oppenheimer L, Stephens B, et al. Epidemiology of trauma deaths. Am J Surg 1980; 140:144–150.

Lansink KWW, Gunning AC, Leenen LPH. Cause of death and time of death distribution of trauma patients in a level I trauma centre in the Netherlands. Eur J Trauma Emerg Surg 2013; 39:375-83.

Trunkey DD. Trauma. Accidental and intentional injuries account for more years of life lost in the U.S. than cancer and heart disease. Among the prescribed remedies are improved preventive efforts, speedier surgery and further research. Sci Am 1983; 249:28–35.

Related topics of interest

Near infrared spectroscopy

Key points

- Near infrared spectroscopy (NIRS) provides a noninvasive, real-time, continuous measure of local tissue oxygenation (Sto_2)
- Sto_2 values correlate well with compartment pressures in patients with compartment syndrome and muscle injury is associated with an increase in Sto_2 values, presumed to be due to hyperaemia
- NIRS can be used to accurately monitor the response to initial resuscitation in trauma subjects, and has significant advantages over conventional assessments of physiology in the clinical environment

Introduction

Spectroscopy is a method for assessing the absorption or emission of light (or other radiation) by matter. The technique is most commonly used to identify unknown compounds or measure the concentration of known compounds in solution based upon their absorption spectra. In clinical medicine, NIRS uses infrared light to determine the relative concentrations of oxygenated and deoxygenated haemoglobin in tissues to provide a measure of local tissue oxygenation (Sto_2 – expressed as a percentage).

In clinical practice, NIRS is almost exclusively used with a reflectance technique, so that the light source and receptor lie in the same plane, and the light follows a parabolic, or banana-shaped, course through the tissues (see **Figure 61a**). Infrared light is able to penetrate tissue to a depth of several centimetres and can therefore obtain readings from deep muscle. It can also penetrate bone to provide measurements of cerebral oxygenation. One of the problems with the technique is that the overall NIRS signal is an amalgamation of the tissues traversed by the light, meaning the Sto_2 measurements from a deeply placed muscle may be attenuated by the signal from overlying skin or fat. To overcome this problem, some systems use a dual-beam technique, shining two beams of light through the tissue: one deep and one superficial. The signal from the superficial beam is then subtracted from that of the deep one that theoretically provides an isolated Sto_2 reading from the deep tissue of interest (see **Figure 61b**).

NIRS has similarities to pulse oximetry (used to measure arterial oxygen saturation – Spo_2), although it should be appreciated that Spo_2 and Sto_2 are fundamentally different measurements. Spo_2 is a systemic measurement and a reflection of global oxygen delivery – it should be the same regardless of monitoring site. Sto_2 is a local measure of tissue oxygenation and is influenced by the global haemodynamic state and local tissue conditions.

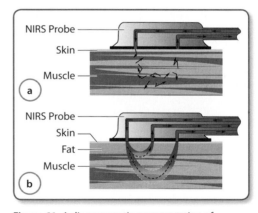

Figure 61 A diagrammatic representation of reflectance spectroscopy. The near infrared spectroscopy (NIRS) probe is attached to the skin overlying a section of muscle, and light traverses the tissues in a parabolic course. (a) A single beam NIRS device – the resulting Sto_2 is amalgamation of all tissues in the optical path (e.g. skin, fat and muscle). (b) A dual beam NIRS device – two beams of light are shone through the tissue and superficial signal subtracted from the deep one to isolate the Sto_2 measurement from the deep tissue.

General considerations in applying near infrared spectroscopy to trauma monitoring

Sto_2 measurements can be used to assess the trauma patient in two conceptually different ways:

- To assess local tissue ischaemia, for example in compartment syndrome or arterial thrombosis
- To reflect the state of global oxygen delivery in cases where local vascular supply is not impaired

The range of normal Sto_2 values is wide and varies significantly between monitoring sites and NIRS devices. While Sto_2 values below the normal range indicate impaired systemic or local oxygen delivery, the upper range of values is often limited by the NIRS machine, although there is no practical clinical significance to 'high' Sto_2 values.

Infrared light is absorbed or scattered by a variety of compounds found in human tissues and both melanin (in dark-skinned individuals) and dark tattoos have been reported to interfere with Sto_2 measurements. Methylene blue is known to absorb infrared light and may theoretically affect Sto_2 values in patients to whom this is administered, although this is unlikely to be a common problem and there are no case reports. Soft tissue injury has been shown to cause an increase in Sto_2, presumably as a result of the hyperaemic response to injury.

Near infrared spectroscopy in trauma resuscitation

In the hypovolaemic patient skeletal muscle Sto_2 falls as a result of inadequate tissue perfusion and sympathetically mediated vasoconstriction. As the patient is resuscitated, tissue perfusion is restored and Sto_2 rises. NIRS has been shown to detect reductions in blood volume as small as 470 mL in subjects donating blood; however, this depends upon a knowledge of the subject's baseline Sto_2, a luxury that is rarely available in the trauma patient.

In human and animal trauma studies skeletal muscle Sto_2 has been shown to accurately track the response to haemorrhage and resuscitation (see **Figure 62**) and correlate with conventional measures of haemodynamic status and systemic oxygen delivery. Sto_2 measurements have been shown to correlate well with base excess and lactate with Sto_2 typically phase leading the

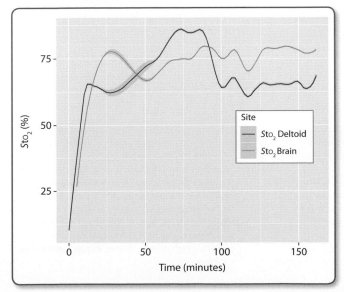

Figure 62 Sto_2 recording from the deltoid and frontal lobe of the brain from a patient experiencing extensive lower limb and chest injuries. Note the initially low Sto_2 in both the deltoid and brain that respond rapidly over initial resuscitation in the first 20 minutes. Once the patient has been resuscitated to normal Sto_2 value absolute Sto_2 values are less useful in guiding resuscitation although changes in Sto_2, such as the drop in the deltoid at approximately 90 minutes, may indicate deteriorations in physiology.

changes in arterial blood gas parameters by 30–35 minutes. StO_2 recorded from injured peripheral muscle sites performs similarly to uninjured muscle in tracking the patient's volaemic state, although there might be differences in the absolute StO_2 values.

Most human trauma studies have recorded StO_2 from the thenar eminence. This site has been used largely for reasons of practicality – the thenar eminence is easily accessible, has little overlying fat, and low levels of pigmentation – rather than any inherent technical superiority of this site. Animal studies have demonstrated that StO_2 recorded from visceral organs (e.g. the liver or stomach) is a poor indicator of haemorrhage, presumably due to preservation of central organ blood flow in the face of hypovolaemia. Current evidence suggests that of the potential monitoring sites in the upper limb, the forearm (over flexor digitorum profundus) is the most sensitive to changes in volume status.

Experience of using NIRS in trauma suggests that it provides a useful tool for the initial triage or assessment of patients and for monitoring their response to resuscitation. Once patients have been resuscitated to within normal StO_2 values, NIRS is less useful in guiding further therapy, and changes in StO_2 measures are generally more useful than absolute values. Although NIRS is not demonstrably better than a combination of heart rate and blood pressure in assessing trauma patients, it has several practical advantages; principally that is it quick and easy to use, noninvasive and provides a continuous real-time assessment of patient physiology.

Near infrared spectroscopy in acute compartment syndrome

In animal and human models of compartment syndrome, StO_2 has been shown to correlate well with lower limb compartment and perfusion pressures and may potentially outperform them in the detection of compartment syndrome. In patients with established compartment syndrome, StO_2 values in affected limbs are significantly lower than those of control limbs, but rise rapidly to near normal values following fasciotomy.

Both compartment pressures and StO_2 rise with soft tissue injury. However, it seems likely that the simple linear relationship between compartment pressures and StO_2 described in experimental studies does not exist. Rather both compartment pressures and StO_2 are increased soon after injury, but as compartment syndrome develops, the relationship is reversed and StO_2 falls while compartment pressures continue to rise. If this is true then NIRS should provide an easy way to distinguish between the hyperaemia associated with an injured limb and the ischaemia of compartment syndrome. Unfortunately, there are no reports of StO_2 monitoring of a compartment syndrome in evolution, and the true nature of StO_2 changes in this condition have yet to be established.

Further reading

Barker T, Midwinter M, Porter K. The diagnosis of acute lower limb compartment syndrome: applications of near infrared spectroscopy. Trauma 2011; 13:125–136.

Barker T, Spencer P, Kirkman E, Lambert A, Midwinter M. An evaluation of the normal range of StO_2 measurements at rest and following a mixed exercise protocol. J R Army Med Corps 2015; 161:327–331.

Cohn SM, Nathens AB, Moore FA, et al. StO_2 in Trauma Patients Trial Investigators. Tissue oxygen saturation predicts the development of organ dysfunction during traumatic shock resuscitation. J Trauma 2007; 62:44–54.

Crookes BA, Cohn SM, Bloch S, et al. Can near-infrared spectroscopy identify the severity of shock in trauma patients? J Trauma 2005; 58:806–813 (discussion pp 813–816).

Ward KR, Ivatury RR, Barbee RW, et al. Near infrared spectroscopy for evaluation of the trauma patient: a technology review. Resuscitation 2006; 68:27–44.

Related topics of interest

- Damage control resuscitation and surgery (p. 83)
- Metabolic responses to trauma (p. 182)
- Viscoelastic assessment of coagulation in trauma (p. 318)

Neonatal trauma

Key points

- A detailed birth history is mandatory in all injured or potentially injured neonates, including their vitamin K status and whether there was an instrument-assisted delivery
- Neonatal injuries presenting to the emergency department should raise the possibility of nonaccidental injury (NAI)
- Neonatal abusive head trauma may present with a variety of symptoms making diagnosis difficult

Birth trauma

Birth trauma is relatively uncommon, complicating <1% of all live births. However, it is an important diagnosis to consider in any neonate presenting to the emergency department with an injury. The most common birth-related bony injuries are fractures of the clavicle, humerus and femur. Clavicular fractures are the most common, with an incidence of 2–3 per 1000 live births. Another common group of injuries involves the brachial plexus, affecting 0.4–4 infants per 1000 live births. Factors associated with birth trauma include a birth weight >4000 g, breech presentation, shoulder dystocia and a prolonged or difficult labour or delivery.

Brachial plexus injuries

The brachial plexus provides the nerve supply to the upper limb from roots C5 to T1. It is injured during birth when the neck–shoulder angle is increased, as occurs with shoulder dystocia. Brachial plexus injury can be associated with both clavicular and humeral fractures.

Erb's palsy (affecting C5–6 and occasionally C7) characteristically presents with the neonate holding the affected arm in an adducted position with an internally rotated shoulder, extended elbow, pronated forearm and flexed wrist and fingers (the waiter's tip position). The bicep's reflex is absent and the Moro reflex is asymmetrical. The mainstay of treatment is physiotherapy

and the prognosis is good, with isolated injuries having a reported 94% rate of spontaneous resolution, 98% when they occur in conjunction with a clavicle fracture.

Injury to the lower plexus (C8–T1) causes Klumpke's paralysis, affecting the intrinsic muscles of the hand and resulting in flaccid paralysis and localised wrist drop. Damage to the T1 nerve root before it separates into sympathetic and motor fibres causes a Horner's syndrome (ptosis, meiosis and anhydrosis). The grasp reflex will be absent. Klumpke's paralysis is also treated with physiotherapy. Spontaneous recovery takes longer than with Erb's palsy (usually 6–18 months), and although functional outcome is good, full neurological recovery is infrequent. Isolated injury to C7 root can cause the elbow to be held in a flexed position. A pan-brachial plexus injury causes a flail limb with no motor function.

Fractures

Fractures commonly present as an infant not moving the affected limb, often without a history of witnessed trauma. Parents often notice discomfort when changing clothes (or nappies in the case of femoral fractures). Babies may also have an evident bony deformity or swelling.

Clavicular fractures usually affect the middle third of the clavicle. Clinical features include swelling and tenderness over the clavicular line, pain with movement and an inability to abduct the arm. Management is conservative with immobilisation of the arm under baby clothes for 2–3 weeks to restrict movement and limit pain. The commonest complication is malunion of the fracture, causing a palpable or visible protuberance, which reduces over time due to remodelling. Neurovascular complications and nonunion are both rare.

Humeral diaphyseal (shaft) fractures are the second most common bony birth injury, occurring as a consequence of either a rotational force (as seen in spiral fractures), or levering force (oblique fractures) (**Figure 63**). The arm will be swollen and tender. Management of these fractures is

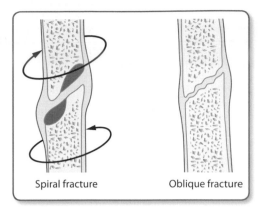

Spiral fracture   Oblique fracture

Figure 63 Spinal and oblique fractures.

also supportive, with arm immobilisation. Associated radial nerve injury is uncommon.

Femoral diaphyseal fractures caused by birth trauma are extremely rare with a reported incidence of 0.13/1000 live births. The association between femoral fractures in premobile infants and abuse is highly significant, and exclusion of NAI in these cases is mandatory. The thigh is usually swollen with bony deformity, and associated pain on movement. Specialist orthopaedic treatment with a hip spica is required with fracture healing usually established by 4 weeks. Complications include malunion and leg length discrepancy – femoral diaphyseal fractures can overgrow up to 2 cm in the subsequent 2 years – or the fracture may heal in a shortened position. Rib fractures at birth are rare and usually associated with large birth weight babies or shoulder dystocia.

Asymptomatic subdural haemorrhage

Subdural haematoma can be caused by birth trauma, especially with vacuum assisted delivery: most resolve by 1 month of age.

NAI in infants

Approximately 1 in 880 babies are seriously physically abused in the first year of life. All neonates presenting to the emergency department with injuries should raise the possibility of NAI. A family history of bleeding

disorders and bone fractures following minimal trauma should be sought, in addition to careful documentation of any history of easy bruising or prolonged bleeding (from the umbilical stump or postneonatal blood spot test). Osteopenia of prematurity (present in most infants born at <32 weeks' gestation), osteogenesis imperfecta, bone dysplasia and rickets should be considered as part of the differential diagnosis.

Fractures

Fractures occur in up to 55% of physically abused children. Rib fractures and classic metaphyseal lesions (CMLs) are highly suggestive of NAI (**Figure 64**). CMLs (also known as bucket handle or corner fractures) are the result of a shearing force, either from the child being lifted by that limb or the limb flailing whilst the torso is shaken. Most heal completely, and growth disruption is rare.

Considerable force is required to break an infant's soft and malleable ribs, usually as a consequence of compressive injury rather than a direct blow. In the absence of a metabolic disorder or major trauma, inflicted injury is the most common cause. These injuries do not occur during cardiopulmonary resuscitation in neonates.

Bruises

Bruises are extremely rare in normal, nonambulant children, occurring in <1% of infants aged <6 months. They are, however,

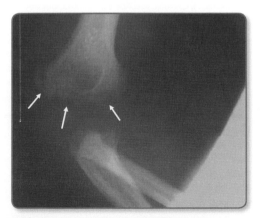

Figure 64 Classic metaphyseal lesion: bucket-handle fracture right distal humerus.

the most frequently found injury in physical child abuse, with the head and soft parts of the body (ear, face, neck, torso, buttocks) being the most commonly affected. Facial bruising has been observed in instrumental-assisted delivery, so a clearly documented birth history is important. Bruises should not be confused with Mongolian blue spots, which are benign, flat, congenital birthmarks most commonly found on the buttocks or lumbosacral area, although they can appear anywhere on the body.

Facial and intraoral trauma

Injuries to the face and mouth have been described in up to 49% of infants who have been physically abused. A torn labial frenulum is the most common abusive intraoral injury, often caused by forcing a teat, pacifier or fingers into the mouth. Any unexplained torn labial frenulum should be fully investigated to exclude the presence of other occult injuries.

Head injuries

Abusive head trauma is defined as inflicted cranial injury, whether shaking or impact or both have been found to be the cause. This has replaced the term shaken baby syndrome that was used to describe the clinical features of subdural haemorrhages and retinal haemorrhages with little or no external evidence of inflicted injury. Abusive head trauma is the commonest cause of death in physical abuse (35/100,000 infants <6 months old, with a mortality of up to 35%). Up to 70% of infant subdural haemorrhages occur as a result of NAI.

Subdural haemorrhages can present in many ways, from mild irritability, poor feeding, vomiting or lethargy, to neurological symptoms such as seizures, or obvious injury. Diagnosis is therefore difficult and a detailed birth history is essential, including neonatal vitamin K administration. Neuroimaging and a formal ophthalmology assessment (for retinal haemorrhages) should be performed in all suspected cases.

Investigations

The diagnosis of suspected fracture is by plain X-ray; both anteroposterior and lateral views should be requested including the joints above and below the suspected fracture site. Preterm babies have a higher incidence of fractures. Absence of callous formation at 11 days or more excludes a birth-related injury. For suspected head injuries, CT head scanning is the imaging of choice, rather than skull X-ray.

Laboratory investigations should be guided by the history and clinical findings, and expert paediatric advice should be sought. Basic tests should include full blood count and coagulation studies, calcium, phosphate, ALP, 25 (OH) vitamin D, parathyroid hormone, copper and ceruloplasmin. Urine organic acids should be assayed to exclude Glutaric Acidaemia Type I.

Further reading

Wall L, Mills JK, Leveno K, et al. Incidence and prognosis of neonatal brachial plexus palsy with and without clavicle fractures. Obst Gynaecol 2014; 123:1288–1293.

Rosenberg D, Mok J, Meadow R. ABC of child protection, 4th edn. London: BMJ Books, 2007.

Related topics of interest

Nonaccidental injury

Key points

- Nonaccidental injury (NAI) is not common but is likely underdiagnosed
- The mortality rate of children sustaining NAI is significantly higher than in children who sustain accidental injuries
- The history is more often than not the most important factor in raising the suspicion of NAI

Introduction

In 2012–2013 there were 69 child homicides, 44 further deaths where intent was not clear, 23,663 sexual offences against children and 7964 cruelty and neglect offences recorded in the United Kingdom. A number of serious case reviews and Lord Laming's two reports outline requirements and suggested improvements across all organisations involved in child protection, following several high-profile child deaths from NAI.

The mortality of children sustaining NAI is significantly higher than of those with the same burden of injury sustained accidentally. The sequelae of NAI are more than the acute injuries noted on presentation – developmental delay, psychological difficulties and lifelong social problems can result from childhood abuse. Certain patterns of injury suggest NAI and clinicians need to remain alert both to these patterns of injury and to inconsistent explanations for them. Beliefs or practices from different cultures, such as rituals of witchcraft or female genital mutilation should be understood in the context of UK law and child protection practice, and although the context may be important, may still present risks to children.

While it is not the clinician's role to undertake legal investigation, there must be a consistent approach to evaluating paediatric injury in order to minimise undetected NAI and neglect. Effective management of NAI involves a multidisciplinary team including the surgical and medical specialties, paediatrics, social services and sometimes the police, mental health teams, substance abuse teams and charities. While the underpinning principles are the same, there exists different legislation within the various constituent countries of the United Kingdom and clinicians should be familiar with that covering their region.

Whilst neglect or poor parenting are semantically different to NAI, they should be dealt with in the same way to it, as the end result remains avoidable injury or suffering to vulnerable children.

Important features in the history

The history is more often than not the most important factor in raising the suspicion of NAI. Many physical findings on examination become suspicious or concerning because of inconsistencies or details in the history. In particular, it is essential to establish whether the history offered is consistent with the injuries sustained and with the developmental age of the child. Injuries in a nonmobile 5 months old may be perfectly innocent in an adventurous toddler. The history should also establish whether there is an acceptable level of adult supervision or the child is being exposed to unacceptable risk (e.g. playing near an unwatched cooker).

The carer should be expected to be able to give a reproducible and consistent account of events and if the events were unwitnessed because the child was alone, an assessment of the appropriateness of this for the child's age is essential. If the incident was witnessed by two people, the descriptions should be consistent with each other. Care must be taken to decide whether any description of a mechanism of injury correlates to radiographic evidence. A description of axial loading to account for a spiral fracture, for example, should provoke further enquiry. Unfortunately, this decision is not always straightforward.

Features of the past medical history that need to be established include previous attendances at hospital, particularly for injuries, whether the child is up to date with immunisations, height and weight recordings and developmental milestones. It is also essential to establish whether there are any siblings and whether the state or social services are already involved with the child or other members of its family (e.g. is the child a looked after child, or is there a protection plan in place).

Risk factors for NAI

Risk factors for NAI include preterm birth, developmental delay or other disability, having a sibling with existing child protection issues, drug or alcohol misuse in the parents or carers and parents, or carers with mental health problems.

Key physical examination signs

A detailed examination (which must be carefully recorded) is essential. Photographs are very useful in recording transient abnormalities such as bruises. The child's overall physical condition, including their cleanliness and the state of their clothes, and whether they are well nourished should be assessed. A detailed all over assessment for the following should be performed:

- Bruising – Is there any patterning (such as partial hand-prints, regular outlines suggestive of an object)
- External genital trauma, signs of infection or perioral manifestations of sexually transmitted infections
- Characteristic wounds such as those from dipping in hot water or cigarette burns (although these are uncommon)

Patterns of injury

It is important to note that although no pattern of injury is exclusive to NAI and therefore diagnostic of it, some are highly suggestive. By the same token, an injury commonly sustained in children should still prompt queries if other elements of the history or physical examination raise questions. Nonphysiological patterns of stress in bone can indicate pulling, twisting

or application of other unusual forces, such as a spiral fracture in the femur. Some injuries that occur at some of the strongest points of a bone, such as metaphyseal corner fractures, are very unlikely to occur naturally.

Processes for raising concern

Consultants should be involved at an early stage in the management of any concerns identified by junior members of their team. In most cases of concern raised by members of the emergency department staff, the first point of contact is usually with the on call paediatric team. Each trust will also have a named doctor, who will be available on-call and will act as advisor and liaison point in the initial stages of the process. A designated doctor additionally provides strategic advice at board and healthcare organisation level but may not be first on-call for individual advice.

The fact that concerns have been identified should not be hidden from the parents or carers, although the timing of this discussion should be carefully considered. They should have the opportunity to discuss the issues with the senior team and occasionally the information gained may be enough to resolve any concerns. Only if sharing this information with them is considered likely to significantly increase the risk of harm to the child should it be withheld.

Information sharing and confidentiality

Serious case reviews have identified a number of preventable incidents in which failure to appropriately share information was a significant contributing factor, sometimes due to unfounded concerns over data protection. In general, risk to a child will override legal requirements for data confidentiality.

Consent for sharing information should be obtained from the child if they have capacity, or their parents. What information will be shared, and with whom, should be explained clearly and the discussion documented. However, the right to confidentiality is not absolute and if either parent or child refuses consent for sharing, their reasons should be considered in the context of potential risk to the child. If their wishes do not outweigh this, then information should be shared with clear documentation of the rationale. If a clinician or clinical department chooses not to pass on information, they are obliged to set in place a system of regular review of both the situation and this decision. Clearly this creates a single point of failure in protecting the child, and a decision not to share should, for this reason, be unusual.

Further reading

General Medical Council (GMC). Protecting children and young people. London: GMC, 2012.
Jütte S. How safe are our children? London: NSPCC, 2014.

Royal College of Anaesthetists (RCA). Child protection and the anaesthetist. London: RCA, 2014.

Related topics of interest

- Neonatal trauma (p. 202)
- Paediatric trauma (p. 215)
- Pregnancy and trauma (p. 233)

Nutrition in trauma and burns

Key points

- Trauma is associated with catabolism, proteinolysis and insulin resistance. Immune activation followed by the development of systemic inflammatory response syndrome (SIRS) leads to fever, high cardiac output and increased basal metabolic rate
- The provision of early enteral nutrition (EN) in patients with a functioning gut is associated with a significant reduction in infection and mortality
- Careful attention to nutrition is an essential component of trauma and burn care

Introduction

Trauma is associated with significant changes in energy expenditure, catabolism, proteinolysis and insulin resistance. Immune activation followed by the development of the SIRS, leads to fever, high cardiac output and increased basal metabolic rate. This is further supported by the stress hormonal response, with high levels of catecholamines, cortisol and glucagon. The net catabolic state results in the breakdown of muscle to provide energy substrate for the immune system and the healing processes. These catabolic changes may last from days to weeks depending on the type and severity of injury.

The provision of early EN (within 24 hours of admission to critical care) in patients with a functioning gut is associated with a significant reduction in infection and mortality. The provision of sufficient energy substrates and micronutrients is vital to the patient's survival and healing processes. However, it is also clear that overfeeding can be detrimental and result in fatty liver infiltration, hyperglycaemia and infectious complications.

Delivery route

The gastric route is the easiest and quickest route of administration, whether by oral intake in patients who are awake or naso- or orogastric tube in the unconscious. Postpyloric feeding should be considered in patients who have gastroparesis after administration of prokinetic agents such as metoclopramide and erythromycin. Enteral feeding itself promotes gut motility. Gastric residual volumes of >250 mL (assessed by aspiration of the gastric tube every six hours) are traditionally considered to represent intolerance and put the patient at high risk of regurgitation, aspiration and pneumonia. However, recent studies have shown that residual volumes of up to 500 mL could be tolerated and feeding continued.

There is little evidence regarding the appropriate use of prokinetic agents, but a general rule may be to start with metoclopramide and to change to or add erythromycin if there is no observed effect within 48 hours. There is little benefit in prolonged treatment (>5 days) with metoclopramide.

The timing of parenteral nutrition (PN) in cases of gut failure remains controversial. Early administration of PN (initiation time <48 hours compared to after 8 days) is associated with a greater incidence of infectious complications and longer periods of mechanical ventilation and organ support. Furthermore, trophic enteral feeding (<500 kcal/day) was noninferior to normal feeding (20–25 kcal/kg/day) in critically ill patients with severe respiratory failure. Therefore, PN should be considered in patients who do not have intact gastrointestinal tracts or patients with persistent gut failure 3–5 days following start of EN.

Calorie requirements

The European Society of Enteral and Parenteral nutrition (ESPEN) recommend a daily calorie input of between 20 and 25 kcal/kg/day and an aim of achieving the target feed within 72 hours. This can be stepped up to 25–30 kcal/kg/day in the recovery period. However, gastrointestinal intolerance, combined with frequent interruptions to feeding (preparation for surgery and anaesthesia), or lack of access to the gastrointestinal tract can result in significant caloric and protein deficit. Local protocols and policies, such as continued feeding in intubated patients having repeated trips to the operating theatre (if not contraindicated by the surgical procedure), as well as addition of catch-up and supplemental night-time feeding help to avoid problems of underfeeding.

Mathematical formulae used to calculate basal metabolic rate based on age, sex, height and weight such as the Harris-Benedict equation allow more precise calculation of daily calorie requirements. The application of correction factors for degree of injury, systemic disturbance (such as pyrexia), treatments administered (inotropes and renal replacement therapy) can further individualise nutritional support.

Protein and immunonutrients

An individual's protein requirement has been estimated to be 1.2–2 g/kg/day in critically ill patients. This is likely to be higher in polytrauma patients and burns, although there is no evidence for benefit from high protein diets unless the patient is on renal replacement therapy. Higher protein delivery may also be beneficial during the recovery period.

Glutamine is a conditionally essential amino acid following major trauma, burns and critical illness. It is important for immune function, antioxidant defences, mucosal integrity and wound healing. Whilst a recent large trial in ventilated patients with multiorgan failure showed higher mortality in patients supplemented with glutamine, there is evidence to support enteral supplementation with glutamine (0.3–0.5 g/kg/day) in trauma and burns patients who do not have multiorgan failure. Patients on PN and not in multiorgan failure should receive 0.35 g/kg/day of glutamine. Other immunonutrients (e.g. omega-3 fatty acids), antioxidants (selenium) and trace minerals are also recommended in polytrauma and burns patients, although the evidence for these is contentious.

Nutrition in burns

Early establishment of EN in burns (**Table 26**), as for all critically ill patients, is recommended. However, more attention should be paid to fluid administration and glycaemic control, in particular over the first few days. The Parkland Formula is often used to calculate fluid requirements in the first 24 hours.

Burns patients have a sustained significantly higher basal metabolic rate, which is proportional to the burnt body surface area. Calorie input should be adjusted by using indirect calorimetry (if available), or by using predictive equations such as the Toronto or the modified Harris-Benedict equations.

Protein requirements are 1.5–2 g/kg/day and intakes of >2.2 g/kg/day show no further benefit. Glutamine supplementation at 0.3 g/kg/day is also recommended. Micronutrients such as vitamin B1, C, D and E, as well as

Table 26 Summary of nutritional guidelines (based on ASPEN and ESPEN guidelines)	
	Recommendations
Timing	Patients with functioning gut should be enterally fed within 24 hours
How much	Dependent on type/severity of injury and degree of systemic upset and gut tolerance
	In early phase no >20–25 kcal/kg/day
	In the recovery phase can be stepped up to 25–30 kcal/kg/day
	Protein supplementation 1.2–2.0 g/kg
Route	Enteral as much as possible using nasogastric tube
	Parenteral nutrition reserved for when the gut cannot be used or there is continued intolerance
Adjuncts	Intravenous metoclopramide or erythromycin can be administered for gut intolerance (high gastric residual volumes)
	Stress ulcer prophylaxis if not enterally fed and stopped when feed established
	Glycaemic control aim 110–180 g/dL (6–10 mmol/L)
ASPEN, American Society of Parenteral and Enteral Nutrition; ESPEN, European Society of Enteral and Parenteral nutrition.	

copper, zinc and selenium are recommended to augment wound healing. These should be added early.

Early debridement and dressing of wounds, as well as nursing patients at higher than usual ambient temperatures (28–30°C) limit the hypermetabolic and catabolic response in burns. If possible, nonselective b-blockers and anabolic steroids (oxandrolone) should be administered after the first week. There is evidence that oxandrolone reduces mortality and length of stay in severe burns.

Adequate hydration and electrolyte replacement forms another major part of daily nutritional requirement. In major burns and complex polytrauma where there are significant fluid losses, intravenous supplementation and close monitoring of renal function and electrolytes is essential. In particular, hypophosphataemia should be avoided.

Close attention to glycaemic control is crucial for wound healing and avoiding infectious complications. Earlier promising survival and infection data using tight glycaemic control of 80–110 mg/dL (4–6 mmol/L) were challenged by a large multicentre study that showed a potential risk from harm from tight glycaemic control, mainly as a result of hypoglycaemia (NICE-SUGAR 2009). These may be even more pronounced in brain-injured patients. A blood glucose target of 110–180 mg/dL (6–10 mmol/L) represents good glucose control with a lower incidence of hypoglycaemia. This is usually achieved by using an insulin infusion according to a sliding scale whilst patients are fed. A summary of nutritional guidelines is detailed in **Table 59.1**.

Stress ulcer prophylaxis

Whilst proton pump inhibitors and histamine-2 antagonists reduce gastrointestinal bleeding in those who are not enterally fed, no benefit is seen in those who are. As a result, most units stop their administration once full feeding is established as there is an increased incidence of pneumonia and a higher mortality associated within this group.

Monitoring nutrition

Simple methods such as taking the patient's weight on a weekly basis are useful, although they can be difficult to do in ventilated patients and are also affected by fluid retention as a result of the inflammatory process. Serum albumin is also affected by the inflammatory process but may be more useful in the recovery phase. Urinary nitrogen excretion tends to wane as the initial catabolic process resolves and may help with calculating protein requirements.

Further reading

Heyland DK, Dhaliwal R. Role of glutamine in critical illness given the results of the REDOXS study. JPEN Parenter Enteral Nutr 2013; 37:442–443.

Marik PE, Vasu T, Hirani A, et al. Stress ulcer prophylaxis in the new millennium: a systematic review and meta-analysis. Crit Care Med 2010; 38: 2222–2228.

McClave SA, Martindale RG, Vanek VW, et al. Guidelines for the provision and assessment of nutrition support therapy in adult critically ill patients: society of Critical Care Medicine (SCCM) and American Society of Parenteral and Enteral Nutrition (ASPEN). JPEN J Parenter Enteral Nutr 2009; 33: 277–317.

NICE-SUGAR Study Investigators; Finfer S, Chittock DR, et al. Intensive versus conventional glucose control in critically ill patients. NEJM 2009; 360: 1283–1297.

Rousseau AF, Losser MR, Icahi C, et al. ESPEN endorsed recommendations: nutritional therapy in major burns. Clin Nutr 2013; 32: 497–502.

Related topics of interest

Ophthalmic injury

Key points

- The possibility of globe penetration or rupture, which may not be immediately apparent should always be considered
- Significant ocular trauma requires specialist input. Early intervention before such help arrives reduces any further damage and is likely to improve the chance of saving the sight of the affected eye
- Retrobulbar haemorrhage is an acute surgical emergency

History

A detailed and careful history is essential in case of injury to the eye or its surrounding structures. It is important to be particularly vigilant with contact lens wearers.

Background information

The following information must be recorded:
- Time and date of injury and attendance at the casualty centre
- List of injuries to eye, its adnexae and any associated injuries to the rest of the body
- Whether any eye protection or eyewear was in use at the time of injury
- Whether any first-aid treatment was given

A careful past medical history must establish the presence of any pre-existing eye disease; including whether the eye had vision before the injury. Other important details include a general medical and allergy history, the previous use of topical drugs to the eye and the patient's tetanus status.

History of the accident

The mechanism and circumstances of injury must be clearly established including the presence of hammering metal or machine tool use, the involvement of broken glass and any exposure to acid, alkali or detergent chemical agents.

Symptoms

The patient may present with a range of symptoms including loss or blurring of vision, pain, the sensation of a foreign body, photophobia or visual impairment. If the vision is impaired, the degree of impairment must be determined as well as the time after injury to the onset of impairment and whether it is was of immediate onset or is progressive.

Examination

Eye trauma patients are likely to be anxious and should be made as comfortable as possible. The possibility of associated cranial trauma should be confirmed or excluded. Visual assessment is carried out using a Snellen chart with spectacles if the patient wears them, or a pinhole to correct mild refractive error or media opacity. If no letters can be read, the ability to count fingers is recorded as CF, the ability to see hand movements as HM, and the ability to perceive light as PL (perception of light) or NPL (nil perception of light). If the patient is only able to perceive light, the quadrants from which light is perceived should be determined. Eye movements must be tested and double vision recorded.

The eyelids

The eyelids should be examined for swelling, bruising, lacerations or burns and lid contour asymmetry. Any wounds should be assessed for depth or contamination and any tissue loss (corneal exposure) identified and recorded as should involvement of the lacrimal/canalicular apparatus (epiphora) ptosis and subtarsal foreign bodies (which should be identified and removed on lid eversion, unless globe rupture is suspected).

The face

The face must be examined for cheek swelling, flattening or asymmetry from a malar fracture and horizontal and vertical alignment of the pupils/canthi from the bridge of the nose (an increase indicates a midfacial fracture. An inferiorly displaced lateral canthus indicates a zygomatic fracture). Careful palpation of the orbital margins should establish the presence of a 'step' deformity indicating an orbital rim fracture or periorbital crepitus indicating a fracture of ethmoid or maxillary air sinuses – infraorbital hypoaesthesia indicates infraorbital nerve involvement.

The globe

The eye ball itself should be assessed for proptosis. A bulging eye suggests an orbital haematoma; if combined with loss of vision and a tense orbit, a retrobulbar haemorrhage should be diagnosed (see below). A sunken eye (enophthalmos) suggests a blow-out fracture, usually of the maxillary floor. Posterior or inferior displacement of the globe suggests the possibility of an orbital fracture. Elution of fluorescein during corneal examination suggests penetrating injury to the globe. A ruptured globe should be gently padded, avoiding pressure, and ophthalmic advice sought.

The pupil

The pupils should be examined for shape, symmetry, red reflexes and reactions to light. A distorted pupil suggests anterior segment trauma. The pupillary red reflex is tested using an ophthalmoscope; it is absent with cataract, vitreous haemorrhage or total retinal detachment. Iris transillumination may detect iris root tears or passage of an intraocular foreign body. Notching of the pupil margin indicates significant ocular trauma.

The cornea

Assessment of the cornea, which is best achieved under magnification using anaesthetic drops and fluorescein, includes a search for corneal opacity and infiltrate for signs of inflammation or infection, for abrasions that stain green with fluorescein under a blue light and for foreign bodies that are intensely painful with conjunctival injection and a swollen eyelid. Superficial foreign bodies can be removed using topical anaesthetic, but embedded foreign bodies and rust rings require ophthalmic intervention. If there is a chance of an intraocular foreign body, radiographic investigation is mandatory.

The conjunctiva

The conjunctiva are examined for chemosis, subconjunctival haemorrhage, superficial foreign bodies, subconjunctival haemorrhage (without a posterior margin this suggests basal skull fracture) and subconjunctival emphysema, suggesting orbital fracture into the ethmoid or maxillary air sinuses.

Anterior chamber

Hyphaema is a visible level of blood in the anterior chamber. In its early stages, it may appear as clouding of the anterior chamber on ophthalmoscopy. A shallow anterior chamber suggests the possibility of an anterior penetrating wound, whereas a deep anterior chamber suggests a posterior penetrating wound.

Lens

The clarity of the lens is assessed by the red reflex; or if it is white and opaque. The lens may be displaced (subluxation) by trauma, usually inferiorly. If this happens, the lens edge may be seen in the pupil.

Vitreous

An ophthalmoscope is used to examine the vitreous for haemorrhage and loss of the red reflex and for intraocular foreign bodies.

Retina

The ophthalmoscope may demonstrate the presence of retinal tears, retinal detachment (leading to a shadow over, or loss of, vision and loss of red reflex if extensive) and preretinal/retinal/subretinal haemorrhage.

Specialist referral

Nonspecialists should have a low threshold for referral for a specialist ophthalmological review. Specific problems requiring such a review include lacerations involving the lid margins, levator muscle, tear glands, or tear ducts (medial part of lid), penetrating foreign bodies, which should not be removed prior to referral and actual or suspected globe rupture or penetration.

Ocular burns

Thermal burns are often from contact with hot liquids, hot gases, or molten metals. Tissue damage is usually limited to the superficial epithelium, but thermal necrosis and ocular penetration can occur.

Ultraviolet burns

Ultraviolet burns occur as a result of exposure to sources including sunlamps and welding arcs. Patients present with a superficial punctuate keratitis and pain may be delayed but is intense. Topical cycloplegics and antibiotic ointment are prescribed and an occlusive patch is applied.

Chemical burns

These are blinding emergencies. Alkaline agents such as lye or cement penetrate cell membranes and cause more damage than acids, which precipitate on reaction with ocular proteins.

In all burns, corneal epithelial defects range from superficial epitheliopathy to total epithelial loss. Limbal ischaemia is a whitened area without blood flow around the eye: the whiter the eye, the worse the burn. Other signs include focal areas of conjunctival chemosis, hyperaemia, conjunctival haemorrhages, eyelid oedema, mild iritis and periocular burns. Management of burns to the eye is with immediate copious irrigation with lactated Ringer's solution for 30 minutes (normal saline or even tap water are alternatives). The pH should be measured after 5 minutes on ceasing irrigation and if it is not neutral (pH 7.0) then irrigation repeated must be repeated until it is. A specialist opinion is essential.

Ocular/periocular foreign bodies

Superficial foreign bodies on the surface of the cornea or conjunctiva can be irrigated or removed using a slit lamp, and a bud or needle deep corneal foreign bodies if inert (e.g. fragments of stone) can be left in situ. After removing iron foreign bodies, the surrounding rust ring also requires removal.

Subconjunctival foreign bodies can be left in situ. Topical antibiotics are given for a week. Intraorbital foreign bodies are diagnosed on CT scan and can usually be left in situ; removal is a complex major specialist procedure. Intraocular foreign bodies require surgical removal and must be suspected in all cases where there has been a high-velocity injury, especially hammering on metal. These patients should be transferred as stretcher case to an ophthalmic unit. Large, protruding foreign bodies should be stabilised and left in situ pending specialist intervention. Further investigations include CT scan, ultrasound and facial X-ray. Prophylactic systemic and topical antibiotics are given.

Acute visual loss following trauma

Acute loss of vision following trauma has many causes and does not necessarily mean there will be no recovery. Diagnosis is with visual acuity and relative afferent pupillary testing, ocular imaging and electrodiagnostic testing. The causes of acute visual loss include:

- Retrobulbar haemorrhage
- Cataract
- Retinal detachment
- Vitreous haemorrhage
- Commotio retinae
- Optic nerve avulsion

Any treatment should be performed in a timely fashion and directed at the cause.

An accurate final visual prediction can be given only after around 4 weeks.

Orbital blow-out fractures

The symptoms and signs of orbital blow-out fractures include:

- Periorbital bruising
- Subcutaneous emphysema
- Infraorbital anaesthesia
- Double vision, usually worse on upward gaze
- Enophthalmos

Evidence of a fracture and soft tissue herniation is provided by CT scanning or plain radiographs. Where the diagnosis is suspected, systemic antibiotics should be given and the casualty instructed not to blow their nose. Management is not urgent but orbital reconstruction is usually performed within 2 weeks to reduce scarring.

Penetrating injuries/globe rupture

This diagnosis should always be considered if there has been a high-velocity activity such as hammering on metal, or when examining a lid injury. Conjunctival swelling may hide a penetrating globe injury. All injuries should be assumed to have a retained intraocular foreign body.

Fine slice CT and or ultrasound 'B' scan of the eye and orbit will determine if there is evidence of a penetrating eye injury such as an intraocular foreign body, intraocular air, a collapsed globe, or obvious eyewall rupture. Occult signs of globe rupture following blunt or penetrating injury include:

- A soft eye
- Total hyphaema
- Abnormally deep anterior chamber
- Restriction of eye movement
- Chemosis (conjunctival swelling)
- Subconjunctival haemorrhage

Surgical repair should be performed within 24 hours and topical medication must not be applied. The wound should not be explored or suture of iris/uveal tissue attempted. The eye should be covered with a protective eye shield, not a compressive eye patch and the casualty nursed sitting up. Systemic antibiotics, an antiemetic, pain relief and a tetanus booster (if required) should be given.

Retrobulbar haemorrhage

Pain is severe in and around the eye with proptosis. There is a fixed dilated pupil with an afferent defect, paralysis of eye movements and visual loss. Retrobulbar haemorrhage must be operated on within 100 minutes of injury. Lateral canthotomy and cantholysis allow the retrobulbar blood to escape anteriorly from the retrobulbar space

Ocular blast injury

The common presentation of ocular primary blast injury is a soft eye without evidence of globe rupture. Conjunctival lacerations and subconjunctival haemorrhages are common. Traumatic cataracts occur, but may spontaneously resolve. Posterior segment involvement includes commotio retinae, vitreous haemorrhage, retinal tears and detachment. Unless there is a surgical indication such as globe rupture or retinal tear/detachment, supportive treatment is best, as the signs spontaneously resolve over 7–10 days.

Secondary ocular blast injuries are due to the impact of fragments propelled by the explosion. Foreign bodies are common and debris can impact and remain buried in the eye wall, especially the cornea. Secondary tattooing of the skin around the eyes and face is common and can be disfiguring and requires early thorough cleaning.

Further reading

Harlan J, Ng E, Pieramici D. Evaluation. In: Kuhn F, Pieramici D (eds), Ocular trauma: principles and practice. New York: Thieme, 2002:52–72.

Scott R. Eye trauma. In: Smith J, Greaves I, Porter K (eds), Oxford desk reference: major trauma. Oxford: Oxford University Press, 2011:313–328.

Scott R. Eyes. In: Brooks A, Clasper J, Midwinter M, Hodgetts T, Mahoney P (eds), Ryan's ballistic trauma, 3rd edn. London: Springer, 2011:349–378.

Related topics of interest

Paediatric trauma

Key points

- Trauma is the commonest cause of death in children between the ages of 1 and 16 years in the developed world. This predominance of trauma deaths continues until well into the fourth decade of life
- There are specific and important differences between children and adults during resuscitation
- Optimal early trauma management may reduce the incidence of late trauma deaths

Epidemiology

Trauma is the commonest cause of death in children between the ages of 1 and 16 years in the developed world. This predominance of trauma deaths continues until well into the fourth decade of life. Traumatic death accounted for approximately 200 child deaths in England and Wales in 2012 (Office of National Statistics Mortality Statistics: Deaths Registered in 2012). The Trauma Audit and Research Network publication England and Wales Severe Injury in Children 2012 identified 737 children under the age of 16 years with major trauma presenting that year with an injury severity score >15. Children who died at the scene or were not transported to hospital were excluded. Head injuries were the predominant cause of morbidity and mortality.

Road traffic collisions (RTC) accounted for the single largest group with 284 (38.5%) children sustaining their injury from this cause; of these 23 died (9.4%). Approximately two thirds of RTC deaths (23/61) occurred at the scene or before arrival at hospital. Penetrating trauma accounted for only nine cases (1.4%). Seventy four cases (10%) were due to nonaccidental injuries in the under 2 years age group.

The number of trauma deaths in children in the United Kingdom has reduced by 50–70% over the three decades between 1980 and 2010. This decline is accounted for by a reduction in unintentional injuries.

Many children form injury patterns or injury severities which are currently unsurvivable, even if early expert intervention is readily available. These deaths, if they do not occur at the scene, will occur shortly after arrival at hospital. Modern medical technology can contribute little to the prevention of the majority of such deaths. Current strategies (which have been very successful over the past 30–40 years) to reduce such deaths rest on the application of the three E's: engineering (better car and road design), education (road safety and seatbelt campaigns) and enforcement (e.g. speed cameras or fire retardant clothes).

Many early deaths still result from causes such as airway obstruction, breathing problems, circulatory insufficiency and neurological injury and are amenable to simple interventions. The majority of such deaths are preventable if early access to the skills and equipment required to treat the underlying cause are facilitated either by up skilling first responders or by early access to an appropriate level of prehospital or hospital care. Prompt resuscitation and expert surgical intervention reduce mortality in this group.

Late deaths are caused in the majority of cases by multisystem failure or sepsis and usually occur days or weeks after the initial injury. However, there is evidence that expert early management and high-quality intensive care might significantly reduce the numbers of such deaths.

Resuscitating the injured child

The initial management priorities for paediatric trauma are the same as for adult trauma and follow the <C>ABCDE protocol. Children who are victims of trauma are prone to hypoglycaemia, and an early estimation of blood glucose is essential. Hypoglycaemia should be corrected with an initial dose of 2 mL/kg of 10% glucose. The response to this dose should be assessed and further doses given as required.

There are a number of differences between adults and children which must be taken into account during trauma resuscitation which is modified accordingly.

General considerations

Children's weight, linear and volume proportions vary within and between age groups. A number of reference charts and tapes (e.g. the Broselow tape) are available which give an estimate of the 50th centile weight for boys for a particular age or body height. These aids are useful for determining the correct dosage of drugs and fluids. To avoid the need for calculation, many of these charts give the correct volume of drug or fluid to be administered for a standard drug concentration.

If such a chart is not available, a simple formula relating age to weight in the over-1 year age group is:

$$\text{Weight (kg)} = 2 \times (\text{Age} + 4)$$

A child's surface area to volume ratio varies with age and is at its maximum in the infant. As a result children lose heat more rapidly than adults and are more prone to hypothermia during resuscitation. Similarly, the relative body surface areas of different body parts vary with age. Age specific charts are available for the calculation of burn area in the child, which reflect these changes.

Catastrophic external haemorrhage (<C>)

When present, this is managed in exactly the same way as in adults.

Airway (A)

An obtunded child is more prone to airway obstruction than an adult due to the following differences in upper airway anatomy:

- A larger head and shorter neck, leading to neck flexion
- A larger tongue
- A compressible floor of mouth
- Loose primary dentition
- Adenotonsillar hypertrophy

Intubation is more difficult in children, due to the large tongue, horseshoe-shaped epiglottis and the high anterior larynx.

Intubation poses problems due to age-related differences in the dimensions of the airway in the child. The correct tube size for a particular age can be estimated by reference to a standard chart. If no chart is available, the tube size may be approximated to the diameter of the child's little finger or nostril. Alternately the formula, Tube diameter = Age/4 + 4, can be used. Although cervical spine injury is uncommon in children, all children who have suffered major trauma or who have a history of an appropriate mechanism of injury should be treated as if they have a spinal injury until proven otherwise. There are occasions when this is not possible, e.g. the agitated child when the risk of exacerbating a spinal injury is greater if the child moves the body against a fixed immobilised head than if a lesser degree of immobilisation is accepted. In such circumstances, the child should be left in a semirigid collar with manual immobilisation if tolerated, or manual immobilisation alone while urgent radiographs are completed. Sedation, paralysis and intubation may be necessary depending on the associated injuries.

Spinal cord injury can occur in the absence of bony injury. Spinal cord injury without radiological abnormality (see p. 273). In all cases where there is a strong suspicion of an injury, the cervical spine should remain immobilised until cleared by an experienced doctor. In the child, the majority of bony cervical spine injuries occur in the upper cervical spine. Children should be kept on long spine boards for the shortest period of time.

Breathing (B)

The chest wall of the child is very compliant and tends to deform more under stress than an adult's, this leads to the possibility of significant damage to the underlying lung even in the absence of rib fracture.

Circulation (C)

The child's circulating blood volume (80 mL/kg) is greater per kilogram body weight than the adult's. Children may be significantly hypovolaemic before clear clinical signs of shock are evident due to their greater capacity to compensate for circulating volume loss than adults. The corollary of this is that the decompensation phase tends to be of rapid onset and may be catastrophic. Early fluid resuscitation in the presence of signs of circulatory impairment combined with frequent reassessment is therefore imperative. Signs of potential or actual circulatory failure include:

- Mental impairment
- Cold peripheries
- Absent or weak peripheral pulses
- Pale or mottled extremities
- Delayed capillary refill

The normal physiological ranges for the commonly measured parameters (blood pressure, pulse, respiratory rate) vary with age and are available on standard reference charts (**Table 27**). A simple formula for estimating the ninetieth and fifth centile values for systolic pressure in the over 1 year age group is:

- Ninetieth centile systolic blood pressure = 90 + (age × 2)
- Fifth centile systolic blood pressure = 70 + (age × 2)

A value below the fifth centile level indicates that decompensated shock is present and that urgent, fluid resuscitation is required. It is vital not to wait for a fall in blood pressure before diagnosing decompensated shock in a child. Replacement fluids are usually given in boluses of either 10 mL/kg or 20 mL/kg. Best practice follows the adult protocol of using blood components rather than crystalloids.

Disability (neurological assessment – D)

During the initial phase, the AVPU (alert, voice, pain, unresponsive) scale (**Table 28**) along with an assessment of pupillary size and response provides sufficient information on which to base management decisions. A formal assessment of conscious level using the Glasgow coma scale can be deferred until the patient is fully assessed and stable following the primary survey.

Exposure (E)

Full assessment requires removal of the child's clothes. As mentioned above, this should be done only to the extent, and for the minimum time required, so as to reduce heat loss and save embarrassment.

Nonaccidental injury

Major trauma in any child under the age of 1 year should raise the strong suspicion of the possibility of nonaccidental injury (NAI). This age group has the highest homicide rate of any age group in England and Wales at 20.1 per million compared to 9.7 per million for the whole population and 15.1 per million for the next highest age group, the 16–29 age range. NAI should be considered in any child who presents with an injury, particularly in the under 2 age group with major trauma. If there is a suspicion of NAI, the appropriate safeguarding agencies should be contacted in line with local policies and procedures as a matter of

Table 28 The AVPU scale	
A	Alert
V	Responds to voice
P	Responds to pain
U	Unresponsive

Table 27 Normal values of commonly measured parameters in the child			
Age (years)	Respiratory rate (breaths/min)	Pulse rate (beats/min)	Systolic blood
Newborn	–	160	60–80
<1	30–40	110–160	70–90
1–5	25–30	95–140	80–100
6–12	20–25	80–120	90–110
13+	–	60–100	100–120

urgency. Early consideration should be given to the safety of any siblings.

Future developments

Although the establishment of major trauma centres in England and Wales appears to have led to improvements in in-hospital mortality and morbidity for children sustaining major trauma, the simultaneous development of trauma networks should be seen as critical in ensuring that 55% of children with major trauma who are initially seen in a trauma unit have the same level of initial assessment and resuscitation as those taken directly to a trauma centre. Trauma networks should have systems in place to ensure that transfers are undertaken in a timely manner and that those undertaking transfers have the knowledge and skills to undertake such transfers safely. With over a quarter of children with major trauma being brought to hospital by means other than ambulance or helicopter, it is likely that a considerable number of children will continue to be initially managed in trauma units.

It should be noted that improvements in factors other than quality of medical care such as improvements in safeguarding systems and a reduction in prehospital road traffic deaths are likely to be required to sustain the fall in injury mortality in children.

Further reading

Advanced Life Support Group. Advanced paediatric life support: the practical approach (APLS), 5th Edition. London: John Wiley & Sons, 2011.

The Trauma Audit and Research Network (TARN). Severe injury in children: England and Wales 2012. Salford: TARN, 2012.

Related topics of interest

Pathological fractures

Key points

- Pathological fractures may be the first presentation of previously undiagnosed malignancy
- Suspected malignancy must be managed by an appropriately skilled multidisciplinary team from the outset
- Managing an impending pathological fracture prophylactically confers prognostic benefit over therapeutic management of a completed one

Common sites of pathological fracture

The sites of pathological fracture tend to relate to two factors; load transmitted through them and vascularity. On this basis, the axial skeleton is more commonly affected than the appendicular skeleton as it transmits load from cranial to caudal. Vascularity is especially a factor in haematologically disseminated metastatic malignancy; metaphyseal bone in particular tends to have a rich blood supply. These two factors explain why the proximal femur is an especially common site of pathological fracture (around 40% of metastatic tumours in bone), as it has a very good blood supply and transmits very

large loads. It is therefore under significant stress by comparison with the proximal humerus, for example.

Processes causing pathological fracture

Strictly by definition, osteoporosis is the most common disease process causing pathological fractures – this subset is more commonly termed fragility fractures (see p. 110) The commonest fractures of the elderly, distal radius, femoral neck and vertebral compression fractures are all in this group. Similarly, osteomalacia and osteopenia can cause structurally weak bone. Less common causes include disorders of bone production such as osteogenesis imperfecta or remodelling (e.g. Paget's disease).

Malignancy is a common cause. This may be from multiple myeloma or metastatic deposits commonly from breast, prostate, renal (**Figure 65**), lung or thyroid malignancy. Primary bone tumours are substantially less common but also carry a risk of pathological fracture. A more recently emerging cause of pathological fracture is bisphosphonate medication – its mechanism of action, inhibition of osteoclastic activity, prevents bone resorption and hence

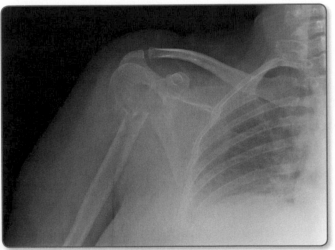

Figure 65 Pathological fracture of the proximal humerus in a patient with metastasis of renal cell carcinoma.

reduces osteoporosis, but also prevents the remodelling process by which bone manages the numerous microfractures which initiate within it every day.

Workup of pathological fractures

Every patient suspected of having sustained a pathological fracture must have a detailed history and examination. In vertebral fractures, the neurological status must be fully evaluated with magnetic resonance imaging of the spine if there is any suggestion of deficit or retropulsion of vertebral fragments visible on plain radiography. Radiography of the complete limb with the fracture should be performed together with biochemistry tests including calcium and alkaline phosphatase looking for evidence of increased bone turnover. A full blood count with particular attention to the differential white cell count should be taken as should an erythrocyte sedimentation rate and specific markers if a malignant disease process is suspected, such as prostate specific antigen for prostate cancer. A serum or urine electrophoresis should be performed if there is a possibility of myeloma. Nuclear bone scanning may demonstrate multiple hotspots due to secondary deposits (**Figure 66**).

Biopsy is contraindicated without clear discussion with a multidisciplinary team including specialist surgeons and oncologists. Reamings from intramedullary nailing may be sent for histological diagnosis if the primary tumour is unknown.

Decision-making in incomplete or impending pathological fractures

Impending or incomplete pathological fractures due to metastatic malignancy may benefit from early surgery to provide pain relief or palliation, improve patient mobility and avoid physiological impact of completion of the fracture. Recent research has demonstrated a more than twofold increase in mortality when femoral nailing was performed therapeutically rather than

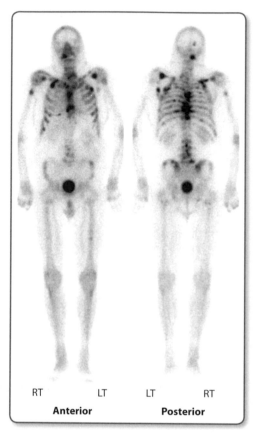

RT   LT   LT   RT

Anterior   **Posterior**

Figure 66 Nuclear bone scan showing multiple malignant hotspots.

prophylactically. Mirel's scoring system (**Table 29**) provides a means by which fractures can be scored based on site, pain, type of lesion and percentage of cortical involvement. A score >8 indicates the need for prophylactic fixation.

A common conundrum is that of the terminally-ill patient with an impending fracture in whom the perceived anaesthetic risk can result in reluctance to offer surgery. In such situations, fixation is palliative in the same way as hemiarthroplasty in hip fracture and to withhold surgery is to guarantee pain, immobility and probably terminal decline.

This approach should not be confused with that for primary bone tumours, which usually require complete resection with as great a margin of clearance as possible and often adjuvant therapy. Any lesion suspected

Table 29 Mirel's criteria for prediction of impending pathological fracture			
Score	1	2	3
Site	Upper limb	Lower limb	Peritrochanteric
Pain	Mild	Moderate	Severe
Percentage cortical involvement	<33	33–66	>66
Type of lesion	Sclerotic	Mixed	Lytic

to be a primary bone tumour should therefore be referred to the regional bone tumour service urgently with no preceding interventions which could disrupt the tumour or disseminate metastasis.

Ongoing management

Benign causes of pathological fracture may need ongoing management for secondary injury prevention. The sentinel event of a first fragility fracture should prompt some investigation of bone health; many institutions now have dedicated referral pathways for this incorporating bone densitometry. Remobilisation is important to prevent further resorption of under-loaded bone and decline from distal radius fractures to hip fractures.

New diagnoses of bone diseases such as osteogenesis imperfecta or Paget's disease should be referred to the appropriate secondary care team. In osteogenesis imperfecta, fracture fixation may best be performed in conjunction with deformity correction surgery such as the modified Sofield–Millar intramedullary rodding procedure.

Further reading

Arvinius C, Parra JL, Mateo LS, et al. Benefits of early intramedullary nailing in femoral metastases. Int Orthop 2014; 38:129–132.

Mirels H. Metastatic disease in long bones: a proposed scoring system for diagnosing impending pathologic fractures. Clin Orthop Relat Res 1989; 249:256–264.

Thompson RN, Phillips JR, McCauley SH, et al. Atypical femoral fractures and bisphosphonate treatment: experience in two large United Kingdom teaching hospitals. J Bone Joint Surg Br 2012; 94:385–390.

Related topics of interest

Pelvic trauma

Key points

- Pelvic ring injuries may be associated with life-threatening bleeding and should be promptly identified by appropriate imaging
- Multiply-injured patients with pelvic injuries have a greater mortality reflecting high-energy mechanisms and associated injuries
- Acetabular fractures carry an increased risk of post-traumatic osteoarthritis

Anatomy and pathology

The pelvis is an osteoligamentous ring with two hemipelvices joined anteriorly at the pubic symphysis and posteriorly via the sacroiliac joints and sacrum. The acetabulum is supported between anterior and posterior columns of bone: anterior extending from ilium to pubis; posterior extending from the greater sciatic notch down into the ischium. The pelvis is closely related anatomically to organs, blood vessels and nerves, all of which are at risk of injury in displaced fractures.

Disruption of the rigid pelvic ring tends to cause injury at two or more sites. For example, superior and inferior pubic rami fractures are typically associated with a sacral fracture. An injury that disrupts the posterior weightbearing complex may cause hip instability and osteoarthritis, sacroiliac pain and instability or pelvic deformity resulting in leg length discrepancy.

Mechanism and classification

Pelvic ring injuries

Typical high-energy mechanisms include road traffic collisions and significant falls. Front-to-back forces [anteroposterior compression (APC)] tend to open the pelvis up anteriorly [e.g. a motorcycle collision which drives the pelvis forward onto the tank, forcing the anterior pelvis apart – the open book fracture (**Figure 67**)]. Side-to-side forces [lateral compression (LC)] such as side impact motor vehicle collisions, or heavy falls onto the side tend to reduce the pelvic volume (**Figure 68**). Vertical forces to one side of the pelvis, e.g. resulting from a fall from a height onto one buttock, cause vertical shear (VS) injuries (**Figure 69**). VS injuries are associated with the highest risk of hypovolemic shock (63%) and have a mortality rate of up to 25%.

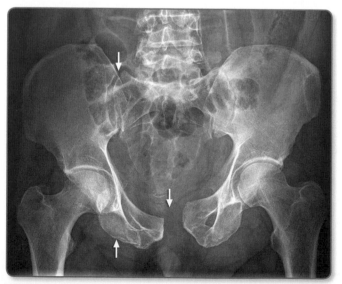

Figure 67 An open-book pelvic ring fracture.

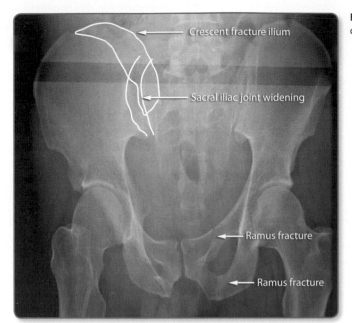

Figure 68 Lateral pelvic compression injury.

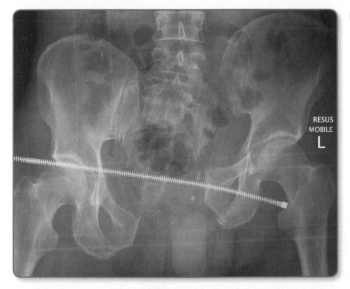

Figure 69 A vertical shear injury.

Two classifications of pelvic ring fractures which are in common use include:

- The Young–Burgess classification is based on mechanism of injury. Fractures are divided into: APC graded I–III, LC graded I–III, VS and combined mechanical injury types (**Table 30**).

- The AO/OTA (Orthopaedic Trauma Association) classification based on the type of instability:
  Type A: stable injuries such as avulsion fractures (e.g. of the anterior superior iliac spine) or isolated pubic symphysis disruption (APC-I), type B: rotationally

Table 30 Young Burgess classification

Anteroposterior compression	
APC I	Symphysis widening <2.5 cm
APC II	Symphysis widening >2.5 cm. Anterior SI joint diastasis. Posterior SI ligaments intact. Disruption of sacrospinous and sacrotuberous ligaments
APC III	Disruption of anterior and posterior SI ligaments (SI dislocation). Disruption of sacrospinous and sacrotuberous ligaments APCIII is associated with vascular injury
Lateral compression	
LC Type I	Oblique or transverse ramus fracture and ipsilateral anterior sacral ala compression fracture
LC Type II	Rami fracture and ipsilateral posterior ilium fracture dislocation (crescent fracture)
LC Type III	Ipsilateral lateral compression and contralateral APC (windswept pelvis)
Vertical shear	
Vertical shear	Posterior and superior directed force

APC, anteroposterior compression; SI, sacroiliac; LC, lateral compression.

unstable injuries such as APC-II and LC-I or II injuries and type C: rotationally and vertically unstable such as APC-III or VS.

Acetabular fractures

These usually result from forces directed along the femur. The direction of the force and femoral position determine the injury pattern. For example, where the knee hits the dashboard in a head-on collision force transmitted along the femur against the seated acetabulum causes a posterior hip fracture–dislocation.

The most widely used classification of acetabular fractures (the Letournel classification), is divided into five elementary and five associated types according to involvement of the columns and walls. Accurate classification guides definitive treatment as the type determines surgical approach.

Emergency assessment and management

General assessment and initial management should follow standard trauma resuscitation guidelines. Specifically, all patients should be examined carefully for evidence of:

- *Open pelvic injuries:* These fractures have a high mortality. The presence of perineal wounds, vaginal and rectal bleeding should be established
- *Urethral trauma:* It is essential to look for blood at the urethral meatus and scrotal or labial swelling. Catheterisation in pelvic injury should be a single gentle attempt by an experienced practitioner
- *Pelvic instability:* Examination may identify pain on movement, leg length discrepancy and rotational deformity of the lower limbs

Management by injury type

There are four main acute presentations:

Mechanically stable pelvic ring without haemodynamic instability

This is the most common presentation and includes pubic rami fractures in osteoporotic patients and most acetabular fractures. Such fractures are managed nonoperatively unless hip stability or congruity is affected by an acetabular fracture. In such cases, the early advice of a pelvic surgeon should be sought in order to plan treatment. Hip dislocations must be reduced promptly to reduce the risk of sciatic nerve injury and femoral head osteonecrosis. Distal femoral skeletal traction may be required to maintain reduction and protect injured articular cartilage.

Mechanically stable pelvic ring fractures with haemodynamic instability

In these cases, the pelvic injury must not distract from the search for the source of bleeding. Haemorrhage control takes precedence over specific management of the pelvic injury.

Mechanically unstable pelvic ring fractures without haemodynamic instability

These fractures require specialist management. If there is vertical instability of the pelvis then skeletal traction, via a distal femoral pin, can help prevent shortening. The use of external fixation should be discussed with a pelvic surgeon.

Mechanically unstable pelvic ring with haemodynamic instability

A key concept in managing pelvic haemorrhage is preservation of primary clot by promoting mechanical stability and prevention of coagulopathy. Measures should be applied early (beginning in the prehospital setting) when pelvic injuries are suspected based on mechanism and pain. Rolling a patient with suspected pelvic injury or 'springing' to detect instability must be avoided. A noninvasive pelvic binder should be applied at the level of the greater trochanters, apposing bleeding bony surfaces and stabilising clot. Binders carry a risk of skin necrosis and should be replaced, if necessary, with alternative fixation as soon as practicable and safe. Tranexamic acid, packed red blood cells, clotting factors, platelets, and patient warming help prevent coagulopathy.

If haemodynamic instability persists, further treatment depends on injury context and the availability of interventional radiology. Active arterial bleeding identified on the trauma computed tomography (CT) should be managed by embolisation if it is available and the patient can be safely transported for angiography. Alternatively and where a patient is in extremis or requires surgery for other reasons, surgical tamponade by packing of the stabilised pelvis is appropriate. Resuscitation should continue in the critical care until definitive management is considered safe.

Investigations

Plain radiographs are used to diagnose isolated low-energy injuries. Selected cases require CT to plan treatment. High-energy injuries in major trauma centres are routinely assessed with a contrast-enhanced trauma CT often as part of a head to femurs protocol. This can identify haemorrhage and associated haematoma by visualisation of contrast extravasation, which may guide therapeutic embolisation. CT is essential when internal fixation is being planned. Trauma CT will identify associated organ injuries but separate investigations such as urethrography or cystography may be required.

Definitive treatment

Commonly, LC injuries are very stable owing to impaction of the associated sacral fracture. Minimally displaced fractures and stable injuries of any mechanism can be considered for nonoperative management consisting of a variable period of rest and analgesia with mobilisation when the pain permits and restricted weightbearing in potentially unstable, but minimally displaced, injuries. Frail patients may have to be permitted to weightbear on a pragmatic basis and the risks of prolonged recumbency must be balanced against the risks of fracture displacement. Rarely, bed rest and traction may be necessary.

Where the position is unacceptable or instability so great that rehabilitation risks displacement, surgery should be considered. If there is any doubt, the plan should be discussed with a pelvic surgeon at an early stage. There are three main strategies:

External fixation

This is primarily used in pelvic ring injuries often used temporarily as postbinder stabilisation until the patient is fit enough for definitive fixation.

Percutaneous fixation

Where closed reduction is achievable, percutaneously inserted screws can be used to stabilise certain pelvic and acetabular fractures. One common example is percutaneous stabilisation of an unstable sacroiliac joint with a screw passed from the ilium across the joint into the sacrum.

Open reduction and internal fixation

Direct visualisation and reduction of fragments with plate and screw stabilisation are sometimes necessary, particularly for displaced acetabular fractures where accurate reduction and rigid fixation are required to reduce the risk of osteoarthritis.

Further reading

British Orthopaedic Association (BOA). BOAST 3: pelvic and acetabular fracture management. London: BOA, 2008.

Eastern Association for the Surgery of Trauma (EAST). Pelvic fracture hemorrhage – update and systematic review. J Trauma 2011; 71:1850–1868.

Mayo K, Oransky M, Rommens P, Sancineto C. Acetabulum - Reduction & Fixation - Kocher-Langenbeck - T-type. Davos: Arbeitsgemeinschaft für Osteosynthesefragen (AO) Foundation, 2007.

Related topics of interest

Penetrating neck injury

Key points

- Assessment of penetrating neck injury should be performed by clinical examination in conjunction with computed tomography angiography (CTA) and estimation of wound trajectory
- Control of external bleeding should be by direct digital pressure over the area of the vessel injury, which may be distant from the surface wound
- Hard signs for mandatory surgical exploration include bleeding from the neck region that is not amenable to pressure, expanding haematoma, a bruit or a thrill in the neck

Epidemiology

Penetrating neck injuries account for 5–10% of traumatic injuries in adults, with a mortality ranging between 3% and 10%. Low-energy bullets or impaling objects tend to cause fewer aerodigestive and vascular injuries, but unsurprisingly, high-energy injuries carry a greater likelihood of serious injury (particularly to the spinal cord) and death.

Pathophysiology

A penetrating neck injury is defined as one in which platysma is breached and which has the potential to cause damage to one or more of the following groups of structures within the neck:

- Airway
- Blood vessels
- Upper gastrointestinal tract
- Neurological structures

Clinical features

Traditionally, the entry wound location of penetrating neck injuries has been described using the zonal system originally described by Monson and based on surface markings:

- Zone I is the area of neck between clavicles and cricoid cartilage
- Zone II between cricoid cartilage and the angle of the mandible
- Zone III up to the skull base

Although this is less relevant for treatment decisions nowadays, it is still important in communicating between colleagues and for judging the appropriateness of investigations.

Signs of damage are listed in **Table 31**, with those hard vascular signs mandating surgical exploration highlighted. Hypopharyngeal or oesophageal penetration is difficult to diagnose preoperatively. Major digestive tract injuries are often accompanied by pneumomediastinum and missed injuries can lead to spreading infection in the chest. A gross neurologic examination is essential as hemiplegia may herald inadequate collateral cerebral blood flow from a damaged

Table 31 Signs of penetrating neck injury			
Vascular	**Airway**	**Digestive tract**	**Neurological**
* Ongoing bleeding from the neck region that is not amenable to pressure	Dyspnoea	Dysphagia	Hemiplegia from carotid artery or vertebral artery damage
* Expanding haematoma	Stridor	Odynophagia	Tetraplegia from high-cervical transection
* Bruit or thrill in the neck	Crepitus or subcutaneous emphysema	Haemoptysis	Paraplegia from low-cervical transection
Hemiplegia	Hoarse or abnormal voice	Haematemesis	Arm weakness from brachial plexus damage
	Air bubbling from wound	Subcutaneous emphysema	
* Hard signs mandating surgical exploration			

carotid system and may greatly influence the operative decision-making.

There is very limited evidence to suggest that cervical spine immobilisation is required in penetrating neck injury compared to blunt. Large studies of military casualties with penetrating neck wounds give incidences of unstable cervical spine injuries in fewer than 2% of casualties, whereas the rate of life-threatening injuries missed as a result of having a hard collar applied may be in excess of 20%.

Investigations

With the widespread availability of CTA, there has been a clear shift away from the use of zone-based algorithms, with the belief that this leads to an increased reliance on invasive diagnostic modalities. For example, it was previously mandatory that endoscopy and angiography be performed for zone I and III penetrations with significant associated risks. In addition, mandatory neck exploration was advocated for zone II injuries, with a resultant high incidence of nontherapeutic neck exploration. Current protocols suggest that in a haemodynamically stable patient, a comprehensive physical examination, combined with CTA, is adequate for triage to effectively identify or exclude vascular and aerodigestive injury.

Marking entry wounds with radio-opaque markers improves the determination of projectile paths and thereby improves predictions regarding which anatomical structures may be damaged, thus guiding diagnostic evaluations. Compared to missiles that do not cross the midline, transcervical gunshot wounds are twice as likely to injure vital structures in the neck. This has led some authors to suggest that these wounds mandate surgical exploration. If a penetrating trajectory is highly suspicious of a vertebral injury, angiography should be performed if at all possible before operative exploration.

Treatment

Immediate

Initial management will follow the <C>ABCDE system. With the exception of

providing digital pressure on any areas of haemorrhage, assessment initially revolves around whether an airway is required and needs to be performed rapidly. Since an expanding haematoma makes endotracheal intubation more difficult as minutes pass after an injury, an experienced anaesthetist should attempt intubation as soon as possible. A rapid sequence technique should be employed using cricoid pressure, liberal suctioning, sedatives and paralytics to afford the best opportunity of success on the first pass. The surgeon should be at the head of the bed ready to perform a cricothyroidotomy if endotracheal intubation fails. Jet insufflation is not recommended except in extremis.

Once the airway is secure, other manoeuvres can be performed, including control of nonlife-threatening haemorrhage and assessment for other injuries. Control of external bleeding should be by direct digital pressure over the area of the vessel injury, which may be some distance away from the surface wound, allowing blood to exit. Simply plugging the surface wound will not slow bleeding and has the potential to cause an expansion of the haematoma over the area of vessel injury exacerbating compression of other structures.

The exact area of vessel bleeding is not always obvious, and pressure should be applied to different areas until it appears that the bleeding is reducing. Clamping of exposed vessels should only be carried out if the vessel is identified clearly and a vascular clamp is available. Blind clamping in an open wound often leads to associated nerve damage, increased vessel wall damage and ineffectual haemorrhage control. Digital control should continue if necessary into the operating theatre where surgical control can be obtained.

Surgical

The treatment of haemorrhage currently remains primarily surgical. The role of endovascular stents in managing cervical vascular injuries continues to evolve and is likely to increase in the future. Proximal vascular control of zone I injuries is difficult and often involves an approach through a sternotomy or thoracotomy. Zone III injuries pose problems with distal control and special techniques such as mandibular subluxation may be needed. Carotid injuries should be repaired unless the surgeon is faced with uncontrollable haemorrhage, ongoing haemodynamic instability or a devastating vessel injury that prevents use of a temporary vascular shunt. In these circumstances, ligation should be employed. Control of haemorrhage from the vertebral artery is surgically exceedingly difficult. Unless the clinical situation precludes it, the most successful way to control bleeding from a vertebral artery is by angiography and embolisation. Temporary methods of control include balloon tamponade with a Fogarty type intraluminal catheter or packing.

Most laryngeal and tracheal defects from penetrating trauma can be repaired primarily. Small defects noted on endoscopy can usually be managed nonoperatively with airway protection and elevation of the head of the bed. Oesophageal wounds are generally managed operatively by a layered closure method but pharyngeal wounds can often be managed conservatively unless gross when similar surgical repair is indicated.

Complications

Immediate or early death is from exsanguination or airway compromise, either from bleeding into the airway or direct compression from an expanding haematoma. Immediate death from spinal cord disruption is rare except for high-energy injury, but carotid or vertebral injury may lead to stroke. Missed oesophageal and pharyngeal damage can lead to significant morbidity and sometimes death, from spreading infection.

Further reading

Demetriades D, Theodorou D, Cornwell E, et al. Transcervical gunshot injuries: mandatory operation is not necessary. J Trauma 1996; 40:758–760.

Shiroff AM, Gale SC, Martin ND, et al. Penetrating neck trauma: a review of management strategies and discussion of the 'No Zone' approach. Am Surg 2013; 79:23–29.

Related topics of interest

Peripheral nerve injuries

Key points

- Nerves are particularly sensitive to compression and stretching
- Differing patterns of nerve injury are seen with differing mechanisms
- Delay in diagnosis and treatment of nerve injury leads to poorer outcomes and early expert advice must be sought

Anatomy

The cell bodies of motor neurones are located in the anterior horn of the spinal cord and of sensory neurones in the dorsal root ganglion. Axons can be over 1 m in length. In myelinated nerves, Schwann cells provide a layer of lipid-rich myelin around each individual axon insulating the nerve and significantly enhancing the speed of conduction. Nerve trunks are organised morphologically by three distinct connective tissue layers:

- *Endoneurium:* The innermost layer which forms a sheath around individual nerve fibres consisting of the Schwann cell, basement membrane, collagen and capillaries.
- *Perineurium:* A dense, strong fibrous connective tissue sheath surrounding individual fascicles.
- *Epineurium:* A loose connective tissue matrix with a well-developed vascular plexus provides cushioning between fascicles. Superficially the epineurium condenses to form the external nerve sheath.

Pathology of nerve injury

The severity of nerve injury varies with the type, magnitude and duration of trauma. A number of different pathological mechanisms are recognised.

Conduction block

Compression and stretching cause a temporary 'physiological' conduction block. The anatomical structure of the nerve is preserved and spontaneous, full recovery normally occurs rapidly (type a), but may be prolonged for several weeks (type b).

Demyelination

Sustained compression or ischaemia causes loss of the myelin insulating the nerve resulting in a block to conduction. Such a block will persist until the myelin can be repaired, a process which requires weeks or months.

Nerve degeneration

Severance of the axon will result in degeneration. Degeneration of the entire axon distal to the lesion occurs (Wallerian degeneration) as well as for a short distance in a retrograde fashion in the proximal stump. The degenerative process takes several weeks. Recovery relies on the nerve cell regenerating a new axon. However, axonal severance may result in neuronal cell death (apoptosis). Nerve cell depletion peaks at around 2 weeks. Early surgical repair protects surviving cells. Surviving nerve cells are capable of regenerating a new axon with growth rates being between 1 and 4 mm/day. The integrity of the connective tissue framework of the nerve is key to successful routing of axons to their target end organ.

Mixed

Continuity nerve lesions often have mixed elements of conduction block and degeneration.

Classification of nerve injury

Seddon described three grades of nerve injury: neurapraxia (conduction block/demyelination), axonotmesis (axonal discontinuity) and neurotmesis (complete nerve discontinuity) (**Table 32**). Sunderland described five grades of injury in which grades I and V correspond to Seddon group's neurapraxia and neurotmesis, respectively. The axonotmesis group is subdivided based upon the connective tissue layers of the nerve.

Table 32 Seddon and Sunderland classification of nerve injury			
		Pathology	Prognosis/recovery
Neurapraxia	I	Conduction block/demyelination	Reversible within weeks to months
Axonotmesis (axonal discontinuity)	II	Loss of axonal continuity. Endoneurium, perineurium and epineurium intact	Preserved endoneurial tube supports accurate axonal regeneration to the correct targets resulting in effective, near full reinnervation
	III	Loss of axonal continuity and endoneurium. Perineurium and epineurium intact	Endoneural pathways are disrupted leading to axonal misdirection, increased intraneural scar may block axons regeneration. Variable reinnervation seen. Surgery may be required
	IV	Loss of axonal continuity, endoneurium and perineurium. Epineurium intact	Total disorganisation of guiding elements of the nerve trunk leading to marked misdirection. Dense intraneural scar leads to neuroma in continuity. Poor recovery. Surgery required
Neurotmesis	V	Complete nerve discontinuity	Recovery requires surgical repair or grafting

Initial assessment

A history of the mechanism of injury will help distinguish the depth of the nerve injury. Careful assessment of the nervous and vascular systems and recording of the results is crucial prior to intervention. All nerves within the zone of injury should be examined for motor, sensory and autonomic functions:

- Motor power is graded according to the system described by the Medical Research Council (MRC) (**Table 33**)
- Sensation is best tested by comparing light touch with the normal side. Any difference, even slight, suggests an injury
- Autonomic function is assessed by looking for reddened and dry skin. This indicates dysfunction of vasomotor and sudomotor systems, respectively

Tinel's sign is invaluable in both initial assessment and subsequent surveillance of nerve recovery. Percussion is performed over the course of a nerve in a distal to proximal direction. Pronounced tingling in the cutaneous distribution of that nerve is a positive sign indicating that there is discontinuity of axons. The sign is present immediately after injury and should progress distally over ensuing weeks as the axons regenerate. A Tinel's sign which fails to progress indicates that axons are caught in scar forming a neuroma. The presence of neuropathic pain in the distribution of

Table 33 MRC grading of muscle power	
Grade	Description
0	No movement
1	Flicker is perceptible in the muscle
2	Movement only if gravity eliminated
3	Can move limb against gravity
4	Can move against gravity and some resistance exerted by examiner
5	Normal power
MRC, Medical Research Council.	

a nerve following injury or surgery implies ongoing injury to that nerve.

A diagnosis of conduction block should not be made if there is autonomic dysfunction or a positive Tinel's sign or neuropathic pain is present.

Investigation

Neurophysiological investigation is the most useful adjunct to clinical assessment.

Nerve conduction studies

Nerve conduction studies are performed 10 days or more after injury to allow for Wallerian degeneration to occur. If conduction in the nerve distal to the site of injury is preserved at this stage, then axons are present and the injury is in one of the conduction blocks.

Electromyography

Electromyography (EMG) studies are performed at a minimum of 3 weeks postinjury. Fibrillations and positive sharp waves are evidence of muscle denervation and will be present at this stage if there has been loss of motor axons. Additionally, reinnervation is apparent on EMG before it is clinically evident, making it a useful tool in monitoring recovery.

Surgical exploration

Surgical exploration of a nerve allows for direct assessment, intraoperative nerve stimulation and decompression of haematoma or fracture fragments. Exploration is indicated when:

- Open wounds are in the territory of a major nerve trunk
- A nerve injury is associated with a fracture or dislocation that requires operative fixation
- A nerve injury occurs following intervention (e.g. manipulation of a fracture of the humerus)
- There is worsening of a neurological deficit while under observation
- There is persisting neuropathic pain
- There is failure of progression during surveillance for recovery (e.g. neuroma in continuity)

Surgical repair and nerve grafting

Early repair leads to superior results. Surgery aims to:

- Restore vascularity to the limb in cases where it has been compromised
- Stabilise the skeleton in cases where it is unstable
- Place repairs into a healthy surgical bed and cover repairs with good quality full-thickness skin
- Achieve coaptation without tension and with correct orientation of nerve ends

Microsurgical epineural or grouped fascicular repairs are performed with 8/0 or 9/0 monofilament sutures. Tissue glues are an acceptable alternative.

Where retraction of nerve ends has occurred or segments of nerve have been lost, mobilisation of a nerve (e.g. anterior transposition of the ulnar nerve at the elbow) may allow direct repair. Autologous nerve grafting is used when direct repair cannot be achieved. Donor nerves include the sural and cutaneous nerves of the arm and forearm. Grafts are reversed and interposed as loosely laid cables of sufficient number to match the calibre of the nerve trunk being reconstructed. Synthetic conduits have been used as alternatives to autologous graft in small defects.

Prognosis

Key factors in prognosis following nerve injury include delay in treatment (the interval from injury to repair should be as short as possible for optimal results), age (normal function can be achieved in children following major nerve repair but this is rarely seen in adults), the level of the lesion (more proximal injuries have greater regeneration distances and a poorer prognosis) and the mechanism of injury (high-energy injuries having a poorer outcome).

Further reading

British Orthopaedic Association (BOA). BOAST 8: the management of nerve injuries: a guide to good practice. London: BOA, 2011.

Lundborg G. Nerve injury and repair: regeneration, reconstruction, and cortical remodelling, 2nd edn. Edinburgh: Churchill Livingstone, 2005.

Related topics of interest

Pregnancy and trauma

Key points

- Pregnancy must be considered in all female trauma patients of childbearing age
- Survival of the fetus depends on optimal resuscitation of the mother
- All pregnant trauma patients should undergo an urgent assessment by obstetrics and gynaecology in order to identify any obstetric complications

Epidemiology

Deaths in pregnant women following trauma are commonly caused by road traffic collisions, domestic violence, or self-harm due to psychiatric disorders. Injuries from road traffic collisions arise due to failure to wear a seatbelt or as a result of incorrect positioning of the seatbelt over the pregnant abdomen.

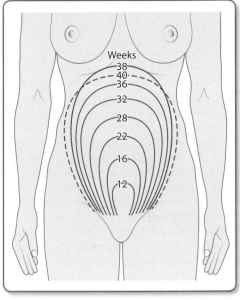

Figure 70 Fundal heights.

Anatomy

The uterus is protected within the bony pelvis for the first 12 weeks of pregnancy. At 12–14 weeks, the uterus becomes palpable above the pelvis, at 20–22 weeks it is at the level of the umbilicus and by 34–36 weeks the uterus reaches the costal margin (**Figure 70**). In early pregnancy, the muscular uterus is thick walled, and the fetus is protected by a large volume of amniotic fluid. As pregnancy proceeds, the uterine wall becomes thinner and the relative volume of fluid is less reducing the cushioning effect provided to the fetus. The placenta is a relatively inelastic structure and is vulnerable to shearing forces to the abdomen in blunt trauma, resulting in placental abruption.

Physiology

Airway

The risk of regurgitation and aspiration is increased due to relaxation of the gastro-oesophageal sphincter by pregnancy hormones, delayed gastric emptying and increased intragastric pressure from the pregnant uterus. Intubation with a cuffed endotracheal tube is preferred over a laryngeal mask airway, with the use of cricoid pressure after induction of anaesthesia and early decompression of the stomach with a naso- or orogastric tube. Intubation may be more difficult due to soft tissue oedema, and enlarged breasts may impede laryngoscopy.

Breathing

Hypoxia is more likely in pregnant women because of increased oxygen consumption. Oxygen must be administered to all pregnant women regardless of measured saturations. Rapid desaturation may occur during intubation attempts. Ventilation may be more difficult due to weight gain, breast enlargement and increased intra-abdominal pressure.

The physiological hyperventilation of pregnancy caused by increased tidal volume, leads to a respiratory alkalosis with a Pa_{CO_2} below 4 kPa and a higher Pa_{CO_2} may indicate ventilatory failure.

The diaphragm rises by up to 4 cm as the uterus enlarges. Any thoracostomy or chest drain insertion may be performed in a higher space (e.g. the 3rd or 4th intercostal space) to reduce the risk of abdominal or diaphragmatic penetration.

Circulation

After 20 weeks, compression of the inferior vena cava by the pregnant uterus in a supine position may lead to a reduction in venous return, and therefore cardiac output, by as much as 40%. This can be prevented by a left lateral tilt or manual displacement of the uterus across to the left side.

By the third trimester of pregnancy, the resting heart rate is increased by 15–20 bpm; systolic blood pressure, which falls in the second trimester by 10–15 mmHg, has returned to near normal and the blood volume has increased by up to 50%. Significant haemorrhage (>1.5 L) may occur before signs of hypovolaemic shock become evident. Blood may be shunted from the uterine and placental circulation into the maternal circulation to mask signs of maternal hypovolaemia to the detriment of the fetus. The uterine circulation is entirely dependent on the maternal blood pressure so a target systolic blood pressure of at least 90 mmHg must be maintained with fluid resuscitation.

Examination

The primary survey should proceed as in the nonpregnant trauma patient. The pregnant abdomen should be palpated for tenderness, rigidity, contractions and fetal movements. External inspection for any bleeding or fluid loss from the vagina should take place as part of the circulatory assessment.

Investigations

Clinically indicated chest/pelvic X-rays or a CT scan should not be withheld because of concerns about radiation exposure to the fetus. At the time of phlebotomy, additional blood should be taken for a Kleihauer test to estimate the amount of fetal blood cells present in the maternal circulation and guide the administration of anti-D IgG. Fetal assessment should include an early Doppler or ultrasound as an adjunct to the primary survey.

Management

In general, management proceeds as for the nonpregnant trauma patient. Pregnant patients with a suspected pelvic injury should have a pelvic splint applied. Tranexamic acid should be given to all pregnant trauma patients showing signs of hypovolaemia or who have suspected internal haemorrhage. Prescribed analgesia should be carefully checked for any contraindications in the appropriate trimester of pregnancy. All pregnant women suffering trauma, no matter how apparently trivial their injuries, require assessment by the obstetrics and gynaecology team before discharge.

Resuscitation of a hypovolaemic woman who is >24 weeks pregnant and who is unresponsive to fluids or blood or in traumatic cardiac arrest may require an immediate resuscitative hysterectomy. In stable patients, fetal distress may be an early indicator of placental abruption or uterine rupture requiring urgent delivery.

Obstetric complications after trauma

Placental abruption

Placental abruption is the premature separation of the placenta from the uterine wall. It may occur after relatively minor trauma and can present late (days) after the initial incident. There may be severe abdominal pain with premature contractions. Bleeding can be concealed with no external loss from the vagina and signs of hypovolaemic shock may present with very few other signs.

Uterine rupture

The uterus can be torn after blunt trauma to the abdomen. Uterine rupture is usually associated with older gestational age with or without a previous Caesarean section. The patient may present with severe abdominal pain, hypovolaemic shock and palpable fetal parts in the abdomen.

Premature labour

Trauma to the uterus may injure the myometrium causing cells to release prostaglandins which stimulate uterine contractions. This may progress to premature labour if there is significant uterine damage and a more advanced pregnancy. In most cases, the contractions resolve without treatment.

Fetal death

Direct fetal injury is rare. Indirect injury may occur due to hypoxia or hypotension in the mother, the conditions described above, or a placental or cord injury. In stable patients, a vaginal delivery will normally be induced a day or two after diagnosis to deliver the dead fetus.

Fetomaternal haemorrhage

Even minor trauma may cause transplacental haemorrhage from the fetal to the maternal circulation. All Rhesus negative mothers who are >12 weeks pregnant will require anti-D IgG injection within 72 hours of injury.

Penetrating injury to the uterus

As pregnancy progresses, the uterus acts as a shield for the maternal abdominal organs but this means a poor prognosis for the fetus. The uterine muscle and amniotic fluid reduce energy transfer from higher-energy missiles. Penetration of the umbilical cord or placenta may cause placental abruption or life-threatening haemorrhage.

Further reading

Barraco RD, Chiu WC, Clancy TV, et al. Practice management guidelines for the diagnosis and management of injury in the pregnant patient: the EAST Practice Management Guidelines Work Group. J Trauma 2010; 69:211–214.

Grady K, Howell C, Cox C. Managing obstetric emergencies and trauma. The MOET course manual, 2nd edn. London: RCOG Press, 2009.
Smith J, Greaves I, Porter KM. Oxford desk reference major trauma. Oxford: Oxford University Press, 2011:374–382.

Related topics of interest

- Abdominal trauma (p. 1)
- <C>ABCDE resuscitation (p. 63)
- Pelvic trauma (p. 222)

Prehospital blood product resuscitation

Key points

- The accepted treatment for bleeding trauma patients in trauma-induced coagulopathy (TIC) is haemostatic resuscitation. This involves resuscitation with appropriate ratios of blood products, rather than crystalloid or colloid, in combination with permissive hypotension and rapid transfer for damage control surgery
- Prehospital packed red blood cells (PRBC) and fresh frozen plasma (FFP) are currently available to a number of military and civilian services
- Dried blood products such as freeze-dried plasma are logistically attractive for remote locations. Further research is required, although freeze-dried plasma is already available to selected services

Introduction

Uncontrolled haemorrhage is still responsible for >50% of all trauma deaths within the first 48 hours after hospital admission and is thought to be the most common cause of preventable deaths. Several studies have demonstrated that one out of four severely injured patients presents to the emergency room with haemodynamic depletion and TIC. In addition to the 'primary' effects of TIC that are unrelated to any medical intervention, there are also the 'secondary' effects of dilution, acidosis and hypothermia which can worsen this primary insult.

Haemostatic resuscitation is the accepted treatment for bleeding trauma patients in TIC. This involves resuscitation with appropriate ratios of blood products, rather than crystalloid or colloid, in combination with permissive hypotension and rapid transfer for damage control surgery. The overarching term given to this is damage control resuscitation (DCR) and the prehospital period of this has recently been described as remote DCR or RDCR. Integral

to RDCR is the provision of prehospital blood products, the availability of which varies across the world depending on logistics and timelines for individual services. This key topic contains an overview of currently available prehospital blood products and potential products requiring further research.

Prehospital blood component provision

PRBC require refrigeration, FFP requires freezing and a time-consuming thawing process, platelets are stored at 22° on special agitators and cryoprecipitate is also frozen. The prehospital use of haemostatic resuscitation as described is therefore logistically challenging.

Some prehospital services carry PRBCs with or without thawed FFP in specially manufactured thermal boxes (golden hour boxes), which maintain the temperature of the blood products for a specified period of time, usually between 24 and 72 hours. The box contains a continuously monitoring temperature tag. After the specified time period, if unused, the boxes are returned to the laboratory and the temperature tag within the box is checked to ensure that the products have been maintained in the required temperature range before they can be put back into the blood bank stores. If the FFP has been thawed by dry heat then it is usable for 5 days post-thawing, whereas if it was thawed by wet heat as in most hospitals in the UK, then it cannot be used after 24 hours. This means that it is not logistically and economically possible for a number of prehospital services to carry thawed FFP as it would result in unnecessary wastage due to low demand.

The UK and the US forces in Afghanistan have projected PRBC and thawed FFP forward to the point of wounding, which from a UK point of view is with the helicopter borne Medical Emergency Response Team (MERT). A number of civilian Helicopter

Emergency Medical Services (HEMS) teams such as London's Air Ambulance and the Norwegian Air Ambulance are now also carrying PRBC and FFP to the prehospital scene. For this process to be viable, significant and regular demand for blood products is essential.

Whole blood

In some deployed or remote situations, whole blood may be taken from an emergency donor panel. It is categorised according to the temperature and duration of its storage. The term warm whole blood is used when the blood is maintained at 22–26°C after donation. If the donated blood is cooled to 2–6°C, it is referred to as cold whole blood (CWB). In the future, refrigeration of CWB after pathogen reduction could ensure wide availability, haemostatic efficacy and enhanced safety in far forward settings, but its potential advantages must be weighed against its logistic burden.

Currently, the position of the Trauma Haemostasis and Oxygen Research (THOR) Network is that whole blood should be used only for life-saving emergency transfusions if there are no acceptable alternatives. In a situation where it is not possible to determine the ABO type of the donor or recipient, then type O donor should be used as a last resort if the benefits of providing whole blood are perceived to be higher than the risk of a severe haemolytic reaction.

Current options for maximising blood safety include the use of pretested donors and rapid testing at the time of donation. WHO standards demand that blood samples should be sent for nucleic acid testing for HIV, HBV surface antigen, HCV and syphilis. Testing may be enhanced to conform to national standards and may include additional testing such as for West Nile virus, malaria, dengue and Chagas disease. Donor testing, while logistically challenging, should be repeated at preagreed intervals such as every 90–180 days.

Dried blood products

While in some services the logistics of carrying the golden hour boxes described above is possible, technical, regulatory and logistical limitations may prohibit the use of blood components in some of the prehospital settings.

Dried blood products (freeze- or spray-dried) capable of being stored at room temperatures for extended periods of time, offer the potential for blood products to be administered more easily in the prehospital environment. The ideal solution would be freeze-dried whole blood, in the form of a unit of autologous whole blood, precollected, dried and carried by each medic; however, this is still a long way from being commercially available.

At the time of writing, freeze-dried plasma (FDP; see p.42) is the only field-ready freeze-dried whole plasma product that offers freedom from some of the logistical constraints described. FDP is authorised for use by the Israeli Defence Force, a few other international military special operations units and the Norwegian Air Ambulance; however, there are still a number of unanswered questions regarding its efficacy and safety.

Fibrinogen is available as a concentrate. As one of the main substrates of the coagulation system, it is vulnerable to rapid depletion in the setting of massive trauma and haemorrhage due to haemodilution, consumption and fibrinolysis. Fibrinogen concentrates appear to be safe even when given in high doses, and may rapidly restore haemostatic function, therefore reducing bleeding and blood product requirements. Randomised trials especially in the primary health care setting are still awaited to guide appropriate use in trauma resuscitation.

Prothrombin complex concentrates are also available and commonly used for bleeding patients who are on warfarin, especially those presenting with head injuries and high likelihood of intracranial haemorrhage. Although potentially useful, their broader use in trauma patients has not been evaluated adequately and so they cannot be currently recommended for the wider trauma population.

Summary

Blood products are a vital component of prehospital resuscitation of the bleeding trauma patient. Some products such as

PRBC and FFP, as well as whole blood are available to a number of military and civilian prehospital services. Significant logistical constraints still exist, especially in more remote locations. Further research into the use of freeze-dried blood products is required which may be useful adjuncts in overcoming these constraints.

Further reading

Glassberg E, Nadler R, Gendler S, et al. Freeze-dried plasma at the point of injury: from concept to doctrine. Shock 2013; 40:444–450.

Holcomb JB, Donathan DP, Cotton BA, et al. Prehospital transfusion of plasma and red blood cells in trauma patients. Prehosp Emerg Care 2015; 19:1–9.

Strandenes G, De Pasquale M, Cap AP, et al. Emergency whole-blood use in the field: a simplified protocol for collection and transfusion. Shock 2014; 41:76–83.

Related topics of interest

- Blood product (1:1:1) resuscitation (p. 42)
- Lyophilised plasma in trauma resuscitation (p. 176)
- Recombinant factor VIIa (p. 242)

Psychological aspects of trauma

Key points

- Post-traumatic stress disorder (PTSD) is not the single most common psychological condition after trauma
- Treatment of post-traumatic conditions should be evidence-based or evidence-informed whenever possible
- Human resilience is the norm

Epidemiology

Trauma is an overused word in the public and psychiatric domains. Everyday adversities are not traumas. The term should be used to describe those events which overwhelm or threaten to overwhelm the coping resources of individuals, families, organisations or communities. Traumatic events may be relatively restricted in their effects (e.g. motor vehicle, domestic and industrial incidents) or they may be very extensive (e.g. floods, earthquakes and terrorist incidents). Some authorities distinguish between natural and man-made events: individuals tend to cope less well with the latter, but the distinction is not always so clear. Earthquakes themselves, while appearing to be natural events, kill relatively few people: bad building construction is the cause of most deaths. Floods may be mainly due to poor flood planning.

About 90% of the victims of contemporary military conflict are civilians and not combatants. The traumatic events with which the civilians have to cope include horrific scenes, multiple losses, dreadful injuries to themselves and their loved ones, grotesque deaths, further threats of violence (including mass rape) and displacement of thousands of persons.

The figures for combatants who are suffering from post-traumatic conditions are often exaggerated. Recent studies of combat troops returning from Iraq and Afghanistan suggest that about 7% may have been suffering from PTSD. Figures for reservists tend to be higher than those for regulars. The figures reported in American combatants tend to be higher.

Many common, normal reactions are observed in the short term in those exposed to different traumas. These must not be medicalised and regarded as symptoms.

Pathophysiology

There is no common pathophysiology in post-traumatic conditions, although symptoms associated with hyperarousal represent an over stimulation of the autonomic nervous system. Chronic PTSD has been linked to atrophy of the hippocampus, but the significance of this is yet to be determined.

Clinical features

Common normal reactions include shock, denial, anxiety, guilt (shown by those who survived when others perished or by those who believe that they could have done more to help others), helplessness, impaired memory and concentration, anger, intrusive memories (flashbacks) of the trauma, hyperarousal and hypervigilance (an exaggerated sense of risk), social withdrawal, insomnia (particularly associated with nightmares) and loss of appetite and energy. There are two major psychiatric taxonomies (the Diagnostic and Statistical Manual, and the International Classification of Diseases), but they do not have a perfect diagnostic concordance because of slightly different diagnostic criteria. However, they both recognise these core symptoms.

Hyperarousal and hypervigilance

These must have endured for about a month post incident as they are otherwise normal reactions. It should also be noted that a number of persons who have been distressed by the trauma can also come through the stronger for their experience. (This is sometimes referred to as post-traumatic growth).

Investigations

There are no biological markers for post-traumatic conditions. Rigorous history-taking and information from significant others, such as family and colleagues are the keystone to a secure diagnosis.

Diagnosis

The diagnosis of post-traumatic conditions is very dependent on self-reporting. Rating scales and questionnaires can be useful, but they tend to inflate the prevalence of conditions. The gold standard is a standardised, semistructured interview, such as the clinician administered PTSD scale. Several scales are available for screening but these are of limited sensitivity and specificity.

Treatment

In the immediate aftermath of a major trauma, specialist psychiatric treatments are very rarely required. Most reactions are normal. Also, it is important that mental health specialists and counsellors do not intrude and compromise the help available from family, friends, colleagues and the community.

Whenever possible, formal treatment should be delivered by experienced practitioners, familiar with the effects of trauma, and who use evidence-based or at least evidence-informed methods. The National Committee for Health and Clinical Excellence has prepared such guidelines with regard to which treatments represent best practice. For PTSD, it is recommended that psychological methods are the first-line interventions. Medication may be required when such methods have not been successful, when patients are not willing to undergo such treatments and when there are no suitably trained personnel to deliver them. Mirtazapine and paroxetine are recommended for general use, and amitriptyline and phenelzine are proposed for use by mental health specialists.

Although not itself a treatment, psychological first aid (PFA) is widely advocated for use in the acute phase of a major incident. It comprises a number of well-tried interventions, for children and adults. These include provision of physical care (e.g. food, water and shelter), psychoeducation (about normal reactions to trauma), links to sources of further help and triage (to identify those who may require expert assistance).

The military and the emergency services commonly use a method of peer support and assessment: Trauma Risk Management (TRiM). Those exposed to traumatic events are assessed post incident by trained peers at 3 and 28 days (approximately) by means of a 10 item scale. Those apparently in need are referred on for expert evaluation and care. The North Atlantic Treaty Organisation (NATO) guidance advocates a stepped care model of response to those who have experienced a major incident. In summary, this recommends allowing victims the chance to benefit from that support which family, friends, colleagues and the community can provide, supplemented by PFA, before involving the specialist mental health and other services.

Complications

Losses of various kinds are commonly associated with major trauma. Grief reactions must be identified and dealt with as they may interfere with the treatment of post-traumatic conditions. Complicated grief is linked to missing bodies, gruesome and mutilating deaths, concurrent life problems among the bereaved and a lack of support.

Further reading

Alexander DA, Klein S. Human reactions to trauma: their features and management. In: Greaves I, Porter K, Smith J, (eds), Practical prehospital care. The principles and practice of immediate care. London: Churchill Livingstone, 2011:465–475.

Hughes R, Kinder A, Cooper CL. International handbook of workplace trauma support. Chichester: Wiley-Blackwell, 2012.

North Atlantic Treaty Organisation (NATO) Joint Medical Committee. Psychosocial care for people affected by disasters and major incidents. Brussels: NATO Joint Medical Committee, 2008.

Related topics of interest

- Epidemiology of trauma (p. 93)
- Mild traumatic brain injury (p. 188)
- Moderate-to-severe brain injury (p. 191)

Recombinant factor VIIa

Key points

- Factor VII (FVII) is one of the coagulation factors produced in the liver
- Recombinant factor VIIa (rFVIIa) is the physiological initiator of coagulation
- There is no convincing evidence to support the routine use of rFVIIa in trauma

Introduction

rFVIIa has been widely used in bleeding situations, including trauma over recent years, although the evidence for its use is limited. In spite of this lack of evidence, 97% of rFVIIa use is for off label, nonlicensed use.

Mechanisms of action

FVII is one of the coagulation factors produced in the liver with about 1% normally present in its activated form. It is therefore rapidly available to bind to subendothelial tissue factor (TF) after injury to blood vessels. This FVIIa/TF complex is the sole physiological initiator of coagulation generating small amounts of thrombin, which, in conjunction with activated platelets, amplifies to produce a thrombin burst. If the thrombin burst is of sufficient magnitude, fibrinogen will be converted to insoluble fibrin and will form a stable clot.

Administration of rFVIIa increases the concentration of circulating rFVIIa approximately 100-fold resulting in a 'boost' in thrombin production at the site of injury. There appear to be two mechanisms by which rFVIIa exerts its effect. The first is TF-dependent pathway where rFVIIa binds to TF at the site of injury causing clot initiation in a normal physiological way. However, its main effect is a second, TF-independent pathway. rFVIIa weakly binds to an activated platelet directly causing thrombin production. Although the efficiency of this reaction is low, the high concentrations of rFVIIa offset this.

Clinical use

rFVIIa license for use is restricted to congenital haemophilia with inhibitors, acquired haemophilia, Glanzmann's thrombasthenia and congenital FVII deficiency. In spite of the narrow license, up to 97% of rFVIIa use was for reasons outside these licensed (off label) indications in an attempt to control bleeding.

A meta-analysis in 2011 looking at 26 trials where there had been off–label use of rFVIIa showed that there was no significant effect on mortality in either group, and a nonsignificant increase in thromboembolic events. There were decreased blood loss and decreased transfusion requirements. However, studies had widely varied dosing regimens.

The conclusion from this meta-analysis was: 'Clinically significant benefits of rFVIIa as a general haemostatic agent in patients without haemophilia remain unproven. Given its potential risks, such use cannot be recommended, and in most cases, it should be restricted to clinical trials.'

rFVIIa in trauma

The use of rFVIIa in trauma was first documented in 1999 in a case report of an Israeli soldier with uncontrolled haemorrhage from a gunshot wound to the inferior vena cava. Since then its (off label) use in trauma has become widespread and there have been other reports favouring its use in the context of major trauma.

Boffard et al. (2005) studied patients with penetrating and blunt trauma with administration of rFVIIa or placebo at 1 and 3 hours after transfusion of 8 units of blood. There was a significant reduction in the amount of blood transfused in the rFVIIa group for blunt trauma, and a nonsignificant trend in penetrating trauma. There was no difference in hospital length of stay, intensive care unit days, ventilated days or mortality and no difference in the rate of thromboembolic events.

In military trauma, the only evidence available comes from retrospective analyses. Spinella et al. looked at those patients in a combat support hospital who had received massive transfusion (>10 units of blood in 24 hours). The rFVIIa group had a lower mortality at 24 hours and 30 days with no increase in thromboembolic events. There was no difference in survival or adverse events.

CONTROL trial

Following these inconclusive trials, a large multicentre trial (CONTROL) was conducted to look at the role of rFVIIa in traumatic haemorrhage. The study was powered for a mortality of 27.5% in the placebo group. The study was terminated early after interim analysis due to a lower than expected mortality of 10.8% and thus the study was underpowered. In patients who were recruited, there was no difference in mortality and no statistically different number of thromboembolic events. There was a reduction in blood product use in the rFVIIa group.

The effect of abnormal physiology

Acidosis affects enzymatic activity and platelet function but it also affects the activity of rFVIIa. A pH of 7.0 will reduce rFVIIa TF-independent activity by 90% and TF-dependent activity by 60%. However, the large pharmacological dose of rFVIIa (a 100-fold increase) may still have enough activity to exert a significant effect even with a pH below 7.2. Hypothermia has minimal effect on the activity of rFVIIa. Since as the TF-dependent pathway activity drops, so the TF-independent pathway activity increases.

The effect of haemodilution is controversial, with some studies showing decreased effect and others unchanged. Most guidelines for the use of rFVIIa suggest that there should be a minimum platelet and fibrinogen level prior to administration. Recent, unpublished animal work, has demonstrated that administration of rFVIIa causes a boost in clotting with an improvement of clotting indices, followed by a rapid increase in consumption of clotting factors, specifically fibrinogen and to a lesser extent platelets.

Summary

The evidence for when and how to use rFVIIa in trauma remains limited. The evidence is mixed, partly due to the differing methods and end points between studies. rFVIIa use does seem to boost clotting causing a temporary reduction in bleeding and blood product use, combined with an accelerated consumption of clotting factors, specifically fibrinogen. Its use is therefore likely to be limited to resources constrained environments in an effort to temporarily reduce blood product requirement, as long as the ability to administer fibrinogen is present.

Further reading

Boffard KD, Riou B, Warren B, et al. Recombinant factor VIIa as adjunctive therapy for bleeding control in severely injured trauma patients: two parallel randomized, placebo-controlled, double-blind clinical trials. J Trauma 2005; 59:8–15.

Hauser CJ, Boffard K, Dutton R, et al. Results of the CONTROL trial: efficacy and safety of recombinant activated factor VII in the management of refractory traumatic hemorrhage. J Trauma 2010; 69:489–500.

Kenet G, Walden R, Eldad A, Martinowitz U. Treatment of traumatic bleeding with recombinant factor VIIa. The Lancet 1999; 354:1879.

Wade CE, Eastridge BJ, Jones JA, et al. Use of recombinant factor VIIa in US military casualties for a five-year period. J Trauma 2010; 69:353–359.

Related topics of interest

Rehabilitation

Key points

- Multidisciplinary rehabilitation provision, guided by a rehabilitation prescription, is now a core feature of trauma care
- The best outcomes are achieved when rehabilitation is goal-oriented, coordinated and communicated
- Defined rehabilitation pathways, including general, specialised and community provision, are essential to effective trauma networks and patient flow

Rehabilitation definitions

Rehabilitation is a measured process of assessment, treatment and management supporting people and allowing them to achieve their maximum potential. In 2001, the World Health Organization moved away from the medical model within the international classification of impairments, disabilities and handicaps and described instead the international classification of functioning and health, comprising:

- Disorder or disease
- Impairment/activity
- Participation
- Contextual factors – personal and environmental

Within this framework, the focus is on an individual's ability, activity and participation in society. The process is person-centred and aims to address physical, cognitive, social and psychological aspects of function, thus improving quality of life.

Specialised rehabilitation is the total active care of patients with complex disabilities by a multiprofessional team who have undergone recognised specialist training in rehabilitation, led by a consultant trained and accredited in rehabilitation medicine.

Rehabilitation medicine is the application of medical skill to the diagnosis and management of disabling disease and injury affecting any system of the body.

Rehabilitation in trauma care

The prevalence of disability following major trauma is increasing and will continue to do so as survival rates increase. Rehabilitation is an essential component of trauma care. Without effective rehabilitation interventions and pathways, trauma networks cannot succeed. Rehabilitation is critical to optimise functional outcomes and support the individual needs of injured patients, but also to improve patient flow and prevent bottle-necks in acute units.

The National Health Services (NHS) major trauma Clinical Advisory Group (CAG) report to the Department of Health in 2010 highlighted the importance of coordinated rehabilitation. The national service specification for trauma care in England now dictates that a consultant in rehabilitation medicine and an appropriately skilled multidisciplinary team must be present in every major trauma centre.

The rehabilitation prescription, introduced in 2012, is a mandatory requirement for all trauma patients with an injury severity score (ISS) of ≥ 9. It is used to document the rehabilitation needs of patients and identify how they will be addressed. It is part of the patient's medical record and provides information when patients are transferred between services. Patients should receive a copy of their own prescription and it should be available to family or carers where appropriate. It should therefore be written in plain language without abbreviations or medical jargon. The rehabilitation prescription should be reviewed and modified throughout the rehabilitation process until there are no ongoing rehabilitation needs and each version should include a recommended date for further review.

While there is no fixed national format, the rehabilitation prescription should include, as a minimum:

- Demographic data
- A list of injuries, including initial Glasgow coma score
- A list of interventions and procedures
- Information about progress and complications
- Relevant preinjury information (e.g. medical, social, employment and housing details)
- Rehabilitation goals
- Key management plan and advice given (e.g. weightbearing status, aids and driving)
- Services to which the patient has been referred, including contact details and likely waiting times
- Details of who has completed the document and their contact details

Details about functional status and the specific rehabilitation interventions required should be included appropriate to the needs of the patient. Major trauma can result in a complex range of impairments and disabilities, with a mixture of physical, cognitive, emotional, social and behavioural problems. The ISS does not provide a good indication of rehabilitation needs: a patient with an isolated head injury may have highly complex problems in comparison to a patient with polytrauma and a higher ISS. A specialist rehabilitation prescription should be issued wherever the patient's needs are complex.

Specialised rehabilitation

A minority of trauma patients, usually those with brain or spinal cord injuries or, less commonly, those with amputation or complex musculoskeletal injuries, will have complex rehabilitation needs requiring admission to a specialised rehabilitation unit. Specialised rehabilitation units are centrally commissioned in England and must now be registered with the UK Rehabilitation Outcomes Collaborative (UKROC). Not all regions have such units and patients may have to travel long distances from home to access them.

Categorisation tools and validated scores exist to help identify patients requiring specialised rehabilitation, which include features such as the presence of multiple issues (physical + cognitive + psychosocial) or the need for multiple therapy disciplines, intensive therapeutic input or specialist equipment.

Four categories of rehabilitation need are described, A to D, with A being the most complex and D the least. There are three levels of provision. Specialised rehabilitation refers to levels 1 and 2, catering for predominantly category A and B needs.

Recovery, re-enablement and rehabilitation

The majority of trauma patients will have an uncomplicated recovery (category C or D needs) and will progress rapidly down the level 3 or recovery, re-enablement and rehabilitation (RR&R) pathway. Their rehabilitation needs can be met within their local services, which can be located in a wide variety of settings, including acute medical and surgical wards, local hospitals, intermediate care beds and community therapy services. There are no separate commissioning arrangements for this rehabilitation pathway.

The rehabilitation process

Goal planning

Regardless of where it is delivered, rehabilitation requires a process of agreeing and working towards goals. When planning rehabilitation goals, adhering to the SMART structure ensures that the process is objective and that the person's progress can be accurately measured.

- Specific
- Measurable
- Achievable
- Realistic/relevant
- Timed/timely

Patients and families benefit from clear timescales and agreed outcomes. Writing truly 'smart' rehabilitation goals can be difficult and requires training and experience, but is the core activity of a competent multidisciplinary rehabilitation team (**Figure 71a**). Examples of the various professionals in rehabilitation teams are given in **Figure 71b**. Goal planning is enhanced when an

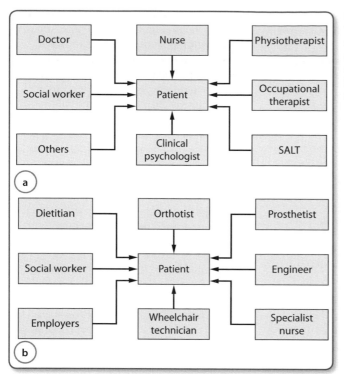

Figure 71 (a) An example of a 'core' rehabilitation team. SALT, speech and language therapist. (b) Examples of the wider multidisciplinary team involved in specialised or longer term rehabilitation.

identified key worker coordinates the process. Goal attainment is a useful outcome measure.

Early trauma rehabilitation

In addition to initiating and delivering the rehabilitation prescription, the input from the acute trauma rehabilitation team includes:

- A detailed assessment of preinjury status
- Communication with families, giving information and managing expectations
- Maximising the potential for future rehabilitation and assisting adaptive recovery
- Organising orthoses, mobility aids, seating and other equipment
- Provision of communication aids and environmental controls
- Prevention of complications, including:
  - Spasticity and limb contractures
  - Postural abnormalities
  - Pressure ulcers
  - Constipation and nutritional problems
  - Post-traumatic agitation and mood disorders

Rehabilitation planning should begin on day 1, with an initial rehabilitation prescription in place within 96 hours of admission. A dedicated rehabilitation coordinator is essential to ensure communication between the rehabilitation team and the various specialties involved in the acute trauma care.

Community rehabilitation

The trauma rehabilitation journey does not stop in the trauma centre or inpatient rehabilitation unit. For every life saved by trauma care, the aim must be to restore the person as closely as possible to their previous functional and social status. This may take months or years. Psychological, vocational and many other issues need to be addressed.

A wide range of services are essential in helping trauma patients return to meaningful roles. These include:

- Specialist community rehabilitation teams
- Wheelchair services and other equipment providers

- Social services
- Employers, job centres and vocational rehabilitation teams
- Age-specific services, e.g. for older adults or children
- Voluntary and third sector organisations

Outcome measurement

Robust measures of outcome are essential to rehabilitation services and should accompany mortality data when assessing the effectiveness of trauma care. A mandatory dataset is required by UKROC for all specialised rehabilitation services, including detailed measures of function and independence such as the functional independence measure and functional assessment measure scores. For less complex rehabilitation pathways, outcomes such as return to work, mobility scores and patient reported quality of life should be measured.

Further reading

British Society of Rehabilitation Medicine (BSRM). Specialist rehabilitation in the trauma pathway: BSRM core standards. London: BSRM, 2013.
Royal College of Physicians (RCOP). Medical rehabilitation in 2011 and beyond. London: RCOP, 2011.

Turner-Stokes L, Nair A, Disler P, et al. Cochrane review: multi-disciplinary rehabilitation for acquired brain injury in adults of working age. Oxford: The Cochrane Database of Systematic Reviews 2009; CD004170.

Related topics of interest

- Immediate trauma care in sport (p. 147)
- Moderate-to-severe brain injury (p. 191)
- Psychological aspects of trauma (p. 239)

Resuscitative balloon occlusion of the aorta

Key points

- Noncompressible torso haemorrhage (NCTH) is defined as vascular injury from or in one or more of a named axial torso vessel, grade ≥4 solid organ injury or the thoracic cavity, with shock or indications for immediate surgery for haemodynamic instability
- Resuscitative endovascular balloon occlusion of the aorta (REBOA) aims to maintain the myocardial and cerebral perfusion and control the source of haemorrhage
- Safe and effective REBOA use is dependent on correct patient selection and a trained operator

Epidemiology

Compressible haemorrhage from extremity injuries can be effectively managed by direct application of pressure, a haemostatic dressing or a tourniquet. The epidemiology of NCTH has been hampered by lack of a consistent definition in the literature with which to characterise these injuries. American and British military surgeons have recently proposed a definition of NCTH to enable analysis of combat-related injuries, which includes:

- Vascular disruption within the thorax, abdomen and pelvis
- Linkage to physiological indices of shock
- The presence or absence of the need for operative haemorrhage control

NCTH has been shown to be associated with a high mortality. In contrast to extremity injury, managing NCTH has traditionally been by conventional operative interventions such as resuscitative thoracotomy (RT).

RT may be performed on trauma patients in haemorrhagic shock who are in cardiac arrest or are periarrest. The aim is to relieve pericardial tamponade, control major vascular injury and air-leaks, allow aortic control and if necessary open cardiac massage, in order to restore spontaneous circulation. The best reported survival rates following RT are observed in patients with thoracic stab wounds and cardiac tamponade. The survival outcomes after RT performed for blunt injuries are much poorer.

REBOA is a technique which can be used to control haemorrhage and as a resuscitation adjunct, prior to further surgical intervention. The first description of REBOA appeared in the literature in the 1950s but its clinical adoption was limited by the technology then available, particularly related to arterial access, suitable balloons and methodology for confirmation of correct placement.

With technical developments driven by endovascular surgery including aortic balloon occlusion during endovascular aneurysm repair, many of these limitations have been resolved. The use of endovascular technology in the management of trauma patients has increased dramatically over the last 2 years. REBOA has been developed to control noncompressible haemorrhage in the torso without the requirement for interventional radiology expertise.

Pathophysiology

Maintaining aortic pressure is important in order to achieve adequate perfusion of the myocardium and brain. Aortic occlusion distal to the origin of the left subclavian artery in order to realise this goal can be a life-saving intervention and is classically performed by aortic cross-clamping either through a left anterolateral thoracotomy or supracoelic occlusion via a laparotomy. The same physiological benefits may be obtained by an endovascular balloon introduced through the femoral artery occluding the aorta without the necessity of an operative approach. REBOA is a technique that can be used in either the thoracic or infrarenal aorta to obtain haemorrhage control and acts as an adjunct to other resuscitative interventions.

In both animal models of uncontrolled haemorrhage and recent reported clinical case series, REBOA is associated with a significant haemodynamic and survival benefit. However, there are adverse consequences related to ischaemia-reperfusion (IR) injury, although this also occurs with surgical aortic clamping. IR injury may be partly ameliorated by adequate resuscitation. IR injury increases with the duration of aortic occlusion and novel methods to ameliorate this will be required in future.

Clinical features

The aorta has been divided into three functional zones for REBOA placement:

- Zone I extends from the origin of the left subclavian artery to the coeliac trunk
- Zone II is the paravisceral aorta from the coeliac axis descending to the most inferior renal artery
- Zone III is the infrarenal abdominal aorta between the lowest renal artery and the bifurcation of the aorta

Zones I and III are the principle REBOA placement zones. Zone I occlusion acts in the same way as clamping the descending thoracic aorta or supracoeliac axis clamp in circulatory arrest for control for abdominal exsanguination. Zone III occlusion is for junctional ileofemoral haemorrhage often associated with pelvic injury. The zone chosen will depend on the specific clinical circumstances.

Investigations

The confirmation of the placement of the wire and consequently the balloon in the desired position may be by plain X-ray. For austere environments without ready access to X-ray, estimates of the distance of these zones from the femoral artery puncture site by morphometric analysis and relation to the individual torso height has been studied. Knowing the torso height from symphysis pubis to the sternal notch allows a calculation of the distance to mid-points of different zones. However, the additional risk in this approach is that the wire may not be in the

aorta but a side branch. Work to develop a truly X-ray free REBOA system with potential for use in the prehospital setting is ongoing.

Placement

The steps to placement of a REBOA device are as follows:

- Micropuncture is performed to access the common femoral artery 2 cm below the inguinal ligament using an 18G femoral arterial line catheter
- An Amplatz wire is advanced into the arterial line catheter to a position proximal to zone 1. An X-ray confirms correct wire placement within the aorta
- An exchange of the arterial line catheter for a 12F sheath is performed over the wire
- The sheath is advanced to the proximal common iliac artery and the dilator removed
- The balloon is advanced to distal zone 1 or 3 and inflated to moderate resistance by feel
- Changes in haemodynamics confirm haemorrhage control
- The sheath, balloon and wire assemble are secured for transport to a location for definitive control of the source of haemorrhage (either in the interventional radiology suite or operating room)
- Once the need for aortic occlusion has passed, the balloon is removed under direct visual control and the artery repaired

Complications

If there exists or coexists an injury proximal to the left subclavian artery such as in the axilla, superior mediastinum, neck or face, this will not be controlled by REBOA and could be exacerbated. In shock, access to the femoral artery may require a surgical approach and the necessary instrumentation should be part of the REBOA minimal equipment set. A diseased vasculature with atheroma may also impede access. Damage to the arterial tree should be minimised by the correct approach and subsequent repair of the femoral artery, avoiding intimal damage, dissection and atheromatous plaque disruption. Ensuring that there is good inflow and back flow at the arterial puncture site at the end of the procedure is vital. Reperfusion injury with metabolic sequel may lead to immediate cardiac instability and combined with inflammatory consequences, later organ dysfunction.

Further reading

Brenner M, Moore L, Dubose J, et al. A clinical series of resuscitative endovascular balloon occlusion of the aorta for hemorrhage control and resuscitation. J Trauma Acute Care Surg 2013; 75:506–511.

Moore EE, Knudson MM, Burlew CC, et al. Defining the limits of resuscitative emergency department. J Trauma 2011; 70:334–339.

Morrison JJ, Rasmussen TE. Noncompressible torso hemorrhage: a review with contemporary definitions and management strategies. Surg Clin North Am 2012; 92:843–858.

Related topics of interest

Road traffic collisions

Key points

- Every year 1.24 million people die and another 20–50 million people are injured in road traffic collisions (RTCs), which are the eighth leading cause of death worldwide
- In the UK in 2012, there were between 630,000 and 790,000 road casualties
- The mechanism of injury is important but should not deflect the clinician from considering all possible injuries

Epidemiology

Every year 1.24 million people die and another 20–50 million people are injured in RTCs, which are the eighth leading cause of death worldwide. The highest proportion of road traffic related deaths are in those countries classified as having middle incomes, which have high volumes of motorised traffic but poor coordination and enforcement of road safety measures. Although low-income countries do not tend to have such high volumes of motorised traffic, inadequate safety measures also result in high death rates. High-income countries usually have high levels of motorised traffic but mitigate the risks linked to this by well-established safety measures including road safety management, safer roads, safer vehicles, safer road users, coordinated post-crash responses and the legislation, policy and enforcement to underpin this.

Worldwide, half of road deaths occur amongst motorcyclists, pedestrians and cyclists with only a third of deaths amongst car occupants. The World Health Organisation is attempting to catalyse change for all road users but particularly vulnerable road users through its Decade of Action for Road Safety.

In the UK in 2012, there were between 630,000 and 790,000 estimated road casualties although only 195,723 casualties of all severities were reported to the police. During this period, an estimated 1754 deaths attributable to RTCs occurred. A cyclist in

Great Britain is 15 times more likely to have a fatal accident than a car driver going the same distance. However, in 2013, there was only one death for every 29 million miles cycled and although the number of cyclists has increased, the number killed continues to decline year on year, despite increasing numbers of road users. Unfortunately, the number of cyclists injured is currently rising, perhaps reflecting medicine's ability to convert yesterday's fatalities into today's injured survivors as well as to the effectiveness of safety measures in force UK wide.

Injury patterns

In an RTC, high-energy levels are transferred over a short distance and the effects of rapid acceleration and deceleration forces on the human body can be catastrophic. Information gleaned at the scene of an RTC gives clues as to the likely injuries of those involved. Key information includes the nature of involved parties (multiple vehicle incident, vehicle versus tree, pedestrian involvement and motorcycle crashes), approximate speeds of the involved parties, orientation on collision, location of involved parties to one another (has a passenger or pedestrian been thrown from a vehicle?), vehicle damage (particularly intrusion into passenger spaces) and the use of restraints such as seatbelts or airbags.

Specific injury patterns are associated with particular types of collision; however, the clinician must always be prepared to encounter a full range of clinical conditions and the importance of reading the wreckage has been over emphasised if it leads to any risk of ignoring the possibility of injuries which do not 'fit' the mechanism. Rote learned lists of possible injuries associated with specific mechanisms are unhelpful and an assessment of possible injuries based on the available information taking into account use of restraint and evident vehicle damage is more helpful. It must also be remembered that medical conditions may be the cause of an RTC and tests such as blood glucose estimation, cardiac enzymes, electrocardiograph or head CT may be required.

Pre-hospital care

Preparation is key prior to attending an RTC and personnel should be properly insured, trained and equipped with appropriate medical kit, communication and personal protective equipment fit for task and with which they are familiar. A vital consideration in attending an RTC is the safety and ingress or egress of emergency response personnel, the casualty and other road users and vehicles should be parked to facilitate both safety and necessary movement.

Multiple casualties are often a feature at RTCs and clinical staff must be prepared to assess the situation and 'read the scene', requesting extra resources at the earliest opportunity and performing triage with life-saving interventions prior to commencing in-depth care of individual casualties. If first on scene, medical personnel must undertake their own dynamic safety assessment and ensure they subject themselves, the casualties and other road users to the minimum risk possible.

The police will be in-charge of the scene, which may be part of a criminal investigation and clinicians must be mindful not to dispose of or tamper with potential evidence when providing care. Cooperation while protecting patient's confidentiality may also represent a challenge. The fire service is generally responsible for scene safety and if in attendance medical personnel should coordinate activities with them. The fire and rescue service will work in six phases in an RTC entrapment:

- Scene assessment and safety
- Stabilisation and initial access
- Glass management
- Space creation
- Full access and immobilisation
- Extrication

Close coordination will be required to ensure optimal outcomes for casualties. A and B extrication plans will need to be formulated and as part of this the consideration of rapid extrication or snatch rescue may be required.

Care must follow the <C>ABCDE paradigm with the focus on minimal interventions to save life and prevent further harm with a view to expediting in-hospital definitive care as soon as possible. C-spine consideration and appropriate immobilisation concurrent with airway assessment are key in patients at RTCs due to the common injury patterns experienced. The patient should be immobilised and packaged for transfer from the scene in such a way as to balance the priorities of injury stabilisation, efficient transfer and transportation and the ability to quickly carry out further assessment and life-saving interventions if required.

Patient transportation options should be considered and requested as early as possible to facilitate the allocation of resources by ambulance control. The more usual transport options are road ambulance or helicopter. When choosing which mode of transport is suitable for a patient, multiple factors require consideration including the limitations or advantages of the vehicle, platform availability, the clinical condition of the patients and the treatment requirements in transit as well as the required crew skill sets. Other considerations include familiarity with the mode of transport, equipment compatibility (helicopters prefer to land prior to performing defibrillation) and destination factors such as communications, trauma capabilities and distance from the scene. Many factors will overlap and there will often be more than one solution to a particular problem.

In-hospital care

On arrival at hospital, the prehospital crew will be required to provide a concise handover and depending on resources may need to assist with initial in-hospital management. It is important that the prehospital crew is both interrogated for any extra information that may prove relevant and thanked for their efforts in often imperfect and difficult conditions, prior to their departure.

In-hospital care will then follow <C>ABCDE guidelines or similar with suitable hospital speciality involvement.

Further reading

Greaves I, Porter K. The Oxford handbook of pre-hospital care. Oxford: Oxford University Press, 2013.

Lloyd D. Reported road casualties in Great Britain: 2012 annual report. London: Department for Transport, 2012.

Toroyan T. Global Status Report on Road Safety 2013: Supporting a Decade of Action. World Health Organization, 2013.

Related topics of interest

- Aeromedical evacuation and retrieval (p. 12)
- <C>ABCDE approach (p. 63)
- Epidemiology of trauma (p. 93)

Selective nonoperative management of penetrating abdominal injuries

Key points

- Not all penetrating abdominal injuries require laparotomy
- In the absence of signs of bleeding and peritonitis, a nonoperative approach should be considered
- CT is recommended for most penetrating injuries, and mandatory for ballistic injuries if nonoperative management is being contemplated. Nontherapeutic laparotomy rates should be minimised – as should delayed laparotomies for missed injuries

Clinical features

Selective nonoperative management (SNOM) of abdominal injury refers to a management strategy where the need for surgical exploration is decided on a case-by-case basis.

During the First World War, it was recognised that penetrating abdominal injuries were associated with high mortality. Mandatory exploration became the standard of care, and remained so throughout the Second World War and beyond. In the 1960s, however, it was noted that many abdominal explorations for abdominal stab wounds were either negative and revealed no injuries at all, or nontherapeutic and revealed injuries which did not require exploration. A seminal study showed that only one third of patients with an abdominal stab wound who underwent mandatory exploration had suffered an intra-abdominal injury, and only one sixth had suffered a hollow viscus injury. It was also noted that many of these procedures were associated with morbidity, either in the short term, e.g. from wound infections or anaesthetic complications, or in the longer term, e.g. from adhesive bowel obstruction, and that the negative laparotomy was not as benign a procedure as had been

assumed. Nontherapeutic laparotomy also increases the length of hospital stays and costs to the health service.

Based on this observation, trauma surgeons began to manage stab wounds nonoperatively: patients who did not exhibit signs of bleeding or peritonitis were observed closely, and only operated on if these signs developed. The safety of this strategy has been confirmed in several retrospective and prospective studies. The selective management of stab wounds is facilitated by their relatively predictable injury pattern, and can be used as a strategy even in resource-limited settings, where cross-sectional imaging is not available. However, when such technology is available, it is often used to delineate the wound track, and corroborate the clinical impression of absence of organ injury. In summary, there is good evidence that many abdominal stab wounds are not associated with visceral injury, and can be managed without laparotomy. The Eastern Association for the Surgery of Trauma (EAST) recently published clinical practice guidelines, recommending that 'A routine laparotomy is not indicated in haemodynamically stable patients with abdominal stab wounds without signs of peritonitis or diffuse abdominal tenderness (away from the wounding site).'

The SNOM of injuries, caused by bullets or fragments originating from explosions, is more contentious, because these injuries are assumed to be associated with higher rates of organ injury requiring operative repair. While this assumption is probably correct, it does not mean that all ballistic abdominal injuries necessitate operation. Nevertheless, mandatory laparotomy remained the standard of care until the 1990s, when several observational studies, from South Africa and the United States, began to challenge this dogma. This paradigm shift was facilitated by the better availability of CT scanning, which permits accurate delineation of the wound track, and identification of organ injuries necessitating repair or resection. Several retrospective and prospective studies have now confirmed the safety of selective management of abdominal gunshot wounds and fragmentation injuries, although most of these originate from a small number of high-volume centres. Nevertheless, the EAST practice management guidelines recommend that 'a routine laparotomy is not indicated in haemodynamically stable patients with abdominal gunshot wounds if the wounds are tangential and there are no peritoneal signs,' and that 'patients with penetrating injury isolated to the right upper quadrant of the abdomen may be managed without laparotomy in the presence of stable vital signs, reliable examination and minimal to no abdominal tenderness.'

Diagnosis

The diagnosis of penetrating injury is usually obvious from the history and clinical examination. Recognition of bleeding is frequently based on abnormal vital signs, but haemorrhage may also be externalised, and is usually relatively straightforward to diagnose. The detection of hollow viscus injury, particularly if signs are slow to develop, is more difficult. There is almost invariably some tenderness around the wound, confounding the assessment, which needs to be distinguished from pain caused by peritoneal irritation. This requires experience, and frequent and diligent examination, ideally by the same surgeon. Patients who are bleeding, or exhibit signs suggestive of a hollow viscus injury, require surgery, and should be managed operatively.

Investigations

CT scanning is mandatory if the nonoperative management of a ballistic injury is being considered. Although perhaps not absolutely essential for the management of stab wounds, CT can add useful information to the decision-making process, and the contemporary management of such injuries – at least in hospitals with reasonable access to cross-sectional imaging – should also include CT. CT evidence of peritoneal violation increases the likelihood of hollow viscus injury, but is not an absolute indication for exploration.

Stab wounds to the thoracoabdominal area, particularly on the left side, deserve particular attention. These injuries may result in violation of the diaphragm, which can lead to herniation and strangulation of abdominal viscera, sometimes months or years after the original injury. Diaphragmatic injury is easily missed on CT, and in the absence of other indications for exploration, these patients should therefore be considered for laparoscopy or thoracoscopy. Although this strategy does not constitute 'nonoperative' management, it still represents a lesser iatrogenic insult than an exploratory laparotomy.

Complications

Missed injuries are the Achilles' heel of selective management. The presence of solid organ injuries will usually be known, if cross-sectional imaging was used, and bleeding from such injuries will usually present with gradual deterioration in vital signs and/or decreasing haemoglobin. Providing patients are adequately monitored, this complication should be detected in a timely fashion.

Undetected, or late-detected, hollow viscus injury presents more insidiously, and thus can be more difficult to diagnose. It also has, arguably, more serious consequences. Established intra-abdominal infection may lead to short- and long-term complications, and may impact on the likelihood of being able to restore gastrointestinal continuity. Concern regarding such injuries should therefore be acted upon promptly.

Most failures of selectively managed penetrating abdominal injuries present within 24 hours of admission. Patients should be observed for this period, but can be discharged thereafter.

In summary, selective management of penetrating injuries is feasible, and has the potential to reduce nontherapeutic laparotomy rates. However, selectivism should not be performed at the expense of safety. When there is concern, patients are usually best served by an operation.

Further reading

Como JJ, Bokhari F, Chiu WC, et al. Practice management guidelines for selective nonoperative management of penetrating abdominal trauma. J Trauma 2010; 68:721–733.

Inaba K, Barmparas G, Foster A, et al. Selective nonoperative management of torso gunshot wounds: when is it safe to discharge? J Trauma 2010; 68:1301–1304.

Inaba K, Demetriades D. The non-operative management of penetrating abdominal trauma. Adv Surg 2007; 41:51–62.

Related topics of interest

Sexual violence

Key points

- Sexual violence is common, but under-reported
- All those who have been sexually assaulted need to be risk assessed for HIV and Hepatitis B
- Emergency contraception is licensed following sexual assault. Levonelle (Levonorgestrel 1500 mg) can be given up to 72 hours following the exposure

Introduction

The British Crime Survey of England and Wales 2012/13 stated that there had been 55,812 cases of sexual offences, including 17,061 cases of rape. Other studies claim that women living in the UK have one in five lifetime risk of sexual assault; however, it appears that only about one in 10 cases are reported to the police. One retrospective study in the US showed that approximately 4% of all assaults presenting to an emergency department were due to sexual assault.

Common injuries

Physical injuries following sexual assault can be extensive or absent. General body trauma occurs more commonly than genital trauma, the extremities being most commonly injured. The prevalence of nongenital injuries ranges between 28 and 97%, whereas anogenital trauma occurs in between 20 and 71%. There is a slightly higher rate of anogenital injury with digital or foreign object penetration. The presence of injury does not imply that intercourse was nonconsensual, nor does its absence mean assault has not occurred.

Initial management

Resuscitation takes priority over forensic examination. The usual process of caring for an injured patient should be undertaken, but any equipment that is used to treat the patient should be preserved after use (e.g. the laryngoscope, endotracheal tube, speculum, sponge holders, gloves or gauze). If stable, the patient can be referred to a sexual assault referral centre (SARC) within England and Wales. However if the patient requires ongoing medical treatment in hospital, a sexual offence examiner (SOE) can be dispatched to carry out a forensic examination in hospital. Similar centres exist throughout the UK and abroad. In the USA, a sexual assault nurse specialist will be available either within the emergency department or by agreement at a nearby facility.

Some emergency departments in the UK have early evidence kits that should be used to preserve evidence in patients wishing to wash prior to the arrival of an SOE. Later, urine will be tested for drugs and a mouth swab for DNA in cases of oral penetration. Any toxicology screens which are done in the emergency department are unlikely to be used in court, as they do not conform to established chain of evidence procedures.

The examination may sometimes be performed without explicit consent, e.g. in the case of a violent assault in an intubated patient. It must only be performed in the best interest of the patient or in the interests of the safety of the public, and always with the consent of the admitting team. In very violent assaults, the police must be contacted in order to ensure that necessary steps are taken to ensure the public safety.

If the patient is fit for discharge, an internal examination should not be carried out, in order to preserve DNA evidence. Minor vaginal or per rectal spotting can be dealt with by a team member at the SARC. Many SARCs offer anonymous forensic services, examination and counselling services for those not wishing to involve the police.

Other actions

Following an initial disclosure of sexual assault, emergency department staff should document the patient's account of events word for word. This account can be called upon in court, as there are normally very few witnesses to a sexual assault. It is important to question the patient about their use of alcohol and drugs and document their response. If the victim did take these it will not necessarily affect the validity of the case, but if it was later found out that these were taken yet not disclosed, then that would reduce the integrity of their other statements.

Definitions

Rape

Rape is the intentional penetration by the penis of the vagina, anus or mouth of another person without consent.

Assault by penetration

Assault by penetration is the intentional penetration of the vagina or anus with a part of the body or anything else without consent.

Sexual assault

Sexual assault is intentional sexual touching without consent.

Consent

A person can only give valid consent if he or she agrees by choice and has the freedom and capacity to make that choice. If a child is 13 – 16-year-old they could have capacity. There is no defence if a child is under 13-year-old.

Follow-up care

All those who have been sexually assaulted need to be risk assessed for HIV. Guidelines from the British Association of Sexual Health and HIV (BASHH) clarify who needs postexposure prophylaxis after sexual exposure (PEPSE) (**Table 34**). It is surprising how few patients are actually at risk, and before commencing a course the patient should be aware of the side effects and long duration of treatment required. Initiation of a hepatitis B vaccination programme or a booster is advised. Hepatitis B immunoglobulin will be needed if the assailant is likely or known to be a hepatitis B surface antigen carrier.

Prior to starting PEPSE, a screen of blood tests should be done to ascertain any contraindications, and to provide a baseline for future side effects of treatment. A baseline serum save should also be taken in case any HIV or hepatitis results become positive at the 3 month check.

Emergency contraception is licensed following sexual assault. Levonelle (Levonorgestrel 1500 mg) can be given up to 72 hours following the exposure. If PEPSE is given, this dose must be doubled. ellaOne (Ulipristal Acetate 30 mg) is licensed for up to 5 days after the exposure but is contraindicated if giving PEPSE. If PEPSE is required, consideration should be given to

Table 34 British Association of Sexual Health and HIV's guidelines for when PEPSE is advised				
	HIV + VL detected	HIV + VL undetected	Unknown HIV status, high risk	Unknown HIV status, low risk
Receptive anal	Recommended	Recommended	Recommended	No
Insertive anal	Recommended	No	Consider	No
Receptive vaginal	Recommended	No	Consider	No
Insertive vaginal	Recommended	No	Consider	No
Fellatio + ejaculation	No	No	No	No
Fellatio – ejaculation	No	No	No	No
Splash of semen to eye	Consider	No	No	No
Cunnilingus	No	No	No	No
VL, viral load; PEPSE, postexposure prophylaxis after sexual exposure.				

arranging intrauterine device insertion, which may be done up to 5 days after the exposure, depending on the patient's menstrual cycle. Recommended medications may vary over time and throughout the world.

Prophylactic antibiotics should be considered; gonorrhoea, chlamydia and trichomoniasis are the most common infections. Ideally these should be tested for specifically rather than giving blind treatment. Patients should be directed to a genitourinary medicine (GUM) clinic. A sexual health screen is recommended 2 weeks after the exposure. Any sooner than this is liable to result in falsely negative results. The patient should be advised to use barrier contraception until they have been fully cleared by a GUM clinic.

A screen for risk of deliberate self-harm is required before discharge. A vulnerable adult assessment or child protection referral may be required.

Professional debriefing in the 1st month following a sexual assault is thought to be unhelpful; in the UK, the guidelines from NICE (National Institute for Health and Care Excellence) recommend watchful waiting for this time. There is an extremely high incidence of post-traumatic stress disorder in sexual assault victims, so the patient should be advised and encouraged to seek professional help if they have flashbacks, recurrent nightmares, hyperarousal or emotional numbing.

Further reading

Basile SL, Mahendra K, Steenkamp R, Ingram M, Ikeda E. National estimates of sexual violence treated in emergency departments. Ann Emerg Med 2007; 49:210–217.

Clinical Effectiveness Group: British Association for Sexual Health and HIV (BASHH). UK National guidelines on the management of adult and adolescent complainants of sexual assault. Macclesfield: BASHH, 2011.

Payne-James J and Beh P. Adult sexual assault. Current practice in forensic medicine. London: John Wiley & Sons, 2011:95–118.

Related topics of interest

Shock

Key points

- Shock is a critical failure of tissue perfusion and oxygenation, resulting in cellular dysfunction
- Common traumatic causes relate to failure of cardiac preload (cardiac tamponade, tension pneumothorax and hypovolaemia), contractility (myocardial contusions) or cardiac afterload (neurogenic shock)
- Without prompt recognition and reversal, shock frequently results in death or serious organ injury

Epidemiology

It is estimated that one in five traumatic deaths is potentially preventable and shock is a presenting feature in 90% of these patients. Shock is a general state that reflects a failure of tissue perfusion and oxygenation and is the final common pathway in several injury processes discussed in this and other key topics. Recognition is important, as the underlying pathology is frequently a threat to life and prompt intervention may save the patient.

Pathophysiology

Tissue oxygen delivery supporting aerobic cellular metabolism is critical to normal cellular function. Shock is the process which occurs when tissue oxygen consumption exceeds tissue oxygen delivery. Conversion of cellular metabolism from aerobic to anaerobic pathways results in a metabolic acidosis and the generation of a myriad of metabolic by-products such as nitric oxide, oxygen radicals and lactic acid. These metabolites drive physiological dyshomeostasis and provoke an innate immune response, driving further haemodynamic instability, tissue ischaemia and systematic inflammation.

This cellular pathway observed in traumatic shock can be initiated by several pathologies, largely mediated by the disruption of cardiac, pulmonary or vascular function. Reduction in preload is the most common cause of shock, which can arise either through obstruction to venous return (cardiac tamponade and tension pneumothorax) or loss of circulating volume (haemorrhage). Hypoxia from airway obstruction or pulmonary parenchymal injury directly contributes to hypoxaemia and shock. Less common causes include reduced myocardial contractility following direct myocardial injury or the sudden loss of cardiac afterload following a cervical cord injury disrupting sympathetic nervous outflow.

Clinical features

General findings

The presentation of shock will vary depending on the severity of metabolic compromise. Patients in the early stage of their clinical course may demonstrate little physiological derangement, whereas patients in advanced shock may well present in extremis with little or no cardiac output. In the majority of cases, significant sympathetic nervous stimulation is a strong feature.

Patients are often anxious, with a sense of impending catastrophe, which may progress to confusion and a reduced conscious level. Significantly hypoxic patients will be cyanosed. The skin of shocked patients is frequently cool and clammy to touch, with a mottled appearance as peripheral perfusion reduces. The exception to this is in the settling of neurogenic shock, where peripheral vasoconstriction is lost and patients generally have warm extremities.

Specific causes of shock

Tension pneumothorax

Tension pneumothorax is less common than recent learning programmes might suggest. It can occur rapidly in the ventilated patient, but may evolve slowly in a spontaneously breathing patient and consequently is sometimes diagnosed on a plain radiograph. Physical evidence of chest injury and pain are common features. In addition to reduced breath sounds on the ipsilateral side, hypotension is a key feature. The classical tracheal deviation is a late sign.

Cardiac tamponade

Tamponade is more common with penetrating injury, but can occur following blunt trauma. Beck's triad, which consists of an elevated jugular venous pressure, hypotension and muffled heart sounds related to preload obstruction, is of little value clinically in a noisy resuscitation room. Cardiac ultrasound is ideal for rapid diagnosis. The blood pressure may also fall on inspiration (termed pulsus paradoxus) but again this is a difficult sign to elicit.

Haemorrhage

In haemorrhage, tachycardia and hypotension predominate as described above. Other clinical features usually relate to the region of injury, e.g. abdominal pain following a liver injury. However, other injuries can distract and some body cavities can be 'silent' in their presentation, e.g. retroperitoneal haemorrhage. Bleeding can also cross anatomical boundaries: a massive haemothorax may drain into the abdomen through a diaphragmatic perforation.

Myocardial contusions

Myocardial contusions are typically seen following blunt trauma and in adults may be associated with a sternal fracture or flail chest. Flail segments, which are exceptionally uncommon in children, are often best identified by observing the chest tangentially from low down at the end of the bed. Early blood gas analysis may show hypoxia with normocarbia. Patients present with chest pain, hypotension and cardiac arrhythmias.

Neurogenic shock

This is associated with severe cervical or upper thoracic spinal injury, which is evident in the history and presentation. Classically patients are hypotensive with warm peripheries.

Investigations and diagnosis

These should be expeditious, focused and must not delay intervention.

Physiological observations

Basic physiological recordings (heart rate, respiratory rate, blood pressure and pulse oximetry) are essential. Shocked patients frequently present with an elevated pulse and respiratory rates along with reduced blood pressure and peripheral capillary oxygen saturation (Spo_2). However, it is very important to be aware of the limitations of these tests.

Pain and anxiety will increase the pulse and respiratory rates, necessitating analgesia and serial measurements. There can be no justification for withholding analgesia in order to avoid masking symptoms. Younger patients may have considerable physiological reserve, preserving relatively normal values until they decompensate. In contrast, elderly patients may have a blunted physiological response, exaggerated by medical comorbidity and polypharmacy (e.g. beta-blockers). Furthermore, measuring devices may have technical limitations. For example, automated pneumatic blood pressure cuffs do not accurately read below 80 mmHg and Spo_2 monitors do not return accurate readings from poorly perfused extremities.

Arterial blood gas chemistry

Baseline lactate or base excess measurements can help identify shocked patients and quantify the degree of shock. Serial measurements will help determine patient's response to treatment. A rising lactate in the face of active treatment is a particularly ominous sign suggestive of an underestimation of the injury or a missed injury. Oxygenation is another useful measure, and a fall may be the first sign of inadequacy of gas exchange.

Imaging

Following the identification of a shocked patient, ultrasound and radiological imaging can be helpful in determining the underlying cause. However, where there is strong clinical suspicion, imaging should not be sought in preference to treatment. Early chest and pelvic films are useful for the identification of life-threatening haemo- or pneumothoraces, pulmonary contusions and pelvic fractures, respectively. Ultrasonography is increasingly available; however, it suffers from interuser variability and with the advent of CT pan-scanning protocols, is probably best used for the identification of cardiac standstill or tamponade, or to assist with venous access. However, the extended focussed abdominal sonography in trauma examination is a well-described protocol that assesses abdominal and pericardial free fluid. This is helpful for identifying abdominal haemorrhage and cardiac tamponade.

CT is the gold standard for the assessment of the traumatised patient. It enables the precise identification of injuries, both clinically evident and occult. Sufficient clinical advantage may be gained that CT pan-scanning is of value in the unstable as well as the stable patient, although clearly such a procedure would be inappropriate in any patient with an identified lesion requiring immediate surgery. The description of the CT scanner as the doughnut of death is obsolete and many shocked patients have had their lives saved by careful management during rapid scanning which has identified the nature of their injuries and facilitated expeditious management.

Treatment
General principles

Patients exhibiting signs of shock following traumatic injury should wherever possible be managed in a major trauma centre by a specialist team. The primary survey should be conducted in accordance with <C>ABCDE principles, where life-threatening problems are identified and treated in parallel. Once a shocked patient is identified, the underlying cause or causes must be sought and promptly corrected.

Specific conditions
Tension pneumothorax

Initially, the tension should be released by a cannula placed in the second intercostal space in the midclavicular line on the side of the tension pneumothorax. An alternative is a finger thoracostomy performed through the fifth intercostal space. The latter is more definitive than a cannula, but is best suited

to ventilated patients or the prehospital environment if the appropriate skills are available. Chest decompression must be followed up by formal chest drainage and repeat thoracic imaging.

Cardiac tamponade

Tamponade requires urgent decompression, especially in the periarrest or arrest situation. Needle pericardiocentesis has no role in a traumatic tamponade, when operative exposure is preferred. In the emergency setting, a clamshell thoracotomy is an effective approach, although in a more prepared setting, a midline sternotomy can reduce incisional morbidity. In patients who recover a spontaneous circulation, a surgical repair of the right atrium or ventricle is usually required.

Haemorrhage

This requires a parallel approach of resuscitation and haemorrhage control. The nature of such approaches will depend on the injury pattern and presentation. Equally, shocked patients responding to damage control resuscitation who become haemodynamically stable, may be managed nonoperatively. Resuscitative endovascular balloon occlusion of the aorta, prior to extensive operative exposure is a novel technique for use in profoundly shocked patients on the cusp of haemodynamic collapse, although its value is yet to be established (see pages 252-254).

Hypoxia

The treatment of hypoxia ranges from the administration of supplemental oxygen by mask to ventilation following endotracheal intubation. Most pulmonary injuries can be managed by chest drainage, although on occasion surgical lobectomy or pneumonectomy is required.

Myocardial contusions

Following the exclusion of other potential causes of shock, most patients can be observed with continuous ECG monitoring. Most arrhythmias are benign and will terminate spontaneously, although intervention is occasionally required. For ongoing hypotension, careful inotrope support may be required.

Neurogenic shock

In the immediate term, spinal stabilisation and pressor support must be provided.

Longer-term care should focus on maximising functional outcome.

Further reading

American College of Surgeons. Advanced trauma life support student course manual, 9th edn. Chicago: American College of Surgeons, 2012.

Cohn SM, Dolich MO, Inaba K. Acute care surgery and trauma: evidence-based practice, 1st edn. London: Informa, 2009.

Rasmussen TE, Tai NRM. Rich's vascular trauma, 3rd edn. Atlanta: Elsevier, 2015.

Related topics of interest

Shoulder, clavicle and proximal humerus fractures

Key points

- Shoulder, clavicle and humerus fractures should be considered following all falls onto an outstretched hand
- There are few absolute indications for surgery. Treatment should be individualised
- CT scanning may assist the planning of treatment in the case of complex fractures

Epidemiology

Fractures of the proximal humerus are common and account for 5–10% of all fractures. Fractures of the clavicle represent 2–5% of all fractures and 40% of all shoulder girdle fractures.

Pathophysiology

In low-energy mechanisms, both proximal humerus and clavicle fractures usually result from a fall onto the affected shoulder. Low-energy proximal humerus fractures are usually associated with osteoporotic bone. Clavicle fractures may also result from a fall onto the outstretched arm. High-energy injuries are often a result of road traffic collisions, leading to significant polytrauma.

Clinical features

Pain, swelling and deformity occur, often instantly and movements are painful. A displaced clavicle fracture may cause overlying skin tenting, leading to skin necrosis if not reduced and stabilised. Even low-energy proximal humerus fractures may be associated with an axillary nerve palsy or vascular damage and the neurovascular status must be assessed.

High-energy injuries should be examined thoroughly for signs of damage to the brachial plexus and the limb vascular status should be assessed. Other fractures of the shoulder girdle or the presence of a 'floating shoulder' should be excluded. Concomitant chest injuries, e.g. pneumothorax or scapulothoracic dissociation may occur and can be fatal if they are missed.

Investigations

Plain radiographs for the proximal humerus include anteroposterior (AP) and lateral views. An axillary view should be taken if possible when glenohumeral dislocation is suspected. For clavicle fractures, in many cases, an AP and cephalic tilt view will suffice. If the fracture is complex, a CT scan with 3D reconstruction further delineates the fracture and may alter management.

Diagnosis and classification

The proximal humerus fracture classification introduced by Neer in 1970 remains the most popular. Neer classified proximal humerus fractures as two-, three-, or four-part fractures. To be considered displaced, there should be 1 cm or 45° of displacement of the fractured part (**Figure 72**). Allman classified clavicle shaft fractures into midshaft, medial or lateral. Neer classified distal clavicle fractures as shown in **Figure 73**.

Management

The rationale for operative fixation of proximal humerus and clavicle fractures is debated and treatment should be individualised. There have been no randomised controlled trials defining best practice. Indications of surgical intervention for both fracture types include open fracture, associated neurovascular injury, floating shoulder, skin compromise and pathological fracture.

Proximal humerus fractures
Nonoperative

Undisplaced (according to Neer), low-energy proximal humerus fractures are

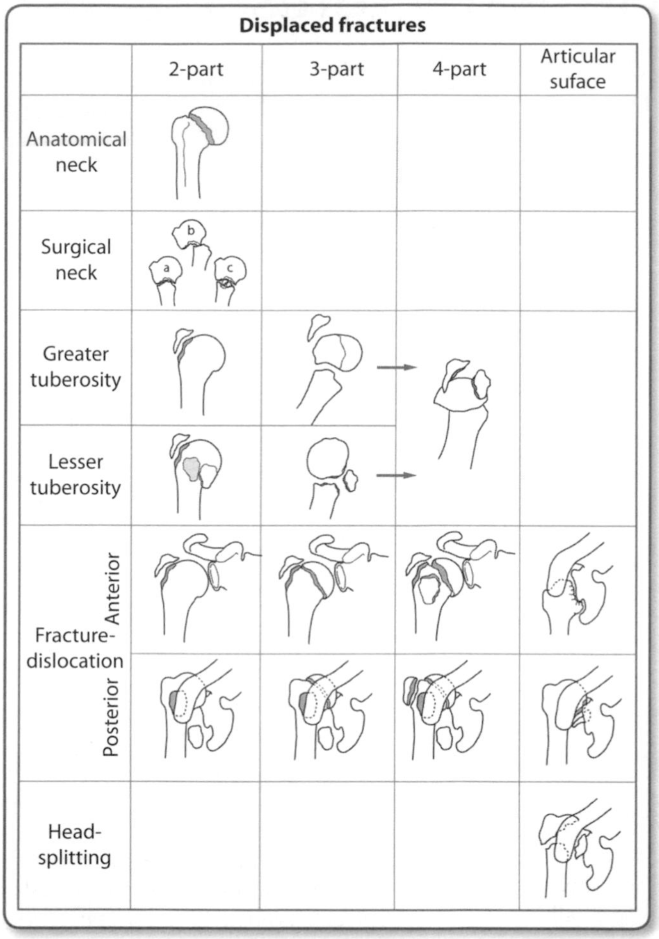

Figure 72 Classification of proximal humerus fractures.

often managed in a collar and cuff. Early pendulum exercises, followed by progressive mobilisation can be commenced from as early as weeks 2 or 3 if radiographs are satisfactory. Patients with significant comorbidity and pre-existing poor function should be managed nonoperatively.

Operative

The objective of operative treatment is to restore the anatomical relationship of the head and tuberosities, and facilitate early mobilisation to prevent stiffness. Displaced fractures in young patients warrant fixation. The optimal management of elderly patients with displaced fractures is uncertain. Hertel identified several predictors of avascular necrosis, which can be used to determine whether to fix or replace the humeral head. Accurate predictors for humeral head ischaemia include integrity of the 'medial hinge', fractures involving the anatomic neck and <8 mm metaphyseal fracture extension.

Plates

Most proximal humerus surgery involves fixation using locking plates. These form a fixed angle construct. Locking plates have advantages in osteoporotic bone; minimising screw cut-out and hardware failure. Screws should be placed in the strong subchondral bone in the humeral head. If there is a fracture of the greater and/or lesser tuberosity, this should be fixed either with screws or sutures – often tied through the eyelets of the plate (**Figure 74a** and **b**).

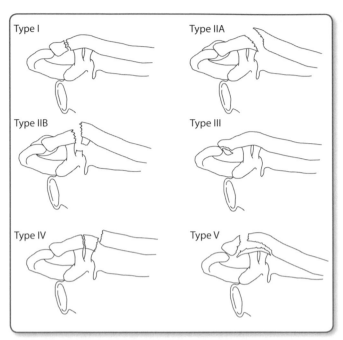

Figure 73 Neer classification of distal clavicle fractures.

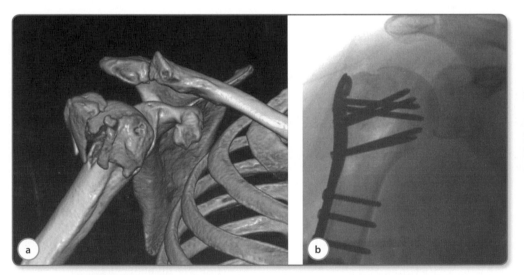

Figure 74 (a) Three-dimensional recon CT image showing a four-part proximal humerus fracture. (b) Intraoperative imaging showing proximal humerus plate fixation using a contoured locking plate.

Proximal humeral nails

These can be used to treat segmental fractures involving the neck and the shaft. Multiplanar screws can capture separate fragments. If the fracture is amenable to closed reduction, the nail can be inserted using a minimally invasive approach.

Arthroplasty

Reconstruction of the humeral head becomes increasingly challenging as comminution increases. Arthroplasty options include hemiarthroplasty or reverse geometry arthroplasty. Hemiarthroplasty often leads to poor functional outcomes. Tuberosity escape is a common complication. Reverse arthroplasty maximises the deltoid lever arm. This improves movement in a cuff which is poorly functioning; either due to coexistent cuff arthropathy, irreparable cuff tear, or unreconstructable tuberosities. Reverse shoulder arthroplasty can lead to improved functional outcomes.

Clavicle fractures

Nonoperative

Clavicle fractures have been traditionally managed nonoperatively. Midshaft fractures with minimal displacement and low-energy mechanisms can be managed in a broad-arm sling for 4–6 weeks with progressive rehabilitation. Minimally displaced lateral end of clavicle fractures can be managed nonoperatively although these are at a greater risk of nonunion.

Operative

Recent meta-analyses have revealed certain fractures which may benefit from plate fixation, including fractures that are high-energy, or those with >2 cm of shortening and 100% displacement. Operative fixation in these cases leads to a higher rate of union and improved functional outcome Displaced distal clavicle fractures have a high rate of nonunion and functional deficit. These fractures may warrant surgery.

Plates

Midshaft clavicle fractures are often treated with small fragment plate fixation. Traditional low contact-dynamic compression plates or contoured clavicle plates can be used. Plates can sit either superiorly, anteriorly, or anterosuperiorly. Anterior placement allows longer screws to be used, which improves the rigidity of the construct. There is also less risk of damage to subclavian vessels which also causes less irritation postoperatively.

For lateral clavicle fractures, contoured distal clavicle plates are available. These provide numerous locking options in the distal part of the plate to stabilise the fracture. Traditional hook plates can also be used (**Figure 75a** and **b**).

Other fixation methods

Displaced distal clavicle fractures involve disruption of the coracoclavicular ligaments (conoid and trapezoid). Devices can be used to reapproximate the clavicle in relation to the coracoid. These include the Tightrope (Arthrex, Florida) and Surgilig (Smith & Nephew, London). In certain patients, these may not provide sufficient strength alone and may need augmentation with other methods of fixation.

Complications

Complications can be divided into immediate, early and late.

Immediate

The standard deltopectoral approach to the proximal humerus risks damage to the neurovascular structures, particularly the axillary nerve, humeral circumflex vessels, and with errant retractor placement; the brachial plexus medial to the conjoint tendon.

The approach to the clavicle risks damage to the supraclavicular nerves and, more medially, damage to the subclavian vessels. Care should be taken when drilling – particularly when drilling in a superior–inferior direction in the medial third of the bone.

Early

Wound infection can occur in 1–2%. Hardware failure, due to weak bone or inadequate fixation, may also occur early, particularly in clavicle fractures.

Late

In proximal humerus fracture fixation, nonunion and malunion are not uncommon. Nonunion may necessitate further intervention using bone graft. Screw cut-out through the humeral head can be a complication. Avascular necrosis is a complication of three- or four-part fractures.

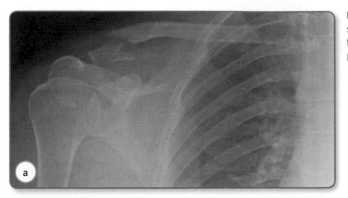

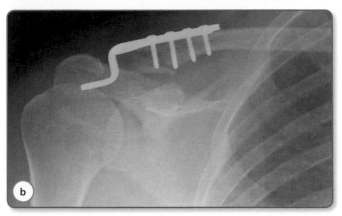

Figure 75 (a) Plain radiograph showing a displaced distal clavicle fracture. (b) Fixation using a hook plate.

Stiffness is a common problem postoperatively and can be difficult to treat. This warrants extensive physiotherapy, and if this fails, cautious manipulation under anaesthesia, and sometimes arthroscopic or open release of the capsule or extra-articular adhesions.

Arthroplasty in the trauma setting may be complicated by escape of the tuberosities, which correlates with poor function. Dislocation, late infection and loosening are difficult problems to treat.

Malunion is the greatest complication in fractures managed nonoperatively. Fractures that are fixed may still lead to nonunion. Revision fixation with bone grafting may be needed.

Scapula fractures

Scapular fractures normally result from high-energy trauma, often a direct blow to the thorax and shoulder girdle after a road traffic collision or fall from a height. Glenoid rim fractures may result from lower-energy injuries and can be associated with glenohumeral dislocation. There is an overall mortality rate of 2–5%. Associated orthopaedic injuries are common; rib fractures in half of patients, clavicle and/or spine fractures in approximately a quarter, and brachial plexus injuries in 5–10%. Injuries to cardiothoracic and other vascular structures may be present. Clinical examination should focus on these associated systems as well as the shoulder girdle in accordance with <C>ABCDE protocols.

Plain radiographs including AP, scapular and axillary lateral views will show most fractures. To delineate fracture fragments and plan reconstruction, or if radiographs are unclear, CT scans and particularly 3D reconstructions are useful.

The classification of scapular fractures is based on the anatomical part of the scapula involved, e.g. the coracoid, acromion, glenoid, scapular neck and scapular body. Glenoid fractures are intra-articular fractures and therefore deserve mention, as anatomical reduction and rigid fixation may be preferred. These injuries have been subclassified by Ideberg.

The vast majority of scapular body fractures heal uneventfully by 6 weeks with nonoperative management in a sling. Scapular fractures, however are uncommon, and indications for operative fixation within the literature are vague. General indications for surgery include open fractures and those with associated neurovascular damage involving the axillary vessels and brachial plexus. Glenoid fractures with associated humeral subluxation or dislocation also warrant operative intervention. Significantly displaced scapular neck fractures may affect shoulder biomechanics as well as rotator cuff function and therefore may warrant surgery.

Further reading

Alentorn-Geli E, Guirro P, Santana F, Torrens C. Treatment of fracture sequelae of the proximal humerus: comparison of hemiarthroplasty and reverse total shoulder arthroplasty. Arch Orthop Trauma Surg 2014; 134:1545–1550.

Cuff DJ, Pupello DR. Comparison of hemiarthroplasty and reverse shoulder arthroplasty for the treatment of proximal humeral fractures in elderly patients. J Bone Joint Surg Am 2013; 95:2050–2055.

Hertel R, Hempfing A, Stiehler M, Leunig M. Predictors of humeral head ischemia after intracapsular fracture of the proximal humerus. J Shoulder Elbow Surg 2004; 13:427–433.

McKee RC, Whelan DB, Schemitsch EH, McKee MD. Operative versus nonoperative care of displaced midshaft clavicular fractures: a meta-analysis of randomized clinical trials. J Bone Joint Surg Am 2012; 94:675–684.

Neer CS 2nd. Displaced proximal humerus fractures. I. Classification and evaluation. J Bone Joint Surg Am 1970; 52:1077–1089.

Parnes N, Jupiter JB. Fixed-angle locking plating of displaced proximal humerus fractures. Instr Course Lect 2010; 59:539–552.

Related topics of interest

Soft tissue knee injuries

Key points

- The history is critical in evaluating knee injuries
- Pain in the knee can be referred from the hip or spine
- The optimal imaging modality for soft tissue knee injuries is MRI

Introduction

The knee is a complex hinge joint primarily allowing movement in the flexion and extension planes but also some rotation. Knee stability is mainly reliant on its soft tissue structures and the complex interplay between passive (menisci and ligaments) and active stabilisers (tendons and muscles) for carrying out its function. Soft tissue knee injuries range from simple meniscal injuries to complex multiligament injuries in the polytrauma setting.

Pathophysiology

The history and mechanism of injury are critical and any trauma should be identified as either high energy (e.g. an automobile collision) or low energy (such as a fall from standing). High-energy trauma should prompt systematic examination of other organ systems. The location of pain is often an indication of the underlying pathology (**Table 35**).

Meniscal injuries

The menisci of the knee are nourished centrally by synovial fluid and peripherally by its vascular plexus. The function of the menisci is to dissipate forces through the knee and they are most susceptible to tears when under abnormal axial and rotational loads. The medial meniscus is less mobile than the lateral meniscus and is therefore more easily torn. Meniscal injury is one of the most common soft tissue injuries affecting the knee joint with acute tears predominating in younger patients and degenerative tears in older patients. The site and configuration of the tear or tears will influence the treatment options and subsequent outcome.

Clinical features

Patients often present with a delayed effusion and symptoms of pain, catching or locking and giving way. The McMurray test can be used to determine the presence of a meniscal tear. To assess the lateral meniscus, the knee is placed in full flexion, and axial loading and valgus stress are applied. The knee is then gradually extended and externally rotated. Positive test findings include pain and a clicking sensation. To assess the medial meniscus, a similar movement is conducted with the knee in internal rotation.

Investigations

The most sensitive imaging modality to confirm meniscal injury is MRI.

Treatment

Asymptomatic tears are treated nonoperatively, whereas symptomatic tears are treated by arthroscopic meniscectomy or repair (for peripheral tears).

Table 35 Approach to knee pain by location			
Medial knee pain	**Anterior knee pain**	**Lateral knee pain**	**Posterior knee pain**
Medial collateral ligament tear	Extensor mechanism dysfunction	Lateral collateral ligament tear	Popliteal cyst
Anserine bursitis	Patellofemoral syndrome	Iliotibial band syndrome	Hamstring tear
Medial meniscal tear	Prepatellar bursitis	Lateral meniscal tear	Deep venous thrombosis
			Popliteal aneurysm

Complications

A significant proportion of patients may develop osteoarthritis as a result of the injury to the meniscus or articular cartilage.

Ligamentous injuries

Collateral ligament injury occurs as a result of varus–valgus stresses and can result in instability. The possibility of associated extra-articular injuries should be considered when anterior cruciate ligament (ACL) rupture is present. Although infrequent, tibiofemoral dislocation is a surgical emergency.

The ACL is the most commonly injured knee ligament. Women engaging in pivoting sports sustain ACL tears significantly more frequently than men. Injury to the posterior cruciate ligament (PCL) is predominantly caused by sports-related activity and motor vehicle collisions, where dashboard injuries are the most common specific cause. Dislocations occur as a result of high-energy injuries including sports injuries and motor vehicle collisions.

Collateral ligament injury usually occurs when a varus or valgus force is applied to the knee. The ACL is the primary restraint to anterior tibial translation and is usually injured as a result of sudden deceleration hyperextension or rotational force. The PCL is the primary restraint to posterior tibial translation. Mechanisms of injury include hyperflexion, hyperextension injuries or direct force to the front of the tibia. Due to the mechanism of injury, knee dislocations cause multiple ligamentous disruption with significant soft tissue and bony damage.

Clinical features

Ligament tears of the knee joint are graded based on clinical and radiological evaluation (**Table 36**). Patients who sustain purely a valgus or varus force may have an isolated collateral ligament injury. Assessing collateral ligament laxity is performed by applying varus and valgus stresses with the knee in full extension (0°) and at 30° of flexion.

If there is varus or valgus laxity at 30° only, there is likely to be an isolated injury to the medial collateral ligament (MCL) or lateral collateral ligament. However if there is laxity also in extension, there is also likely to be injury to posterior capsule, ACL or PCL. In an ACL rupture, the patient classically describes an audible 'pop' following which there is rapid swelling (haemarthrosis) and pain.

The three diagnostic tests for an ACL injury are the anterior drawer, Lachman and pivot shift tests, although these may be difficult to carry out in an acute setting. It is important to examine the knee for injury to other structures in the joint (as in O'Donoghue's triad of ACL and MCL rupture combined with medial meniscus tear). Patients with a PCL rupture often have a classic history of direct injury to the anterior aspect of the flexed knee such as in a dashboard injury or a fall in sport. Specific tests include a posterior drawer and posterior sag sign. Tibiofemoral dislocations are often clinically obvious given the history of acute trauma and gross deformity. As some dislocations may reduce spontaneously, one needs to have a high index of suspicion to avoid missing the potential complications of these injuries. In such cases, there is likely to be an effusion and evidence of gross ligamentous laxity.

Investigations

Plain radiographs of the knee are useful for assessing associated bony injuries and bony avulsions. MRI, however, is the modality of choice for evaluating the location and extent of injury as well as identifying other intra-articular pathology. In the setting of a knee dislocation, the vascular status may need to be assessed by Doppler ultrasound and angiography.

Treatment

Grades 1–2 collateral ligament injuries are treated with physiotherapy and bracing. For more severe injuries or those in association with other ligamentous injuries,

Table 36 Grading of ligamentous injury	
Grade 1	Ligament stretch, but no fibre disruption. No laxity
Grade 2	Partial ligament tear, but no laxity
Grade 3	Complete ligamentous tear, with laxity

consideration needs to be given to repair (acute) or reconstruction (chronic). ACL injuries can be managed nonoperatively (physiotherapy and bracing). Surgical reconstruction is reserved for those wishing to return to pivoting activities, those who have symptoms of instability, meniscal injuries or associated multiligamentous injuries. The majority of PCL injuries are treated nonoperatively with emphasis on rehabilitation and bracing.

Any knee dislocation will need to be reduced. The knee must then be immobilised and associated injuries treated. A vascular surgeon may need to be involved to treat any vascular injury. Early reconstruction of the disrupted ligaments provides the best results when carried out within 3 weeks of the injury.

Complications

Lateral injury may be complicated by common peroneal nerve injury. Severe collateral ligament injuries, if untreated, may lead to chronic laxity with subsequent development of osteoarthritis. The complications of conservative management of ACL injuries include persistent instability with the risk of meniscal tears and articular cartilage injury and subsequent osteoarthritis even after reconstructive surgery. Knee dislocation may be associated with injury to the popliteal artery and common peroneal nerve.

Further reading

Bollen S. Epidemiology of knee injuries: diagnosis and triage. Br J Sports Med 2000; 34:227.

Seroyer ST, Musahl V, Harner CD. Management of the acute knee dislocation: the Pittsburgh experience. Injury 2008; 39:710–718.

Shulz MS, Ruse K, Echhorn HJ, Eichhorn HJ, Strobel MJ. Epidemiology of posterior cruciate ligament injuries. Arch Orthop Trauma Surg 2003; 123:186–191.

Related topics of interest

Spinal cord injury without radiological abnormality

Key points

- Spinal cord injury without radiological abnormality (SCIWORA) is an acute traumatic myelopathy with normal radiographic and CT findings
- MRI is the best clinical tool for assessment of patients with SCIWORA and is helpful in prognosis
- Spinal cord injuries (SCIs) can be missed in the multiple injured patient

Epidemiology

The total incidence of SCI is 19–47 per million population. SCIWORA is commonest in children, accounting for between 20% and 30% of paediatric SCI cases. The majority occur in children under 8 years of age. SCIWORA in adults is less common, accounting for up to 18% of total SCIs. Road traffic collisions, falls and sporting injuries account for most cases in both adults and children.

Pathophysiology

SCIWORA is defined as a traumatic myelopathy (signs of SCI) without concurrent signs of fracture or ligamentous instability on plain radiographs or CT scans.

In children, SCIWORA can be explained by the differential elasticity of the spinal column and spinal cord. The highly elastic ligamentous structures in the immature spinal column can be stretched up to 2 cm without sustaining injury, whereas the spinal cord can only be stretched up to 0.5 cm.

In adults, nonphysiological movement of the spine can distract or compress the spinal cord leading to damage. This is more likely in patients with cervical spondylosis, spinal canal stenosis, ankylosing spondylitis and other degenerative conditions. In these groups, less force is required to injure the spinal cord, without concurrent skeletal injury.

The injury of the spinal cord is due to the initial primary mechanical insult, in addition to critical ischaemia in the surrounding area. Treatment is based on preserving the surrounding critical area by preventing any secondary insults due to poor oxygenation and perfusion, or by further direct damage.

Clinical features

In the multiply injured trauma patient, a spinal injury may not be immediately recognisable. Careful consideration should be given to the possibility of occult spinal injury in unconscious or intoxicated patients or those with pre-existing risk factors, such as cervical spondylosis or other degenerative spinal disease. A thorough neurological examination is needed in order not to miss a spinal injury, and careful senior review of imaging is essential. Any uncertainty requires continuation of spinal immobilisation. Repeated neurological examination is needed in order to detect any extension of the original insult. Accurate and regular recording of examination findings is important, preferably using a standardised assessment form, such as the American Spinal Injuries Association (ASIA) assessment tool. The patient may complain of spinal pain, inability to feel or move their limbs, and burning or an electric shock sensation in the trunk or limbs.

SCI in general will cause a variable degree of motor or sensory abnormality, depending on the level and degree of injury. The neurological level of injury is defined as the most caudal level with bilaterally normal motor and sensory function. It may not correlate with the level of injury. A complete SCI implies that there is no sensory or motor function more than three segments below the neurological level of injury, with no sacral sparing. An incomplete injury has partial preservation of function and sacral sparing. Sacral sparing implies some continuity of long tracts in the spinal cord and gives rise to intact perianal sensation, voluntary anal contraction and great toe flexor activity.

The degree of SCI cannot be determined immediately due to the presence of spinal shock. This is usually a period of up to 72 hours of complete loss of sensation, motor function and reflexes below the level of injury. SCI in an unconscious patient may be suspected if there is evidence of neurogenic shock, diaphragmatic breathing, flaccid areflexia or priapism.

In adults, SCIWORA is associated in 95% of cases with incomplete SCI, of which half have a central cord syndrome. In children under 8 years of age, 70% of cases have a complete injury with an unfavourable outcome. Children over the age of 12 years are more likely to have incomplete injuries and a more favourable outcome.

Central cord syndrome is commoner in adults with pre-existing cervical spine disease. It is due to pinching of the spinal cord between osteophytes anteriorly and a bunched up ligamentum flavum posteriorly. The upper extremities are affected more than the lower, and the distal areas worse than the proximal. It has the most favourable prognosis.

Investigations

The initial investigation of any patient suspected of having an SCI will be plain radiographs or CT scan. By definition, patients with SCIWORA will have no evidence of injury on these investigations. Therefore any patient with continued suspicion of SCI requires MRI of the spinal cord.

An MRI can detect ligamentous and intervertebral disc damage, vascular injury and SCI. The spinal cord may show injury due to haemorrhage, contusion or oedema. The spatial degree and nature of the injury evident on MRI correlate with the eventual outcome. The spatial extent is related to the neurological damage and rate of recovery.

The nature of the injury also relates to the degree of recovery; those with no demonstrable injury or oedema having the best recovery; those with contusion having the worst.

Treatment

The initial treatment of the multiple injured trauma patient proceeds according to conventional <C>ABCDE guidelines, with a rapid overall assessment in order to identify and treat significant injuries. If an SCI is suspected, it is important to prevent further direct injury with spinal immobilisation, and secondary injury by correcting hypoxia and hypoperfusion.

Spinal immobilisation is achieved by ensuring effective manual in-line stabilisation, or by use of sandbags and tape without a collar and standard spinal precautions including minimal handling. Hypoxia is corrected by maintaining oxygen saturations between 95% and 98% with oxygen therapy, establishing and maintaining a clear airway and ensuring adequate ventilation. Early intubation, paralysis and ventilation may be necessary. Shock is most likely to be attributable to haemorrhage and must be actively investigated, controlled and corrected. Neurogenic shock is likely in the presence of hypotension with bradycardia and peripheral vasodilatation, but may be present in combination with haemorrhage.

Incomplete spinal cord lesions with deteriorating or progressive neurological signs may be amenable to decompressive surgery. Steroids are not indicated in SCI and are associated with an increase in adverse events such as sepsis, gastrointestinal bleeding, pancreatitis and pulmonary embolism. The definitive care of patients with SCI by traction, bracing or surgery is best achieved in a specialist spinal injuries unit.

Further reading

Greaves I, Porter K, Garner J. Trauma care manual, 2nd edn. London: Hodder Arnold, 2009:135–145.

Holtz A, Levi R. Spinal cord injury. Oxford: Oxford University Press, 2010:167.

Moss R, Porter K, Greaves I. Minimal patient handling: a faculty of pre-hospital care consensus statement. Trauma 2015; 17:70–72.

Smith J, Greaves I, Porter KM. Oxford desk reference major trauma. Oxford: Oxford University Press, 2011:164–184.

Related topics of interest

Splintage

Key points

- Splintage of fractures is essential for pain relief and haemorrhage control
- Distal neurovascular status must be assessed before and after application of any splint
- The choice of splintage method should reflect the injury type and the clinical environment

Principles of splintage

Analgesia with or without sedation is usually required to facilitate application of the splint. Reduction of any fracture–dislocation should normally take place before splintage, although this may not always be possible or practical. The distal pulses, capillary refill time and sensation of the limb must be assessed before and after application of any splint and ideally fingers and toes should be left exposed to allow examination. If any deterioration occurs, the splint should be removed and the neurovascular status reassessed. Underlying wounds should be photographed and then covered with saline-soaked gauze swabs before splint application in order to reduce the need for repeated removal for inspection. The splint should immobilise the joints above and below the fracture. Padding should be used to protect any vulnerable bony points.

Following immobilisation in a splint, the limb should be elevated to reduce swelling. The complications of pressure sores, skin infection and compartment syndrome must be considered at all times.

Benefits of splintage

Effective application of suitable splintage is a key element of the management of bony trauma. The key benefits are:

- Offers nonpharmacological pain relief by reducing movement of the fractured bone ends
- Acts to reduce bleeding by the anatomical alignment of fractured bones, the reduction of cross-sectional soft tissue area in which bleeding may occur and the prevention of clot disruption
- Reduces the risk of neurovascular or skin damage
- Reduces the risk of fat embolism
- Facilitates patient handling, package and transportation

Types of splintage

The following types of immobilisation may be used:

Manual splintage plus adjuncts

The patient may support his or her own injury (e.g. holding their own arm or supporting it on a pillow), or the practitioner may hold the limb in alignment to provide manual immobilisation. This may be used in conjunction with a broad-arm sling in case of upper limb fractures, or blankets to support a lower limb fracture.

Commercial splints

A variety of types of commercial splints are widely used in the prehospital environment, which are as follows:

Vacuum splints: These are composed of a tough fabric shell filled with polystyrene balls, which mould around the injured body part or whole body when air is extracted. They can conform to any shape and allow support of the bone without pressure at the injury site (**Figure 76**).

Box splints: These are used to provide splintage for lower limb injuries from the knee to the foot. Because of their shape, additional padding may be required to provide comfort. A long leg box splint makes a very effective spinal immobilisation or transport device for a small baby (**Figure 77**).

Pelvic splints: The SAM Pelvic Sling or T-POD pelvic stabilisation devices are commonly used to immobilise suspected pelvic fractures (**Figure 78**).

Traction splints: These can be applied to the lower limb following manual traction to maintain realignment of displaced bony fractures and allow relaxation of muscles in spasm. Traction also reduces the volume of

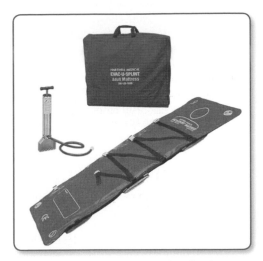

Figure 76 A vacuum splint. Reproduced with permission from MedTree, Telford, UK.

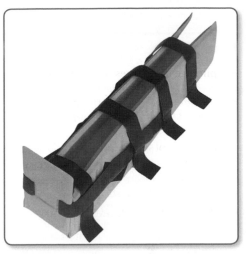

Figure 77 A box splint. Reproduced with permission from MedTree, Telford, UK.

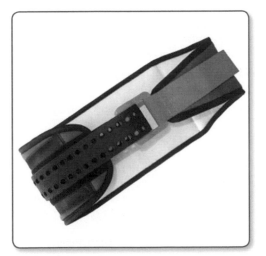

Figure 78 SAM pelvic splint. Reproduced with permission from MedTree, Telford, UK.

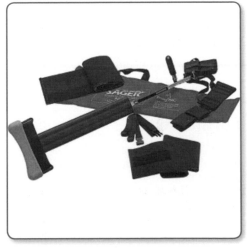

Figure 79 SAM traction splint. Reproduced with permission from MedTree, Telford, UK.

the thigh, which decreases the space available for ongoing internal haemorrhage. The KTD (Kendrick traction device), SAM and Sager splints are commonly used for this purpose in prehospital practice (**Figure 79**). The traction device may remain in situ until the patient goes to theatre or can be replaced by skin traction in the emergency department. Traction devices are contraindicated if there is a coexisting fracture–dislocation of

the knee, fracture of the distal femur or an unstable ankle fracture. Some traction splints which use the pelvis against which to provide traction are contraindicated in established or suspected pelvic fracture.

Plaster of Paris: A plaster of Paris backslab may be applied in the emergency department to provide temporary splintage of a fracture. The cast is not circumferential in order to prevent the adverse effects of ongoing tissue swelling under a complete splint.

Upper limb splintage

In the upper limb, the location of the fracture and the aims of treatment will determine the type of splintage or immobilisation.

- Clavicle/shoulder – broad-arm sling
- Proximal humerus fracture – collar and cuff (provides some disimpaction due to the weight of the arm)
- Elbow – broad-arm sling, vacuum splint or above elbow backslab
- Forearm fracture – broad-arm sling (initially), vacuum splint or backslab
- Wrist or hand fracture – high-arm sling, Futuro splint or backslab
- Finger fracture – neighbour ('buddy') strapping

Lower limb and pelvis splintage

Where there is suspicion of a pelvic fracture (usually due to the mechanism of injury – springing the pelvis must be avoided and an early plain film obtained), a commercial pelvic splint should be applied, ideally with a figure of eight bandage around the ankles to maintain adduction of the hips with internal rotation. Patients with a dislocated hip should be managed by supporting the leg in the most comfortable position (normally flexed) using blankets or pillows for padding.

In the case of neck of femur fracture, the feet can be tied together with a figure of eight bandage with triangular bandages at midfemur and midtibial level and padding in between the legs to prevent movement of the injured leg. Midshaft femur fracture is best treated with traction splintage. Tibial plateau fractures and knee dislocation should be immobilised in a vacuum splint, padded box splint, or above knee backslab and patella dislocations immobilised in the most comfortable position (usually flexed) using blankets or pillows. Midshaft tibia and fibula fractures require a vacuum splint or above knee backslab, ankle and foot fractures require a vacuum splint, box splint or backslab.

Further reading

Boyd AS, Benjamin HJ, Asplund C. Principles of casting and splinting. Am Fam Physician 2009; 79:16–22.

Lee C, Porter KM. Pre-hospital management of lower limb fractures. Emerg Med J 2005; 22:660–663.

Smith J, Greaves I, Porter KM. Oxford desk reference major trauma. Oxford: Oxford University Press, 2011:258.

Related topics of interest

- Analgesia (p. 19)
- Long-bone fractures (p. 171)
- Pelvic trauma (p. 222)

Systemic inflammatory response syndrome

Key points

- Systemic inflammatory response syndrome (SIRS) in trauma is characterised by a three tier response: metabolic, immunological and haemodynamic
- The SIRS diagnostic criteria are core temperature > 38°C or < 36°C, heart rate > 80 bpm, respiratory rate > 20 breaths per minute or $P\text{CO}_2$ < 4.3 kPa and white blood cell (WBC) count > 12 or < 4 (or >10% immature neutrophils)
- Novel hybrid resuscitation may attenuate the post-trauma inflammatory response

Introduction

The impact of the SIRS on the severely injured cannot be overstated. There is emerging evidence that points to an exaggerated SIRS response in some patients, as well as modification of the response in relation to the resuscitation strategy employed. A systemic inflammatory response is not inherently dangerous and is ultimately required for tissue repair, but an unregulated response in extreme conditions can compromise healthy tissue and distant end-organs and further promote inflammation. SIRS in trauma is characterised by a three tier response: metabolic, immunological and haemodynamic.

The SIRS is driven by cytokines and chemokines, as well as damaged tissues (damage-associated molecular patterns, DMAPs). DMAPs are known to release proinflammatory cytokines, but there is evidence that they may also inhibit anti-inflammatory cytokine. The inflammatory response is essential to reduce and remove the results of damage to an organism. A dysregulated inflammatory response can set in motion a dangerous cycle of inflammation–damage–further inflammation. The clinical challenge is to utilise the beneficial effects of this inflammatory response without allowing it to exceed a level that becomes unregulated.

Pathophysiology of SIRS in trauma

Precipitants or exacerbators of SIRS in the severely injured include:

- Tissue trauma
- Shock/tissue hypoxia
- Blood transfusion
- Ventilation
- Sepsis

Metabolic response

Following major trauma there is a hypermetabolic response. Along with this there is increased secretion of adrenaline and cortisol as part of the generalised neuroendocrine stress response and an increase in circulating glucagon, growth hormone, aldosterone and antidiuretic hormone.

The metabolic response is associated with increased oxygen demand in the tissues. This is particularly problematic in the elderly or those with significant underlying chronic disease states, who are unable to tolerate this due to lack of physiological reserve. The presence of a prolonged hypermetabolic state (in excess of a week) indicates a severe SIRS response and raises the suspicion of underlying infection and sepsis.

Immunological response

Local endothelial damage in the area of trauma causes the release of proinflammatory cytokines, notably interleukins (IL-1, IL-6, IL-8) and tissue necrosis factor (TNF-α). IL-6 is detectable very early in trauma and correlates with the degree of trauma. IL-6 further activates neutrophils and promotes hepatic acute-phase protein synthesis.

Haemodynamic response

The haemodynamic response to major trauma is bimodal. There is initial peripheral vasoconstriction, retention of sodium chloride and water and migration of blood from the peripheries to central vital organs. This is the shock phase. There then follows a flow phase whereby the hypermetabolic response leads to increased oxygen and carbon dioxide production. The body responds physiologically by inducing a tachycardia, increased respiratory rate and vasodilatation. This phase lasts 4–5 days; if there is persistent vasodilation and tachycardia, then complications should be suspected.

Clinical course of SIRS

Proinflammatory and anti-inflammatory systems act to determine the time course of the SIRS response. IL-1, IL-6, IL-8 and TNF-α are all involved in the inflammatory response with the anti-inflammatory actions of IL-4 and IL-10 being responsible for a decrease in the production of these proinflammatory cytokines. The physiological and biochemical changes that define SIRS include:

- Core temperature > 38°C or < 36°C
- Heart rate > 80 bpm
- Respiratory rate > 20 breaths per minute or P_{CO_2} < 4.3 kPa
- WBC > 12 or < 4 (or >10% immature neutrophils)

Excessive activity of proinflammatory cytokines leads to severe SIRS with the potential risk of organ dysfunction and death. An excessive anti-inflammatory response leads to immunosuppression and a risk of increased mortality later in the clinical course. (This is due to activation of the hypothalamic–pituitary–adrenal axis with overproduction of glucocorticoids, causing an immunosuppressive effect.)

Damage control strategies to modify the SIRS response

Because of its crucial role in the inflammatory response it has been suggested that IL-6 might have a role as a marker in mapping the response to major trauma. The accepted concept of damage control resuscitation should be utilised to minimise the possibility of an excessive SIRS response. Coagulation derangement, major trauma and SIRS are all linked. The aggressive correction of coagulation disturbance by the early use of blood and blood products, along with tranexamic acid, will reduce the impact of coagulopathy.

Multiorgan distress syndrome

Multiorgan distress syndrome can be the result of a pronounced SIRS reaction after trauma. Organ dysfunction usually involves the lungs, cardiovascular system, kidneys (acute kidney injury), liver and central nervous system. The reasons for this are complex but may be due to the following mechanism:

- Capillary leak and increased interstitial fluid
- Tissue hypoperfusion from vasodilation, which may be refractory due to nitric oxide (NO) production
- Disseminated intravascular coagulation
- Neutrophil-generated reactive oxygen species and proteases

In the respiratory system, this can be seen as capillary endothelial dysfunction resulting in interstitial oedema as endothelial permeability increases in response to proinflammatory cytokines. In the cardiovascular system, SIRS releases vasoactive cytokines and causes synthesis of inducible NO, resulting in a fall in systemic vascular resistance. This may be resistant to conventional treatment with fluids and inotropes. The cytokines and NO also depress cardiac function by reducing contractility and preventing cardiac relaxation during diastole. Renal blood flow is also affected in the SIRS response due to cytokine-induced vasodilation and hypoperfusion. Similar effects are seen in gastrointestinal tract with the possible consequence of sepsis due to translocation of bacteria across an impaired intestinal barrier into the blood stream.

All of the above pathophysiological changes are compounded by tissue hypoxia due to both hypoperfusion and mitochondrial level dysfunction. This is mediated by a block in the electron transfer chain affected by NO.

Emerging concepts

Persistent inflammation, immunosuppression and catabolism syndrome

Advances in intensive care management have meant that some patients survive their initial SIRS (and/or sepsis) only to develop what is being termed persistent inflammation, immunosuppression and catabolism syndrome (**Table 37**).

Novel hybrid resuscitation

There has been an acceptance of hypotensive resuscitation in the initial and prehospital phases of trauma resuscitation over the last few years. This is not without a physiological penalty though, due to reduced tissue perfusion and development of metabolic acidosis. If this is prolonged, it can result in severe lactic acidosis and perpetuates the SIRS response.

An emerging strategy that has potential benefits in terms of modification of the

Table 37 Criteria for persistent inflammation, immunosuppression and catabolism syndrome	
Persistent	Intensive care stay > 10 days
Inflammation	C-reactive protein > 150 mcg/dL
Immune suppression	Total lymphocyte count < 0.80 × 10⁹/L
Catabolism	Plasma albumin level < 30 g/L Weight Loss > 10% during hospital stay or BMI (body mass index) < 18 Retinol binding protein level < 10 mcg/dL
BMI	<18

inflammatory response to trauma involves targeting hypotensive resuscitation for the first 60 minutes, reverting to normotensive resuscitation thereafter. Experimental evidence has shown that targeted resuscitation attenuates the development of metabolic acidosis and improves tissue oxygen delivery.

Further reading

Brochner AC, Toft P. Pathophysiology of the systemic inflammatory response syndrome after major accidental trauma. Scand J Trauma Resusc Emerg Med 2009; 17:43–53.

Doran CM, Doran CA, Wooley T, et al. Targeted resuscitation improves coagulation and outcome. J Trauma 2012; 72:835–843.

Gentile LF, Cuenca AG, Efron PA, et al. Persistent inflammation and immunosuppression: a common syndrome and new horizon for surgical intensive care. J Trauma Acute Care Surg 2012; 72:1491–1501.

Meeran H, Messant M. The systemic inflammatory response syndrome. Trauma 2001; 3:89–100.

Pugin J. How tissue injury alarms the immune system and causes systemic inflammatory response syndrome. Ann Intensive Care 2012; 2:27–32.

Related topics of interest

Tertiary survey

Key points

- The tertiary survey is part of the continuum of trauma care and exists to identify and catalogue all injuries after resuscitation and the first stage of operative management
- The National Peer Review Programme for Trauma has set standard T14-2C-407, dictating that a formal tertiary survey protocol is required in major trauma centres
- If the patient is unable to communicate or has an altered level of consciousness, the process may need repetition, potentially several times

Introduction

The tertiary survey is a complete assessment of the trauma patient designed to ensure that no injury is missed. As a result, it inevitably occurs after the initial assessment resuscitation and immediate management of the patient is complete. The National Peer Review Programme for Trauma has set standard T14-2C-407, dictating that a formal tertiary survey protocol is required in major trauma centres. In the United States, the American College of Surgeons guidelines require this to happen within 24 hours of admission. The process must involve full physical examination and a review of laboratory and imaging studies and should be fully multidisciplinary. Evidence has clearly demonstrated that a substantial number of new injuries are revealed at tertiary survey. Within any trauma system, a single individual must be identified who is responsible for ensuring the tertiary survey has been completed. A 2012 systematic review demonstrated missed injury rates of 4.3% at primary survey and 1.5% after tertiary survey.

Radiological tertiary survey

Although interpretation of images by requesting clinicians is the norm when planning emergent care, definitive reporting by a radiologist should take place as part of the tertiary survey. There is an appreciable rate of missed injury between radiologist and nonradiologist interpretation of images. Incorporating reporting into a multidisciplinary environment such as a trauma meeting may provide a better clinical context and more rapid reporting as well as offering a learning opportunity for the wider team. In paediatric trauma, prospective evaluation of the utility of whole-body plain radiography series has found a low yield, and hence imaging guided by examination findings is advocated, even in infants unable to communicate. Hoff et al. (2004) reviewed 432 consecutive admissions at a level II trauma centre and found that 9.7% of patients had injuries detected by the radiology team on images, which had been missed by the trauma team.

Controversies

Although there is consensus that a tertiary survey is an important component of patient care, there is no unified protocol or standard of documentation. The drawn-out nature of serial re-examination may realistically mean that patients with prolonged sedation, e.g. never receive a full, formal tertiary survey carried out on a single occasion. The survey is regarded as a repetition rather than an escalation, so patients may receive all their full examinations from junior doctors even if the results are reviewed by consultant level clinicians. Similarly, after admission under a specialist team, patients may not always have a tertiary survey performed by a clinician with the breadth of experience required to identify a full range of injuries.

Approach

The tertiary survey must be considered as a consultant-led, multidisciplinary review and should be performed as many times as necessary to ensure that no injury, however trivial, is missed. A possible system is outlined below.

Airway

The status of the patient's airway should be continually reassessed, especially if there has been a head injury or there is any other reason (e.g. drugs or alcohol) for a fluctuating level of consciousness. Consideration should be given to the provision of a more permanent airway such as a tracheostomy if the patient is already intubated.

Breathing

A careful physical examination of chest including a detailed inspection and observation of chest wall movements should be carried out. Particular attention should be paid to the possibility of typically delayed sequelae such as pulmonary contusion and adult respiratory distress syndrome (ARDS), and arterial blood gas analysis is essential. Ventilator requirements should be reviewed.

Circulation

Fluid balance should be reviewed, and changes in haemodynamic status assessed along with changes in serial haematocrit measurement. Concealed haemorrhage must be identified or excluded. Careful attention must be paid to arterial pressure monitoring, lithium dilution cardiac output (LIDCO), central venous pressure (CVP) and ongoing vasopressor requirements. Transfusion requirements should be reviewed, and TEG or ROTEM should be used to guide specific blood component therapy. It should be remembered that a haemoglobin adequate for ward care may be inadequate if further surgery planned, and transfused red blood cells are maximally effective sometime after transfusion due to initially reduced 2,3-diphosphoglycerate levels.

Disability

Thorough scrutiny of neurological observations is essential, and decisions must include the timing of repeat imaging. Any alteration in neurological status should prompt early rescan and neurosurgical review. If the patient has suffered a spinal injury, it is essential to ensure that a spinal injury unit referral be made. Pressure areas must be assessed, and serial American Spinal Injuries Association (ASIA) charts or equivalent are mandatory. Liaison with spinal surgeons is vital to ensure that there is consensus on whether emergency decompression or stabilisation is necessary

Exposure

Every joint must be examined when the patient is conscious, and any necessary imaging is performed. Particular attention should be paid to the hands where injuries are easily missed but can be life changing. Any temporizing hardware must be assessed and frames confirmed to be tightened and functioning correctly, any pin sites to be cleaned. Swelling should be checked where soft tissues are delaying surgery. The chosen definitive fracture fixation strategy should be outlined and updated as necessary.

Serial abdominal examinations should be performed, with repeat imaging being requested if appropriate and with a low threshold. Urinary and faecal continence must be actively managed and nutrition discussed with a dietician. Stoma support referrals should be made for patients who have had an emergency diversion, and a decision should be made regarding whether catheterisation should continue, and if so, whether it needs changing to long-term device.

Psychological aspects

At the earliest, possible contact should be made with psychology and occupational therapy to ensure prompt professional assessment and to commence the recovery process.

Further reading

Hoff WS, Sicoutris CP, Lee SY, et al. Formalized radiology rounds: the final component of the tertiary survey. J Trauma 2004; 56:291–295.

Keijzer GB, Giannakopoulos GF, Del Mar C, Bakker FC, Geeraedts LM. The effect of tertiary surveys on missed injuries in trauma: a systematic review. Scand J Trauma Resusc Emerg Med 2012; 20:77.

Related topics of interest

Therapeutic hypothermia

Key points

- Therapeutic hypothermia has been successfully used for tissue protection in certain patient groups, which in future may include trauma patients
- Non-therapeutic hypothermia is a precipitant of adverse metabolic responses to trauma and must be prevented or treated
- Non-therapeutic hypothermia (defined as a core body temperature < 35°C) occurring in conjunction with trauma is associated with increased morbidity and mortality

Introduction

As a consequence of prolonged scene times or inappropriate exposure, many trauma patients are hypothermic on admission or develop hypothermia during resuscitation, although the incidence of both varies with definition and is not related to the time of year. This hypothermia is associated with the 'ebb' phase of the body's metabolic response where reduction in basal metabolic rate and focus on attaining cardiovascular stability predominate.

As metabolism falls so does body temperature, the degree of hypothermia relating to the severity of the injury with a reported incidence of around one in three severely injured patients (ISS > 15), though this does vary. The fall in temperature may also indicate exhaustion of the body's energy stores of adenosine triphosphate as oxygen demand exceeds supply in the shocked patient. Cool resuscitation fluids and open body cavities during surgery may also contribute.

This hypothermia is typically associated with acidosis and coagulopathy known as the lethal triad where each aspect augments the next in a downward metabolic spiral leading to death. Shivering may worsen the energy supply and demand mismatch with myocardial dysfunction and arrhythmias being induced at low temperatures. This hypothermia is associated with severe injury increased resuscitation requirements,

significant complications and poorer outcomes. In contrast, therapeutic or induced hypothermia has been postulated as a protective mechanism in the management of major trauma.

Therapeutic/induced hypothermia

Therapeutic hypothermia is the controlled reduction in body temperature of a patient to a specified point to generate a reduction in metabolism and in tissue oxygen requirements with the aim of increasing tissue hypoxic–ischaemic injury tolerance and preventing irreversible damage. Therapeutic hypothermia may blunt cellular apoptotic pathways, reduce the body's systemic immune and inflammatory responses and protect against reperfusion injury. Sedation and neuromuscular blockade are employed, the latter to stop shivering.

Therapeutic hypothermia has been increasingly investigated as a method of protecting and preserving tissues that have been subject to insult and is used in a number of types of surgery and some medical conditions. The effect of hypothermia on tissues appears dependent on the degree and duration of cooling as well as the time of starting cooling (before, during or after injury) and the rate of induction and rewarming. The weight of influence of each factor will vary according to the injury type, and thus the ideal techniques to use, which are currently not fully established, are likely to also vary.

Degrees of cooling

Mild hypothermia (33–36°C) has been used in a number of applications following cellular damage and organ injury, such as cardiac arrest and traumatic brain injury (TBI). The effects on metabolic rate appear minimal: more beneficial effects are seen in reduction in immunologically mediated secondary damage pathways, increased production of and prevention of loss of neuroprotectants.

Evidence so far for deeper hypothermia (16–27°C) is predominantly from surgical patients and anecdotal cases of rapid severe hypothermia due to accidental ice water immersion where it is thought to prevent cellular energy depletion and thus tissue ischaemia. Little is known about this degree of hypothermia in the trauma or bleeding patient where ischaemic damage has already been initiated.

Complications of cooling

Potential complications of cooling include immune suppression leading to increased infection rates and impaired coagulation (from fibrinolysis, platelet dysfunction and other mechanisms), although studies show variable results and are often in animal models. Profound hypothermia increases blood viscosity and may increase the risk of microvascular thrombosis. Potential adverse effects include:

- An altered response to drugs, which varies depending on the agent investigated
- Shivering leading to increased oxygen requirements/consumption
- Cardiac dysfunction and arrhythmias, typically at temperatures < 28°C
- Respiratory depression, typically at temperatures < 28°C

Major haemorrhage and hypothermia

Uncontrolled major haemorrhage is the second most common cause of death in the trauma patient and is thought to be the most preventable cause of death in this group. Control of bleeding and reinstatement of the interrupted organ perfusion is required within 5 minutes for the brain and 20 minutes for the heart to prevent ischaemia and possible fatal damage. Animal studies have shown improved survival when mild hypothermia (>33°C) was induced in bleeding subjects whether alone, or in combination with limited fluid resuscitation. A number of cellular and metabolic changes also occur with haemorrhagic shock, which may lead to ischaemic–reperfusion injury and further damage. Hypothermia may blunt this immune activation and prevent against reperfusion damage. It is currently postulated that maintaining mild-induced hypothermia during haemorrhage control and then active rewarming after this has been achieved is likely to be the recommended technique; however, further research is still needed.

Therapeutic hypothermia may be relevant in the severely unstable or arrested bleeding trauma patient to buy time to get to hospital or surgery for definitive haemorrhage control. Penetrating trauma may lead to massive blood loss and hypovolaemic arrest from a potentially reparable wound. There is evidence for successful outcomes in animals where deep hypothermia (10°C) is rapidly induced after cardiac arrest from penetrating trauma, with gradual rewarming after surgical control of haemorrhage. Of note, the rewarming process itself may be significant in terms of the timing and rate of temperature increase. A maximum of 60 minutes hypothermic arrest time was found before outcomes were detrimentally affected. Further investigation is needed to confirm these findings, and the technique requires a cardiopulmonary bypass circuit, which also limits its current applications.

Traumatic brain injury and hypothermia

The role of hypothermia and neuroprotection after TBI has been investigated: the mechanism of action is debated but may include reduced metabolism and oxygen requirements, alterations in biochemical and neurotransmitter levels (namely glutamate), inflammation suppression, and reduction in intracranial pressure and oedema.

Initial studies showed a benefit from moderate therapeutic hypothermia (32–33°C) in patients with TBI; however, they were small studies and varied in terms of the protocols used. Systematic reviews have also shown a mortality benefit with cooling for >48 hours, a neurological benefit with cooling for 24 hours and a neurological benefit with cooling for >48 hours compared with normothermia. However, the best time to cooling, target temperature, time at target temperature and rewarming process are not known, and since the studies were particularly heterogeneous, the authors highlighted caution in result interpretation. A Cochrane review found no evidence of improved mortality or neurological outcome with cooling for TBI and noted significant benefit was only seen in the poorer quality trials. The better quality trials showed no reduced mortality with cooling; however, these results were not significant and thus may have been due to chance. Currently, hypothermia to improve outcome after TBI is not recommended, and further randomised controlled trials are needed.

Summary

Investigation into therapeutic hypothermia in the trauma patient is currently still in the research phase. Whether outcome benefits will be seen, in which types of trauma patients they will occur, and the best method and timing of cooling and rewarming remain unknown. As discussed, potential roles may include neuroprotection and brain injury and the management of haemorrhagic shock in the pre- and inter-hospital settings and limb salvage.

Further reading

Fukudome EY1, Alam HB. Hypothermia in multisystem trauma. Crit Care Med 2009; 37:S265–S272.

Kheirbek T1, Kochanek AR, Alam HB. Hypothermia in bleeding trauma: a friend or a foe? Scand J Trauma Resusc Emerg Med 2009; 17:65.

Sydenham E, Roberts I, Alderson P. Hypothermia for traumatic head injury. London: Cochrane Database of Systematic Reviews 2009.

Related topics of interest

Thoracic trauma

Key points

- Thoracic injuries are common, and the vast majority are managed nonoperatively
- Initial evaluation, in addition to history and physical examination, includes portable chest X-ray (CXR) and computed tomography (CT) scanning
- Associated nonthoracic injuries must be identified as these are associated with very high mortality

Epidemiology

Thoracic trauma is common. Eight per cent of US trauma admissions are for blunt thoracic injury, overwhelmingly the result of motor vehicle collisions. In an urban trauma centre, penetrating thoracic injuries account for up to 20% of admissions for penetrating injury. The mortality is substantially higher for blunt thoracic injury (28%) than for penetrating thoracic injury (7%). This discrepancy is related to the extrathoracic injuries, the presence of which carries a 42% mortality. Overall, approximately one quarter of trauma deaths are directly attributable to thoracic injury, which contributes to about half of all trauma fatalities. Thoracic injury is the second leading cause of death within 1 hour of arrival at a trauma centre.

Approximately 85% of thoracic trauma can be managed nonoperatively. Thus, patients needing operative intervention have significant, complex injuries and may be haemodynamically unstable. Operative mortality has been reported to be as high as 45% and is related to haemodynamic instability, the nature and severity of the intrathoracic injuries and the presence of associated injuries.

Pathophysiology

The thoracic skeleton and chest wall musculature protect the intrathoracic structures, especially following blunt trauma. In adults, who have a less compliant chest wall, rib fractures suggest the presence of pulmonary contusion. In children, pulmonary injury can occur without rib fractures because the chest wall is more compliant. Rib or sternal fractures and flail chest are the result of direct force which, if not dissipated in the chest wall, will be transmitted to the intrathoracic organs. Penetrating trauma results in direct organ injury with haemorrhage as the key feature. Any intrathoracic organ may be involved. Abdominal injuries may be present as well, either from a projectile traversing the diaphragm or from an additional abdominal wound.

Alveoli rupture can result in pneumothorax or tension pneumothorax when increased intrathoracic pressure causes decreased venous return, low cardiac output and if untreated cardiac arrest. Pulmonary contusions are common and vary greatly in severity. Systemic air embolisation is rare but can occur when the injury involves an airway adjacent to a bronchial artery, in which case positive pressure ventilation will cause cardiovascular collapse.

Direct injury, rib fractures with parenchymal impalement, and shear forces can all cause pulmonary lacerations: pneumothorax, haemothorax or both may result and haemorrhagic shock may occur. Thoracic tracheobronchial injuries usually occur within 2 cm of the carina when rapid deceleration with resultant shearing forces disrupts the airway. Less commonly a sudden rise in intrathoracic pressure, especially against a closed glottis, can lead to rupture of the membranous portion of the airway. A persistent pneumothorax following tube thoracostomy, continuous air leak and inability to oxygenate and ventilate suggest the diagnosis. Infrequently, the airway is injured from a penetrating mechanism.

Blunt diaphragm injury is most often the consequence of a rapid rise in intra-abdominal pressure and more involve the left side. Abdominal contents may be located in the chest, and associated abdominal injuries are not infrequent.

Blunt aortic injury is the result of the shear forces that occur in horizontal deceleration.

Typically, the injury occurs in the proximal descending aorta just distal to the left subclavian artery.

Clinical features

An adequate history including from the prehospital providers and a detailed examination are essential. Examination must include the axilla, where small puncture wounds can be easily overlooked. Careful observation of the work of breathing and arterial saturation is essential. Endotracheal intubation should be performed as indicated for respiratory distress or airway protection.

Rib fractures are painful leading to splinting and respiratory distress. Paradoxical chest wall motion is often observed with a flail segment, and sternal instability may be noted with a sternal fracture. Parenchymal lung injuries may present with signs of pneumothorax or haemothorax, such as subcutaneous air, decreased or absent breath sounds and shock. Needle decompression or tube thoracostomy is indicated in unstable patients, especially if tension physiology is present. A small pulmonary contusion may be clinically silent, whereas a larger one may lead to respiratory distress. Their natural history is to increase over time, typically 24–48 hours, and they may be exacerbated by volume resuscitation.

The hallmarks of tracheobronchial trauma are persistent pneumothorax in spite of tube thoracostomy and large, continuous air leaks. Blunt aortic injury may be suspected by mechanism of injury. Generally, physical examination is not diagnostic, but a blood pressure difference between the upper extremities should raise the possibility. Respiratory distress may be the only sign of diaphragmatic rupture.

Investigations

In addition to routine laboratory tests, an arterial blood gas is extremely useful in assessing oxygenation, ventilation and depth of shock. Focused abdominal sonography for trauma (FAST) may be considered as well as a portable chest radiograph. The FAST should image the abdomen for haemoperitoneum and the precordium for haemopericardium. A CXR may demonstrate a haemothorax, pneumothorax or a wide mediastinum, which necessitates additional investigation for blunt aortic injury. A CXR can be rapidly performed and should be done on all patients. A pelvic film should be obtained in those with a blunt mechanism. Multislice CT scanning, even in unstable patients, is an important tool in quantifying the totality of a patient's injuries.

Additional diagnostic studies such as oesophagoscopy, oesophagram, angiography and bronchoscopy should only be performed in haemodynamically stable patients. The combination of a negative oesophagram and oesophagoscopy effectively excludes an oesophageal injury. Similarly, an airway injury can be excluded by a negative bronchoscopy.

Diagnosis

The combination of physical examination and imaging will generally confirm the diagnosis of specific organ injury following thoracic injury. A pneumothorax will be detected on a CXR; the exception is small or anterior pneumothorax only seen on CT. A hazy hemithorax on CXR may be the result of a haemothorax, pulmonary contusion or both. Chest CT can determine the size of the haemothorax, which has implications for treatment. Rib fractures and a flail segment may be identified on examination and confirmed on CXR. Lateral rib fractures are best seen on CT. Pulmonary contusion is better characterised on chest CT.

Tracheobronchial injuries most commonly present with a large pneumothorax or significant residual pneumothorax or a massive persistent air leak following tube thoracostomy. Subcutaneous air may be apparent on examination. Chest CT may suggest the injury, but bronchoscopy is diagnostic. Patients with great vessel injuries can present either in profound shock or be haemodynamically stable. Additional imaging with chest CT angiography is extremely valuable in stable patients as it defines the nature, extent and exact location of the injury. CT angiography has replaced angiography as the modality of choice to diagnose blunt aortic injury.

Large diaphragmatic injuries resulting in abdominal contents displaced into the chest may be suspected on a CXR and a nasogastric tube above the diaphragm is diagnostic. CT scan has a role but small injuries, particularly from a penetrating injury, may be missed on imaging studies. Laparoscopy is diagnostic and potentially therapeutic. On a note of caution, high-quality CT imaging with enhanced resolution is overly sensitive in identifying pulmonary pathology that may be clinically unimportant.

Shock following penetrating injury requires operative management. For a penetrating injury in the 'cardiac box', sternotomy offers the optimal exposure; a clamshell incision can also be used. Suspected injury confined to one hemithorax is best approached through an anterolateral incision; if necessary, the incision can be continued across the sternum as a clamshell.

Treatment

Analgesia, pulmonary toilet, aggressive chest physiotherapy and ambulation are generally all that is necessary to effectively treat rib fractures. Mortality and morbidly increase with both age and number of ribs fractured. Epidural anaesthesia is excellent for pain control and can lower mortality. The same treatment can be used for a flail chest, and mechanical ventilation is reserved for those in respiratory distress. The underlying pulmonary contusion generally contributes more to the respiratory compromise than does the altered chest wall mechanics. Large flail segments markedly displaced rib fractures, and rib fractures hindering ventilator weaning are among the indications for rib plating.

Small pneumothoraces, especially those only seen on CT scan, can be observed unless the patient requires positive pressure ventilation when a chest drain should be inserted. A pneumothorax detected on CXR is treated by tube thoracostomy. Small haemothoraces, those < 300 cc, can be observed; larger ones require tube thoracostomy. Residual haemothoraces, those persisting after a chest drain has been inserted, are best treated by video-assisted thoracoscopic surgery (VATS) within 5 days of injury. Pulmonary contusions are treated with supportive care and careful fluid administration.

Nonoperative treatment with tube thoracostomy and supportive care may be all that is necessary in the majority of cases. Initial chest tube outputs of blood > 1500 cc or 200–300 cc per hour for 3–4 hours are the accepted indications for emergency thoracotomy. Persistent haemorrhage may not be appreciated if the chest drain is clotted or poorly positioned. In this situation, a repeat CXR will detect the increasing haemothorax.

If operative management is indicated, the choice of repair will depend on the location and extent of the laceration, depth of shock, haemodynamic stability and associated injuries. As expected, mortality increases with the magnitude of the repair or resection.

Tracheobronchial injuries are best treated operatively. Distal tracheal injuries are primarily repaired with interrupted absorbable sutures. Every effort should be made to repair the main stem bronchi in the same way. If repair is not possible, pneumonectomy is required, which carries a morality in excess of 75%. More distal airway injuries are treated by primary repair or resection. While lobectomy is often necessary, there is clearly a role for lung sparing procedures such as sleeve resection, if the anatomy is favourable.

In the acute setting, diaphragmatic injuries are best approached transabdominally. Laparoscopy is very useful for penetrating thoracoabdominal wounds, and the diaphragm is examined and repaired if needed. Likewise, if a laparotomy is indicated, the diaphragm can be addressed.

Endovascular techniques are ideal for treating injuries in haemodynamically stable patients. Thoracic endovascular aortic repair has replaced open repair for almost all blunt traumatic aortic injuries. Catheter-based therapies, such as stents and embolisation, can be used in selected patients with great vessel injury. At operation, arterial injuries are repaired primarily or with graft interposition, both vein and prosthetic material are acceptable conduits.

Arterial ligation is reserved for life-saving circumstances. With the exception of the superior vena cava, intrathoracic veins can be ligated.

Penetrating thoracic trauma in a haemodynamically unstable patient warrants operative exploration. The decision regarding surgical exposure may be problematic especially if there is concomitant abdominal injury. Haemodynamic instability following blunt trauma is a more difficult problem as there are multiple locations for haemorrhage in the polytrauma patient. Spinal cord injury with neurogenic shock can further complicate the haemodynamic picture.

Complications

Pneumonia is a common complication following chest trauma and is associated with higher injury severity score (ISS), blunt mechanism and mechanical ventilation. Atelectasis, often the result of splinting from pain, can occur and may lead to pneumonia. Retained haemothorax occurs in approximately 5% of thoracic injuries.

Larger haemothoraces require drainage, generally by VATS, which should be performed within 5 days of injury. The risk of empyema from a retained haemothorax is 26.8%, hence the need for early drainage. Empyema can also be a complication of a thoracotomy performed for trauma. Operative management of empyema is often necessary to control the pleural infection. Chest drainage and antibiotics are generally inadequate. Mediastinitis and sternal dehiscence occur infrequently.

Bronchopleural fistula and persistent air leaks (lasting > 7–10 days) are troublesome. Continued contamination of the pleural space can lead to an empyema. Most air leaks will seal within 7 days, especially if the lung is fully inflated. Air leaks lasting > 7–10 days are usually treated by VATS. Other options include a blood patch and a Heimlich valve.

Another rare complication of chest trauma is chylothorax. Milky chest tube output with a triglyceride level > 6.1 mmol/L (110 mg/dL) confirms the diagnosis. Nutritional depletion and compromised immune function may result. Treatment consists of nothing by mouth except medium chain triglycerides, total parenteral nutrition (TPN) and octreotide. If nonoperative management is unsuccessful, then operative intervention is warranted.

Further reading

DuBose J, Inaba K, Demetriades D, et al. Management and outcomes of retained hemothorax after trauma: an AAST multicenter, prospective, observational trial. J Trauma 2012; 72:11–22.

DuBose J, Inaba K, Okoye O, et al. Development of post-traumatic empyema in patients with retained hemothorax: results of a prospective, observational AAST study. J Trauma 2012; 73:752–757.

DuBose J, O'Connor JV, Scalea TM. Lung, trachea, and esophagus. In: Mattox KL, Moore EE, Feliciano DV (eds.), Trauma, 7th edn. New York: McGraw Hill, 2012

Martin MJ, McDonald JM, Mullenix PS, Steele SR, Demetriades D. Operative management and outcomes of traumatic lung resection. J Am Coll Surg 2006; 203:336–344.

Schuster A, Davis KA. Diaphragm. In: Mattox KL, Moore EE, Feliciano DV (eds.), Trauma, 7th edn. Columbus: McGraw Hill, 2012.

Related topics of interest

Topical haemostatic dressings

Key points

- Catastrophic external haemorrhage is a common cause of death following trauma
- Topical haemostatic dressings are an underused life-saving adjunct in haemorrhage control
- The agent should be chosen to reflect the most probable spectrum of injuries and the operating environment

Introduction

Catastrophic external haemorrhage remains an important cause of death in trauma. Stepwise strategies for control of haemorrhage are employed by both prehospital clinicians and those who care for acutely injured patients in hospital. Topical haemostatic agents should be considered for use when simple strategies for the control of bleeding have failed, particularly in the prehospital environment, where surgical arrest of haemorrhage is not possible.

Whilst tourniquets have proved themselves to be life-saving in catastrophic haemorrhage, there are several types of wound where they cannot be used. Injuries to the thorax, abdomen and those in junctional zones – the neck, groin, perineum and the axillae – clearly cannot be managed with a tourniquet, and it is in these injuries that topical haemostatic dressings prove most useful.

The ideal haemostatic dressing

Attempts have been made to describe the perfect topical haemostatic, and it is widely acknowledged that no such perfect product exists. The characteristics of the perfect dressing include:

- Stops severe arterial or venous bleeding in ≤2 minutes
- No side effects
- Does not cause pain
- Functional at extreme temperatures
- Long shelf life
- Inexpensive

It is important to recognise that the design of these dressings is an important factor in their success. A dressing that provides the perfect scientific basis for haemostasis but is the wrong shape or durability to be used in most wounds will have little clinical impact. In addition, the environment in which these dressings are used is often challenging so products that blow away or require very precise placement in almost surgical conditions cannot be utilised widely. When introducing a new product for use in a medical system, care must be taken to ensure the product best matches the type of injury most commonly encountered, the place where patients are treated, the end users of the product and, of course, its affordability.

When choosing a dressing, attention should also be paid to its form, e.g. small square dressings have a different utility to rolls of haemostatically impregnated bandage.

Types of topical haemostatic dressing

Recent military conflicts have seen significant investment in the design of topical haemostatics. The evidence for their use is based largely on animal in vivo models. Several broad types of dressing have emerged; however, those considered in this topic are the dressings, which are commonly used by civilian and military medical personnel.

Mineral-based agents

Early products (e.g. QuikClot powder) utilising mineral-based technology focussed on the naturally occurring material Zeolite. This worked by providing a cofactor to the coagulation cascade and by causing an exothermic reaction where water was adsorbed from the blood to concentrate the clotting proteins and form a stable clot. Initially, this was delivered in the form of granules that proved problematic in outdoor environments. It was also suggested that the exothermic reaction might pose a risk to patient and care provider, especially in windy conditions. Second-generation products improved the application method of the material and reduced its heat production properties.

More recently, a third generation (QuikClot Combat Gauze) has been developed using kaolin, a similar aluminium silicate compound. Kaolin is an activator of the intrinsic clotting pathway, and a clot forms in and around the dressing. Some studies have suggested that this increases the time to haemostasis compared with adhesive dressings, although this has been improved by producing a larger two-ply dressing.

It should be noted that as all mineral-based dressings work by enhancing or activating the clotting cascade, their effectiveness could in theory decrease in the presence of significant coagulopathy. Despite this, these dressings have been used extensively in recent conflicts, particularly by the US military.

Chitosan-based dressings

An alternative to dressings based on the mineral agent Zeolite is a range of dressings impregnated with Chitosan. Poly-N-acetyl glucosamine is a naturally occurring polysaccharide found in a variety of marine life. When highly acetylated, it is known as chitin, whereas the deacetylated form is called chitosan. This polymer is utilised in a number of delivery platforms by the manufacturers of Celox and HemCon.

On insertion into a bleeding wound, the chitosan dressing swells and becomes sticky. It is thought that the chitosan flakes create clot by ionic interaction with red blood cells as well as further activation of the clotting cascade. Importantly, due to its point of action being at the erythrocyte, the dressing successfully terminates bleeding in patients who have coagulopathy as a result of their injury. It has also been demonstrated to work in hypothermic patients and those on blood thinning agents. There is also some evidence to suggest chitosan provides an antimicrobial effect by disrupting gram-negative bacteria. Celox is currently the prehospital topical haemostatic of choice of the U.K. Armed Forces.

Chitosan is broken down by lysozyme to form glucosamine and as such dressings can be left in place for extended periods of time or washed away with saline at surgery.

Clotting factor-based dressings

The use of fibrin and its precursors has a long history in the control of haemorrhage. Current dried fibrin dressings have been demonstrated to be clinically effective. However, the cost of these dressings is highly prohibitive, and they are not currently in widespread use.

Using a haemostatic dressing

If direct pressure and elevation have failed to control haemorrhage and a tourniquet is unavailable or anatomically inappropriate, a topical haemostatic dressing should be utilised. To be effective, dressings must be used carefully and according to the manufacturer's instructions.

The wound must be fully exposed before the dressing is firmly packed into it. A conventional dressing is then applied over the haemostatic dressing. Different haemostatic dressings require different periods of direct pressure to be applied over the conventional dressing, usually 2-5 minutes.

Use in surgery

As well as prehospital use, haemostatic dressings may have a role to play in management of continued uncontrolled bleeding in surgery. Evidence from case reports suggests that chitosan dressings can be successfully used to help control pelvic bleeding after penetrating trauma, particularly in austere or under resourced environments, where options such as interventional radiology may be unavailable. Chitosan foams have been developed but are not in widespread use.

Conclusion

The last 15 years have seen a significant advance in the technology of haemorrhage control, and the array of commercially available haemostatic dressings reflects this. When choosing which product to use, it is important to balance the available evidence with the suitability of the product for the patient and the nature of the environment and medical system. When used appropriately haemostatic dressings undoubtedly have a key role to play in increasing the survivability of traumatic injury.

Further reading

Kheirabadi B. Evaluation of topical haemostatic agents for combat wound treatment. US Army Med Dep J 2011: 25–37.

Lawton G, Granville-Chapman J, Parker PJ. Novel haemostatic dressings. JR Army Med Corps 2009; 155:309–314.

Smith AH, Laird C, Porter K, et al. Haemostatic dressings in prehospital care. Emerg Med J 2013; 30:784–789.

Related topics of interest

- Tourniquets (p. 295)
- Tranexamic acid (p. 298)

Tourniquets

Key points

- Properly used, tourniquets have a key role to play in the control of life-threatening external haemorrhage
- Tourniquets should be applied approximately 10 cm proximal to the bleeding wound
- Periodic loosening and tightening of a tourniquet may cause rebleeding and must be avoided

Introduction

The use and misuse of tourniquets have been debated since the Greek physicians of antiquity. There is historical evidence that Roman surgeons used tourniquets during amputations, but the first established use of an arterial tourniquet in a prehospital environment is usually attributed to Etienne Morel, a French surgeon in the 17th century. It was Jean Louis Petite in 1718 who first published the description of a device called a 'tourniquet' from the French tourner (to turn) as it was worked by screw compression. Whilst the use of intraoperative pneumatic tourniquets to create a bloodless field in limb surgery is widely accepted in hospitals, the use of tourniquets in the prehospital emergency and military environments has been much more controversial.

Clinical issues

A properly applied tourniquet will occlude arterial flow in a limb by compressive force. This therefore renders the limb effectively avascular, and ischaemic damage will occur in proportion to the duration of the tourniquet application, with irreversible ischaemic damage occurring beyond about 2 hours. Compartment syndrome, nerve injury, thromboembolism, skin and muscle necrosis, increased infection rates in the limb, reperfusion injury, limb loss and death have all been reported following tourniquet use. Furthermore, incorrect application of a tourniquet or insufficient tightening that fails to occlude arterial flow but obstructs venous flow will worsen bleeding.

The benefits and risks of prehospital tourniquet use have caused controversy in every major conflict since the Crimean War. In the First World War, casualties often had to wait hours before arriving at a medical facility, and tourniquets, therefore, caused limb loss, which led Major Blackwood of the Royal Army Medical Corps to describe them as 'an invention of the Evil One.' However, from analysis of casualty data from the Vietnam War, it was estimated that 7% of US fatalities had exsanginated from limb injuries that could have potentially been prevented by the use of a tourniquet.

A number of studies from current military casualties sustained in Iraq and Afghanistan have proved the life-saving efficacy of the issued windlass tourniquets in modern combat operations. Tourniquets were shown to significantly improve survival, the greatest survival benefit occurring if they were used prehospital and before the onset of shock. The rapid evacuation times of coalition soldiers to the field hospital during the Iraq and Afghanistan conflicts meant that a tourniquet was rarely applied for >2 hours. As a consequence, the published complication rate is 1.7% for nerve injuries with no attributed limb loss or death in a US study of 499 major limb injuries in Iraq.

The evidence base for the benefit of tourniquets in a military prehospital environment that has grown over the last 10 of combat operations has meant that their use has now transferred to, and become increasingly common in, civilian practice. The UK Ambulance service guidelines, Trauma Care guidelines and ATLS teaching now recommended a tourniquet for catastrophic haemorrhage from a limb that cannot be controlled by other means.

The most widely used prehospital tourniquet is a one-handed windlass strap design such as the Combat Application Tourniquet (CAT Composite Resources, SC, USA, **Figure 80**), which is issued to most UK and US service personnel and used by

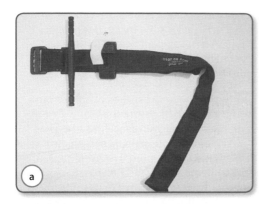

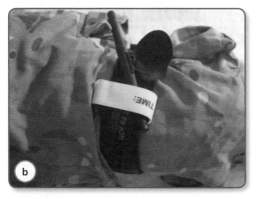

Figure 80 Combat application tourniquet.

many UK Ambulance services. The one-handed design allows for self-application, a skill that is now taught to all British soldiers. Pneumatic tourniquets provide a known and more evenly distributed occlusion pressure; however, the equipment's size, weight and lack of robustness usually limit their use to the in-hospital setting.

Indications

As the use of a tourniquet is not without risk, it should not be a first-line device to stop bleeding. The concept of a 'haemostatic ladder,' details progressive steps for controlling haemorrhage: dressings as a first line, then direct pressure and elevation, then topical haemostatics and finally a tourniquet. The decision to use a tourniquet should be taken when the risk to life from blood loss outweighs the risk to the limb.

Current civilian and military evidence has led to the establishment of a number of

principles guiding the use of tourniquets. Any medical practitioner who may use a tourniquet should be familiar with it and practiced in its correct usage. Windlass tourniquets need to be tightly applied with the straps fastened prior to tightening with the windlass to achieve effective compression. Tourniquets should be applied one hand's width (or around 10 cm) proximal to the injury and directly over the skin. Tourniquets should not be placed over a joint. Some argue that a tourniquet should be placed over a single bone (e.g. the thigh or upper arm) as the artery is more easily compressed; however, the amount of ischaemic tissue is minimised by applying the tourniquet just proximal to the wound.

In the patient with catastrophic external haemorrhage, immediate application of a tourniquet can be life-saving. Following attention to other priorities – airway, breathing, circulation, disability, exposure (ABCDE) – the wound may be packed and a pressure dressing applied. Following this, if the patient is some distance from hospital (suggesting a delay of >2 hours), a trial of tourniquet release may be considered. If further bleeding occurs, the tourniquet must be immediately tightened. Clearly, a tourniquet should not be used for > 2 hours to prevent ischaemic damage to the limb and the subsequent complications of this. If for any reason a tourniquet has been in place for > 6 hours, it should be left and only removed in a suitably resourced hospital because the limb may not be salvageable at this time and the reperfusion injury can be life threatening. Current best practice guidelines suggest a maximum tourniquet time of 2 hours.

If the wound continues to bleed after the application of a tourniquet, then the tourniquet should be further tightened. On the thigh, a second tourniquet placed adjacent and proximal to the first may be required as a result of the larger volume of tissue, which must be compressed to occlude blood flow.

The requirement for a tourniquet should be reviewed as the situation changes. Routine periodic loosening and tightening of a tourniquet is associated with increased bleeding and is not recommended. If a patient remains clinically shocked, then the tourniquet should not be removed. A properly applied tourniquet is very painful and the pain will increase as ischaemia develops in the limb. Patients should be given adequate analgesia.

The threshold for using a tourniquet is dependent on the wider situation. It may be used during triage of a mass casualty situation or to facilitate rapid evacuation of a casualty from a hostile situation.

The tourniquet must be visible and clearly documented in the patient's clinical notes and on the patient. Whilst military issue tourniquets are black, those used in the civilian setting are usually brightly coloured to aid recognition on the patient. The use of a tourniquet should make that patient a top priority category for evacuation and treatment, and the presence of a tourniquet must be included in any handover process.

Conclusion

Tourniquets are a life-saving tool in limb trauma, particularly when used early and in the prehospital setting. Training and research should continue to ensure that their current acceptance does not lead to inappropriate use. The situations and injury patterns in which a tourniquet is indicated are uncommon, particularly in a civilian setting; however, no patient should die from limb haemorrhage that could be controlled by a tourniquet.

Further reading

Kragh JF, Littrel ML, Jones JA, et al. Battle casualty survival with emergency tourniquet use to stop limb bleeding. J Emerg Med 2011; 41:590–597.

Kragh JF Jr, Swan KG, Smith DC, et al. Historical review of emergency tourniquet use to stop bleeding. Am J Surg 2012; 203:242–252.

Lee C, Porter KM, Hodgetts TJ. Tourniquet use in the civilian prehospital setting. J Emerg Med 2007; 24:584–587.

Related topics of interest

Tranexamic acid

Key points

- Tranexamic acid (TXA) is an antifibrinolytic drug, which reduces clot degradation through its role as an inhibitor of both plasminogen and plasmin
- Tranexamic acid has a proven benefit in reducing all-causes mortality in trauma if administered within 3 hours of trauma
- Clinical benefit from TXA mandates administration within 3 hours of injury

Introduction

Tranexamic acid was described in 1966 and given US Food and Drug Administration approval shortly afterwards. Its use in controlling menorrhagia emerged in 1968 and other applications have developed in the years since then, especially in dental, paediatric and cardiothoracic surgery. With the recognition of the acute coagulopathy of trauma as a pathophysiological process, which happens independent of iatrogenic contributions to coagulopathy based on fluid choice, volume and temperature, a further possible therapeutic application for TXA was identified.

The TXA is an antifibrinolytic drug, which reduces clot degradation through its role as an inhibitor of both plasminogen and plasmin. It is important to understand that it does not upregulate the process of clot formation but downregulate clot removal. TXA has a proven benefit in reducing all-causes mortality in trauma if administered within 3 hours of trauma, although administration > 3 hours after trauma appears to increase mortality.

To maximise clinical outcome in trauma, TXA use must form part of a wider blood product resuscitation strategy. Whilst it does not replace blood product administration, it may help reduce the volume of a finite resource needed for any individual trauma patient. TXA has now been included on the World Health Organisation's list of essential medicines and offers a low-cost intervention for trauma in the developing world.

Pathophysiology

The acute coagulopathy of trauma is suspected to be based on activation of the protein C pathway, resulting in the denaturing and inactivation of factors Va and VIIIa and increased fibrinolysis due to reduction of tissue plasminogen activator (t-PA) inhibitor concentration. TXA binds to lysine-binding sites on plasminogen, which prevents it becoming activated to plasmin and displaces it from fibrin if it is already attached. At high concentrations, TXA is postulated to bind similarly to plasmin, and as plasmin activates a number of components of the inflammatory cascade, TXA may also reduce inflammatory response.

Strategies for administration

Patient selection for TXA therapy remains contentious. The main research studies use inclusion criteria based on established shock or fibrinolysis, but this may select out those not yet demonstrated to benefit, and the low side effect profile suggests that wider usage may be more appropriate. A bolus dose of 1 g intravenously is given as soon as possible after injury and within 3 hours with the subsequent infusion of 1 g infusion over the following 8 hours. Repeated dosage may be guided by clinical assessment and thromboelastography. Since TXA is now carried by many advanced paramedics, it is essential that prehospital personnel make it absolutely clear that TXA has been given when they arrive in the resuscitation room.

Key studies

CRASH-2

The 20,000 patient multinational randomised controlled trial, CRASH-2 (Clinical Randomisation of an Antifibrinolytic in Significant Haemorrhage-2), demonstrated that early administration of TXA conferred survival benefit in bleeding events, with a relative risk of 0.68 and absolute risk reduction from 7.7% mortality in placebo group to 5.3% in TXA group. Early administration of TXA was essential, with administration after 3 hours postinjury showing worse outcome than placebo. The inclusion criteria for the study meant that patients needed neither transfusion nor operative intervention to be included

MATTERs

The Military Application of Tranexamic Acid in Trauma Emergency Resuscitation study (MATTERs) was a retrospective observational cohort study of military trauma patients requiring transfusion in a deployed hospital in Afghanistan. Subgroup analysis was performed on those patients who required > 10 units of packed red cells (massive transfusion subgroup). The TXA group had an unadjusted mortality of 17.9% when compared with those who had received no TXA with a mortality of 23.7%. This was in spite of a higher mean injury severity in the TXA group. The massive transfusion subgroup saw mortality nearly halved from 28.1% to 14.4%. Coagulopathy was reduced by TXA, but blood product ratios were similar between two groups, possibly reflecting the increased injury severity score in the TXA group.

It is important to note that CRASH-2 found no increase in venous thromboembolism with TXA, but MATTERs did. The MATTERs authors suggested this might be due to the higher burden of injury in the TXA group causing more profound systemic physiological effects.

Issues yet to be addressed

Whilst the effect of TXA has been demonstrated, the mechanism behind it has yet to be fully understood. Of the larger studies, none report real-time thromboelastography data, which might help illustrate hyperfibrinolysis and its correction. In addition, the potential systemic anti-inflammatory effect may well contribute to survival benefit of TXA, but a study has yet to investigate this. At present, there is no consensus regarding thromboembolic events after administration, despite two large studies failing to show a statistically significant increase purely attributable to the TXA administration.

Although some studies have demonstrated no benefit in non-shocked patients, many departments are now advocating TXA therapy based on the mechanism of injury. Given the relatively low side effect profile, this may be reasonable, but consensus would be beneficial and studies are needed to prove both the benefit and the absence of adverse effects.

The place of TXA in the management of patients with severe head injuries including intracranial bleeding remains to be established; however, the CRASH-3 trial is now being conducted to assess the effect of TXA on the risk of death or disability in patients with traumatic brain injury.

There has been some suggestion that studies failing to show benefit from the early routine administration of TXA may have been confounded by other failings within the resuscitation strategy employed in the protocols.

Further reading

CRASH-2 collaborators, Roberts I, Shakur H, et al. The importance of early treatment with tranexamic acid in bleeding trauma patients: an exploratory analysis of the CRASH-2 randomised controlled trial. Lancet 2011; 377:1096–1101,e1–2.

Morrison JJ. Military application of tranexamic acid in trauma emergency resuscitation (MATTERs) Study. Arch Surg 2012; 147:113.

Napolitano LM, Cohen MJ, Cotton BA, et al. Tranexamic acid in trauma. J Trauma Acute Care Surg 2013; 74:1575–1586.

Related topics of interest

Trauma scoring

Key points

- Trauma scoring is an essential tool for the comparison of different treatment modalities and trauma systems
- An injury severity score (ISS) ≥ 16 is considered the threshold for major trauma; life-changing trauma is defined as an ISS of ≥ 9
- Scoring systems may be physiological, anatomical or mixed

Introduction

Trauma scoring exists principally for the assessment and comparison of trauma interventions and systems by allowing retrospective study of the outcomes of trauma and trauma care. Trauma scoring may also facilitate the triaging of trauma patients to appropriate facilities and the assessment of the survival likelihood of individual patients, although this cannot be used to influence treatment. The first role is particularly important if different levels of trauma facilities are available: since the inception of major trauma networks, efficient dispatching has permitted direct admission to specialist facilities for the most severely injured: trauma scoring has already demonstrated improvements in patient outcomes following these organisational changes

Scoring systems

Scoring systems can be usefully divided into physiological, anatomical and combined scoring systems.

Physiological scoring systems

The first commonly used scoring system was the trauma score developed by Howard Champion in the USA in the early 1980s. The original trauma score used five parameters: respiratory rate, respiratory effort, systolic BP, capillary refill time and the Glasgow coma scale (GCS). The probability of survival (Ps) was found to fall from 99% with a maximum trauma score of 16 to 0% with a score of 2.

Champion revised his original system to produce the revised trauma score (RTS) in 1989. The RTS eliminated the parameters of respiratory effort and capillary refill time from the analysis. The RTS is therefore based on GCS, systolic BP and respiratory rate, with a weighting given to each parameter (**Table 38**).

Each parameter score is multiplied by the weighting and the values added. The relationship between RTS and survival is shown in **Table 39**. The triage RTS (TRTS) uses the unweighted values and is sometimes used as a physiological triage tool. The relationship between TRTS and the Ps is given in **Table 40**. The maximum TRTS is 12 and the minimum is 0. In the USA, a score of ≤3 in any one parameter (e.g. a total score of ≤11) indicates the need for transfer to a level 1 trauma centre.

Problems with physiological trauma scoring include lack of experience amongst clinicians, lack of validation for the very

Table 38 Weighting coefficient

Parameter	Weighting coefficient
Glasgow Coma Scale	0.9368
Systolic blood pressure	0.7326
Respiratory rate	0.2908

Table 39 The relationship between revised trauma score (RTS) and Ps (probability of survival)

RTS (rounded to nearest whole number)	Ps (%)
8	99
7	97
6	92
5	81
4	61
3	36
2	17
1	7
0	3

Table 40 Relationship between TRTS and Ps	
TRTS	Ps (%)
12	99.5
11	96.9
10	87.9
9	70.65
8	66.7
7	63.6
6	63.0
5	45.5
4	33.3
3	30.3
2	28.6
1	25.0
0	3.7

TRTS, triage revised trauma score; Ps, probability of survival.

young or very old and a tendency to underscoring on initial assessment due in part to assessment before physiological compensation has failed.

Anatomical systems

Anatomical scoring systems are based on the location of the patient's injuries. The most widely accepted is the Abbreviated Injury Scale (AIS), which allocates a seven figure code to each injury. The code indicates three aspects of the particular injury using seven numbers (**Figure 81**).

The severity score is based on tables of survival for injuries rather than the clinician's assessment.

In the ISS, the patient's injuries are coded using the AIS severity scores and divided into six body regions. The highest severity score from each of the three most severely injured regions is taken and squared. The ISS is the sum of the three squares and will range from 0 to 75, the maximum individual survivable score in a single region being 5. The New ISS (NISS) uses the three highest AIS scores irrespective of body area (with the proviso that any severity of score of 6 automatically gives an NISS of 75. An example of these calculations is given in **Table 41**. A score of ≥ 16 is considered to indicate major trauma, an ISS ≥ 9 is considered to indicate life-changing trauma.

The NISS does not mandate that each score must come from different systems, and so three mangled limbs can count three times, which may be a more accurate reflection of the burden of injury than the relatively low score assigned to one limb, which would represent maximum scoring under ISS. The NISS might be said to behave in a way that appears more logical than does

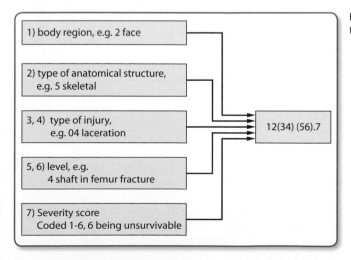

Figure 81 Derivation of the seven figure Abbreviated Injury Scale.

1) body region, e.g. 2 face

2) type of anatomical structure, e.g. 5 skeletal

3, 4) type of injury, e.g. 04 laceration

5, 6) level, e.g. 4 shaft in femur fracture

7) Severity score Coded 1-6, 6 being unsurvivable

12(34) (56).7

Table 41 Comparing ISS and NISS				
Region	Injury description	Abbreviated injury scale code	Abbreviated injury score	Abbreviated injury score (squared)
Head and neck	Depressed parietal skull fracture	150404	3	9
	Subdural haematoma	140652	4	16
Face	Abrasions	210202	1	
Thorax	Three rib fractures	450220	2	4
Pelvic/abdominal contents	Nil			
Extremities and pelvic girdle	Open fracture of radius	04	3	9
	Open fracture of ulna	753204	3	
External (skin)	Nil			

ISS (sum of the square of the three highest scoring injuries in the three highest scoring region) = 16 + 4 + 9 = 29
NISS (sum of the square of the three highest scoring injuries in any body region; may include more than one injury per region) = 16 + 9 + 9 = 34

the ISS: as injuries increase in number, death becomes more likely, even if these injuries are accumulating in the same body region. Similarly, adding a trivial injury (e.g. a distal radial fracture) to a different body region should not significantly affect the likelihood of death.

It is important to remember that the AIS was designed as a measure of health economics rather than prognosis – as a score designed by the insurance industry, severity is assigned by costs rather than outcome. Permanent survivable disability often costs more than death due to on-going care, and so these scores have inherent limitations when predicting clinical outcomes.

Combined systems

Anatomical systems are combined with physiological systems in trauma score ISS (TRISS) methodology.

TRISS methodology

The TRISS methodology combines physiological (RTS) and anatomical (ISS) methods together with the age of the patient and the method of injury (blunt or penetrating). The Ps is defined as follows:

$$Ps = \frac{1}{1 + e^{-b}}$$

where $b = b_0 + b_1\,(RTS) + b_2\,(ISS) + b_3\,(A)$

b_{0-3}: weighted coefficients based on American trauma data and different for blunt and penetrating trauma. A: age (score 0 if < 54, 1 if >55). TRISS methodology originally used data derived from American series, coefficients based on British data are now available.

M statistic

Calculation of the M statistic is used to decide whether comparison between a study survival rate and the American database is valid. The M statistic has a value between 0 and 1, values < 0.88 indicate that comparison of data would be invalid.

Z statistic

The Z statistic is used to compare the outcome of trauma care systems between two groups of patients and hence between two hospitals:

$$Z = \frac{\text{number of survivors} - \text{predicted number of survivors}}{\sqrt{\text{sum of } [Ps - (1 - Ps)]}}$$

The normal range for Z is between –1.96 and +1.96. Z statistics are not valid unless the M statistic indicates that the groups are comparable with the American database. Computer programs are available for the calculation of TRISS methodology.

W statistic

The *W* statistic (*W*s) measures the number of excess survivors or deaths per 100 patients managed at a specific site when compared to the norm. A high value of *W*s indicates more survivors than expected. *W*s is usually shown graphically, with 95% confidence intervals, as a caterpillar plot against all other sites to allow direct visual comparison.

More recently in the United Kingdom, The Trauma Audit & Research Network has developed a new model to overcome the problems of poor recording of RTS data. This model uses age, sex, ISS and GCS (when GCS is missing, intubated is used instead). New weightings have been calculated based on this model.

More recently, comorbidities for individual patients have been incorporated as well as the reporting of a true 30-day outcome (alive or dead) based on information derived from the Office of National Statistics. This new information is used to calculate two Ws charts, one for hospital outcome and one for true 30-day outcome.

Further reading

Association for the Advancement of Automotive Medicine (AAAM). The Abbreviated Injury Scale. Chicago: AAAM, 2004.

Lecky F, Woodford M, Edwards A, Bouamra O, Coats T. Trauma scoring systems and databases. Br J Anaesth 2014; 113:286–294.

Lefering R. Trauma scoring systems. Curr Opin Crit Care 2012; 18:637–640.

Related topics of interest

Traumatic amputation

Key points

- A <C>ABCDE approach is essential as part of damage control resuscitation, which must be with warmed blood products and tranexamic acid (TXA)
- A tourniquet must be applied at the earliest opportunity
- Reimplantation is rarely possible, but even if the part does not seem salvageable, it may be used as a source of nerve (for grafts), skin and bone-graft for other injuries.

Epidemiology

In civilian practice, traumatic amputation commonly follows intended or accidental injury relating to vehicles or dangerous equipment. Scene safety for care providers is paramount. In military or terrorist-related practice, traumatic amputation follows explosive, blast and bomb incidents. Although the injuries in the former may look similar to the latter, in blast-related incidents, particularly in bus, tunnel or tubes – the possibility of blast-lung injury must be considered.

Basic principles

Although conventional protocols may propose an ABCDE approach (airway, breathing, circulation, disability, exposure) experience with traumatic amputations injuries shows that if attention is initially focussed on the airway, then by the time circulation is reached, the patient may have bled out. This has led to the <C>ABCDE paradigm where the first <C> stands for <catastrophic external haemorrhage>, which is dealt with first.

First aid

Wearing appropriate personal protection a tourniquet such as the Combat Application Tourniquet should be applied to the affected limb and the time of application recorded. If the amputation is above the knee a second tourniquet should be applied as a single tourniquet is unlikely to be effective. Pneumatic prehospital tourniquets, such as the Emergency Medical Tourniquet, Delphi Medical, available, are more effective (**Figure 82**). On arrival in the emergency department, these prehospital tourniquets should be changed as soon as practical to padded, operating room standard pneumatic devices.

As soon as stump control is achieved, management priorities return to the airway and chest, particularly the back, to ensure that an injury to the chest or larynx has not been missed. There is a significant association between traumatic lower limb amputation and pelvic fractures (particularly in blast, where the incidence is 40%). Application of a suitable pelvic binder at the level of the greater trochanters should therefore be considered in all cases.

One in 10 traumatic amputation victims (as a result of blast) will have a primary blast lung injury. The history of injury will give significant clues. Explosions in a confined space such as buses, tubes or tunnels cause blast reflection and pressure amplification. Those very close into the blast centre, who remain alive, may present with rib fractures, hypoxaemia and blood-stained sputum. These patients do badly and can have a mortality of over 50%. Lung protective ventilation from the outset of care is key – in-transit, emergency department and the operating theatre – not just eventually in the intensive therapy unit where it may be too late. Low tidal volume ventilation is used. This reduces ventilator-associated lung injury and decreases volutrauma (hyperinflation and shearing injury), barotrauma (alveolar rupture and pneumothorax) and biotrauma (release of inflammatory mediators). Typically, tidal volumes of 6 mL/kg predicted body weight (not actual body weight), plateau pressures of 30 cmH$_2$O and a permissive hypercapnia are used.

The typical baseline resuscitation requirements following traumatic amputation are 4 units of packed cells and 4 units of plasma per limb amputated. These must

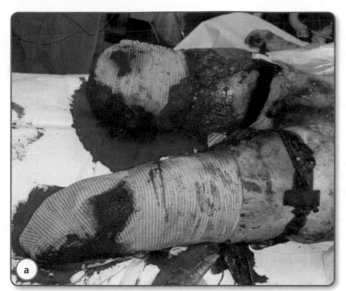

Figure 82 (a) Traumatic lower limb amputation with Combat Application Tourniquet applied; the wound is still oozing.
(b) A pneumatic surgical tourniquet is applied and all the bleeding has stopped.

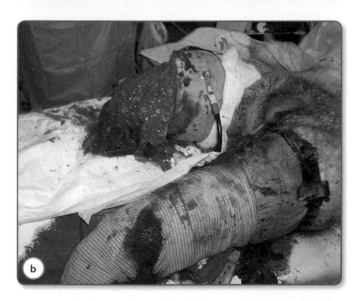

be available in the emergency department before the patient arrives (together with the pneumatic tourniquets). The patient should be assumed to be cold and have a coagulopathy – even without testing. Saline should not be administered as a resuscitation fluid, since the patient's survival in these cases is inversely proportional to the amount of saline given. Resuscitation must be blood product based. Guided where possible by thromboelastography [rotational thromboelastometry (ROTEM) or TEG – see Chapter 92] as soon as possible. TXA and appropriate antibiotics should be given within 1 hour of injury (typically 1 g TXA and 1.2 g of Co-amoxiclav). The pelvis should be X-rayed with the binder on and if normal it can be removed. Photographs of the limb should be taken, and the patient's temperature should be recorded every 30 minutes.

Replantation

Reimplantation is at best only 'moderately' successful, even in clean cases. Nerve regeneration is the major limiting factor, particularly in those over 30 who smoke. A well-functioning prosthesis is often better than a non-functional replanted limb. If a viable body part is brought to hospital with the patient, obvious contamination should be washed off with cold water, the limb rinsed off and then patted dry. A saline-soaked swab should be placed over the cut end, and the part put in a plastic bag, which is then placed into cold water with ice cubes in it. Use of both dry ice and ice cubes alone must be avoided. Kept cold the part may be viable for up to 18 hours. Kept warm it starts to die at 4 hours and is useless at 6 hours. In developed countries even if the part does not seem salvageable, it may be used as a source of nerve (for grafts), skin and bone graft for other injuries.

Surgery

This should be rapid, focussed and efficient. The tourniquet should be kept inflated until the major vessels have been identified and controlled. Initially, trauma shears are used to cut away any loose hanging gobbets and mushed tissue. The limb should be held over a bucket or tray and scrubbed with a dilute povidone-iodine or chlorhexidine solution and a scrubbing brush. The limb is then reprepped and draped. Longitudinal extensile incisions should be made proximally to identify normal tissue, working from normal to abnormal, not the other way around. Scissors are used to remove 1-cm cubes of tissue per cut. Colour, consistency, contraction and capillary bleeding (4 'Cs') are used as a guide. Anything that is clearly massively contaminated or dead should be removed, but the temptation to try to 'tidy things up' should be resisted. The formation of anything that might be considered a definitive flap is absolutely contraindicated at this stage. If the bone is alive and long, it should be left as it will stabilise the soft tissues. If bone is short and tissue long, it should be left, especially in blast trauma, as this is an evolving injury and tissue die-back will occur. A guillotine amputation should not be performed nor an amputation through a fracture. The patient's condition must be continuously monitored, and the surgeon should communicate regularly with the anaesthetist. This initial surgery should take no longer than an hour, leaving 10 minutes at the end to apply a topical negative pressure dressing to the stump.

Postoperative care

The patient should be topped up with blood plasma and continue antibiotic therapy. Further assessment and imaging as required should ensure that no injuries are missed. Late fungal infections are a possibility where incidents have taken place in a highly infectious environment (market places, agricultural areas, woodland etc.).

Outcomes

Isolated transtibial amputations (and most unilateral transfemoral) are associated with 'normal lives'. Most patients will walk with a prosthesis, marry and have children, jobs and a normal life expectancy. Bilateral transfemoral amputees walk less, have greater mobility issues and are less likely to be in employment.

Further reading

Guthrie HC, Clasper JC, Kay AR, Parker PJ. Initial extremity war wound debridement: a multidisciplinary consensus. J R Army Med Corps 2011; 157:170–175.

Parker PJ. Consensus statement on decision making in junctional trauma care. J R Army Med Corps 2011; 157:S293–S296.

Prucz RB, Friedrich JB. Upper extremity replantation: current concepts. Plast Reconstr Surg 2014; 133:333–342.

Related topics of interest

Traumatic cardiac arrest

Key points

- Recent evidence suggests survival rates are approximately 20% in traumatic cardiac arrest (TCA)
- Optimal outcomes are only achievable with aggressive resuscitation based on immediate reversal of the potential causes of TCA
- Traumatic cardiac arrest must be clearly differentiated from medical causes of cardiac arrest

Introduction

Attempts to resuscitate patients in TCA have, in the past, been viewed as futile. However, reported outcomes from TCA in the last 5 years, particularly from military series, are improving. The pathophysiology of TCA is different from medical causes of cardiac arrest, and therefore, treatment priorities also need to be different. The frequency and volume of military casualties from recent conflicts has led to significant improvements in their management. It is clear that a significant proportion of patients deemed to be in TCA by personnel at scene are in fact in a critically low cardiac output state (LCOS) rather than true cardiac arrest. This distinction is extremely important, as patients in an LCOS could be salvageable if offered aggressive, timely and appropriate treatment.

The European Resuscitation Guidelines from 2010 included a review of 18 articles with a total of 3032 patients presenting with TCA following blunt trauma. Of these, 94 (3.1%) survived with only 15 out of 1476 patients (1%) reported to have a good neurological outcome. Of 1136 patients with TCA following penetrating trauma, there were 37 (3.3%) survivors, 19 of whom (1.9%) had a good neurological outcome.

However, in a prospective study involving 52 adult casualties (mean age of 25 years) suffering TCA presenting to a military field hospital in Afghanistan, a rate of return of spontaneous circulation (ROSC) of 27% was recorded, with 8% surviving to discharge. All of the survivors achieved a good neurological recovery. Exsanguination was the most common cause of the cardiac arrest. In another paper describing military outcomes, Russell et al. found that 18 of 78 (24%) patients in their study with TCA survived. The reason for unexpected survival in this group was put down to the advanced resuscitation strategies employed by the UK military and in particular the ability to effectively stop and treat catastrophic haemorrhage following combat trauma. In another paper looking specifically at 65 patients with TCA who underwent resuscitative thoracotomy, Morrison et al. describe ROSC in 33 patients (51%) and overall survival in 14 patients (21%), although this rose to 11 of 26 (42%) patients who underwent thoracotomy in the emergency department.

Management principles

Patients suffering medical cardiac arrest will usually have a full circulating volume, and external chest compressions will restore some cardiac output. In contrast, the majority of patients with reversible TCA will have critical hypovolaemia, tension pneumothorax or cardiac tamponade, the physiology of which cannot be reversed by cardiopulmonary resuscitation (CPR).

In a critically low flow state, although a central pulse may not palpable, organised cardiac electrical activity may still be present (pulseless electrical activity, PEA) with ventricular hyperdynamic contractility, although they appear under filled on ultrasound. In this situation, a degree of organ perfusion may be maintained despite the absence of a central pulse witnessed by the presence of a low end tidal CO_2 ($ETCO_2$) trace. This is a key factor in the first few minutes when interventions may determine the survivability or otherwise of the patient. European Resuscitation Guidelines state that the diagnosis of TCA is a clinical one in trauma victims who are unresponsive, apnoeic and pulseless, with or without organised (electrocardiographic) cardiac activity. The concept of the LCOS means that it is difficult to ascertain the start point of true cardiac arrest.

The team – horizontal resuscitation

Optimal management of TCA requires strict adherence to clearly defined protocols, practice and experience, which is difficult to gain in most civilian settings. The resuscitation of the TCA patient must allow multiple sequences of activity to occur simultaneously.

These resuscitations are very personnel intensive and need senior and experienced staff, ideally at consultant level. Key tasks include rapid intravenous access (8.5F gauge) and management of rapid infusion devices for rapid transfusion of blood products. A consultant radiologist should be part of the trauma team, providing diagnostic information with ultrasound and early visualisation of the heart to guide subsequent targeted treatment if required, e.g. of cardiac tamponade.

Management

Aggressive resuscitation must be directed at the reversible causes of TCA rather than the establishment of CPR. The <C>ABC sequence is a guide, but steps may be simultaneous and not necessarily in the conventional order. Approached logically, the likely causes of TCA are easily identified and managed:

- Catastrophic haemorrhage is controlled with pressure dressings, novel haemostatic agents and tourniquets
- Non-compressible haemorrhage is controlled with a pelvic binder and long bone traction for identified fractures
- Endotracheal intubation and mechanical ventilation are instituted to ensure sufficient oxygen delivery
- Tension pneumothoraces are managed with bilateral open thoracostomies
- Haemostatic resuscitation is established for critical hypovolaemia, with rapid volume replacement using blood products

- Clamshell thoracotomy is performed for cardiac tamponade and proximal control of subdiaphragmatic haemorrhage

Rapid large vessel circulatory access is essential to facilitate rapid infusion. However, if there is any delay, rapid infusion of blood products can still be achieved through an intraosseous needle.

Prehospital management

Many prehospital services now train extensively in providing appropriate interventions to this subgroup of patients in TCA. Rapid infusion of blood products, thoracostomy and thoracotomy are all now performed in the prehospital environment and appear to have led to improvements in survival. The presence of highly skilled clinicians in prehospital care means that the resuscitative process can commence before and continue through the emergency department.

The role of resuscitative thoracotomy

The outcome following emergency department thoracotomy (EDT) in blunt trauma victims with witnessed TCA is poor, with an estimated survival rate of 1.6%. The survival rate is highest, estimated as 31%, following penetrating cardiac injuries with a short on-scene and transport time, witnessed signs of life or electrocardiographic activity. Resuscitative thoracotomy must be considered in every patient presenting in TCA. Similarly, the time-critical 10-minute window from point of witnessed cardiac arrest to thoracotomy is likely to be challenged when current evidence is reviewed.

Thoracotomy is a relatively straightforward procedure, which can be performed with non-specialist equipment in any clinical setting. Existing incisions for bilateral thoracostomies can be extended anteriorly to the midline and slightly posteriorly in a clamshell approach. The main indication for EDT in the management of TCA is to relieve cardiac tamponade, but it will also facilitate control of bleeding from the heart, lungs or great vessels using direct pressure, haemostatic compounds, sutures or surgical clips. Rescue techniques to control bleeding, such as the hilar twist, have also been described. Thoracotomy also enables cross-clamping of the descending aorta, or simply direct pressure applied posteriorly against the vertebrae, to control on-going haemorrhage below the diaphragm.

Irreversible causes of TCA

There are a number of situations where resuscitation would inevitably be futile for example massive head and facial trauma and hypostasis. In addition, resuscitation is deemed futile when there has been asystole for >15 minutes without bystander CPR, or submersion for >1 hour in an adult or 1.5 hours in a child.

Reversible causes of TCA

The reversible causes of cardiac arrest are traditionally described as the 'the 4Hs and 4Ts'. Those specific to TCA are hypoxia, hypovolaemia, tension pneumothorax and cardiac tamponade.

Markers of a low cardiac output state

It is important where possible to rapidly determine whether a trauma victim arriving in suspected TCA still has residual cardiac output with a potentially reversible cause, which might benefit from aggressive resuscitation. The first method is to visualise the rate and quality of myocardial contractility and cardiac filling on ultrasound. In an intubated patient, $ETCO_2$ monitoring provides a surrogate marker of cardiac output enabling the monitoring of trends that may indicate impending TCA. $ETCO_2$ may also be a useful prognostic indicator to guide further resuscitation or to assist in decisions regarding futility. The cut-off value for $ETCO_2$ is 1.3 kPa (10 mmHg), and readings below this suggest futility after all emergency resuscitative interventions have been undertaken and in the absence of organised electrical or mechanical cardiac activity.

Blood product resuscitation

Blood products are the resuscitation fluid of choice in the management of TCA. Early transfusion of packed red blood cells

and fresh frozen plasma is recommended to replace circulating volume, restore oxygen-carrying capacity and maintain coagulation. The use of crystalloids should be limited to avoid exacerbation of traumatic coagulopathy, unless there is no alternative and emergency transport is prolonged.

Ultrasound

Emergency ultrasonography is a proven investigation in trauma resuscitation, and it is a sensitive test for pericardial tamponade. Other important findings, such as haemoperitoneum and haemo- or pneumothorax, can also be diagnosed reliably with ultrasound. As a portable bedside technique, it can be integrated unobtrusively into TCA protocols. Prehospital ultrasound includes simple thoracic ultrasound and focused assessment with sonography in trauma.

Postresuscitation care

Once ROSC has been achieved, access to definitive surgical haemorrhage control is key to optimising outcome. Military experience has emphasised the benefit of having a functional operating theatre adjacent to the resuscitation room. However, physical proximity is only part of the solution – the mindset also needs to be right. Trauma team leaders should recognise when to transfer the patient rapidly to an operating theatre, or even to move directly there on arrival. Surgical control of life-threatening haemorrhage is a key component of damage control resuscitation, and the operating theatre should therefore be seen as an extension of the resuscitation room in cases of TCA. Whole body computed tomography scanning should be considered for diagnostic purposes following ROSC, if the patient is stable enough.

When to stop resuscitation

Cessation of resuscitation is an emotive subject and one of the most difficult decisions in trauma management. In many cases, the nature of the injuries, presentation and comorbidities allow an appropriate decision to be made with confidence. However, there are other features that suggest futility in continuing resuscitation, and guidelines have been published regarding the termination or withholding of out-of-hospital resuscitation for TCA cases, although the general adoption of these remains controversial. In a recent case series of 52 patients, the longest duration of TCA associated with survival was 24 minutes. All of the survivors demonstrated PEA rhythms during arrest, whereas asystole was universally associated with death. Six out of 24 of the patients had ultrasound evidence of cardiac activity during arrest; all six with cardiac activity subsequently exhibited ROSC and two survived to hospital discharge.

Summary

The key to management of patients in TCA is personnel and system familiarity with the underlying pathophysiology and reversible causes of the arrest. Recent evidence suggests that the previously poor survival rates for TCA may gradually improve with the introduction of new protocols and the recognition that such cases do not always result in patient death.

Further reading

Morrison JJ, Poon H, Rasmussen TE, et al. Resuscitative thoracotomy following wartime injury. J Trauma Acute Care Surg 2013; 74:825–829.

Russell RJ, Hodgetts TJ, McLeod J, et al. The role of trauma scoring in developing trauma clinical governance in the Defence Medical Services. Philos Trans R Soc Lond B Biol Sci 2011; 366:171–191.

Sherren PB, Reid C, Habig K, Burns BJ. Algorithm for the resuscitation of traumatic cardiac arrest patients in a physician-staffed helicopter emergency medical service. Crit Care 2013; 17:308.

Soar J, Perkins GD, Abbas G, et al. European Resuscitation Council Guidelines for Resuscitation 2010 Section 8. Cardiac arrest in special circumstances: electrolyte abnormalities, poisoning, drowning, accidental hypothermia, hyperthermia, asthma, anaphylaxis, cardiac surgery, trauma, pregnancy, electrocution. Resuscitation 2010; 81:1400–1433.

Tai NR, Russell R. Right turn resuscitation: frequently asked questions. J R Army Med Corps 2011; 157:S310–S314.

Tarmey NT, Park CL, Bartels OJ, et al. Outcomes following military traumatic cardiorespiratory arrest: a prospective observational study. Resuscitation 2011; 82:1194–1197.

Related topics of interest

Triage

Key points

- Triage is the sorting of patients by priority for treatment or transport
- Triage is dynamic and a patient's triage category may change
- The expectant category has not been used in the United Kingdom and would require authorisation at a very senior level

Introduction

Triage is a process by which patients are grouped by degree of injury severity. The term was apparently first used in a medical context by Baron Dominique Jean Larrey, chief surgeon to Napoleon Bonaparte, to identify those who could be rapidly returned to the battlefield following injury (so-called reverse triage). Triage is an essential part of any emergency department's patient flow management to ensure correct prioritisation and resource allocation and in a major incident is intrinsic to managing scarce resources. Triage is a dynamic process and may need to be repeated as the patient's circumstances, situation or condition change. Patients may be triaged for treatment or transport to medical facilities.

The sorting of patients into priority groups prior to treatment will be required in two situations:

- Where the number of patients and the severity of their injuries do not exceed the available medical resources, but it is necessary to select the more seriously injured for priority treatment (the model used in the emergency departments of UK hospitals)
- Where the number of patients and the severity of their injuries exceeds the available medical resources, and it is necessary to identify those who will be given the best chance of survival with the most 'economical' use of resources (at the extreme end of major incidents, or in battlefield situations)

Triage categories

The commonly used triage categories (P system, T system and colour coding) are given in (**Table 42**).

Patients in the immediate category (P1/T1) are colour coded red and are those in need of immediate medical attention, whereas urgent patients (P2/T2), colour coded yellow, are those requiring treatment within 4–6 hours. Patients allocated to the delayed category (P3/T3) and colour coded green do not require treatment within 6 hours.

The expectant category (T4) is used to identify those patients whose condition is so critical that the effort required to attempt to save them would compromise the survival of larger numbers of less seriously injured patients. In civilian practice, it is important to note that using this category usually requires a decision by the gold commander (the UK term for the commander in strategic control of their organisation's resources during an incident) and the inquiry post 7/7 bombings in London initiated a great deal of discussion regarding the ethical and practical considerations that would have arisen if the expectant category had been used.

There is no 'P' equivalent to T4, although some armed forces use the term P1 hold. This term should not be used in the civilian environment where the T system is preferred.

A number of triage tools have been developed for use in emergency departments –

Table 42 Triage categories			
Colour	P	T	Description
Red	P1	T1	Immediate
Yellow	P2	T2	Urgent
Green	P3	T3	Delayed
Blue*	-	T4	Expectant
White	Dead	Dead	Dead

*Green with folded corners revealing red, using the Cambridge cruciform card.

the Manchester Triage System and National Triage System are amongst them. They tend to assign patients to colour codes, which carry a target time within which the patient should be seen. These systems offer convenient audit standards and form part of many quality metrics by which departments are measured.

Assignment to triage categories

The triage sieve

The triage sieve (**Figure 83**) is an initial triage tool for rapid categorisation, usually of mass casualties; however, there are several potential problems with its use. The pulse may be difficult to elicit due to environmental conditions, it is not strictly applicable to children due to the physiological normal values used, and the reliance on the patient's ability to walk may cause problems with the categorisation of patients with isolated lower limb injuries or conversely in those with critical injuries who remain mobile.

The triage sort – triage revised trauma score

The triage sort [sometimes called the triage revised trauma score (TRTS)] scores the three parameters respiratory rate, systolic blood pressure and the Glasgow coma scale (**Table 43**). The RTS is based on weighted values for the three parameters. The TRTS assigns a triage category based on the total unweighted score (**Table 44**). This method is simple and

Table 43 Respiratory rate, systolic blood pressure and Glasgow coma scale scores and TRTS values			
Score	Respiratory rate (breaths/ min)	Systolic blood pressure (mmHg)	Glasgow coma scale
4	>29	>90	13–15
3	10–29	76–89	9–12
2	6–9	50–75	6–8
1	1–5	1–49	4–5
0	0	0	3

TRTS, triage revised trauma score.

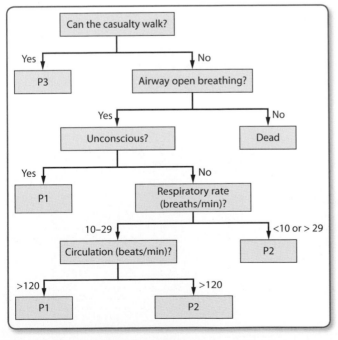

Figure 83 The triage sieve. An initial triage tool for rapid categorisation of casualties.

Table 44 Triage categories based on unweighted score	
TRTS	Triage category
1–9	T1
10–11	T2
12	T3
0	T4
TRTS, triage revised trauma score.	

reproducible: the parameters and their scores are given on standard triage cards.

Because it includes both the patient's Glasgow coma scale score and systolic blood pressure, the triage sort is complex and time consuming and subject to interobserver error. Intended to be used as a secondary triage method once the initial categorisation has been performed using the sieve, and when more assets are available, its use may not always be appropriate and it may be replaced by a repetition of the sieve, or a decision based on clinical expertise and experience by a more senior member of staff.

Triage labelling

Once a patient has been triaged in the mass casualty or prehospital environment, it is essential that he/she is labelled with the appropriate category. A wide range of labels are available such as the Cambridge cruciform triage card. Other systems used are the British Association for Immediate Care (BASIC) card and the Medical Emergency Triage Tag (METTAG) card. If cards are not available, skin marking with indelible waterproof ink may be used.

Further reading

Farrohknia N, Castrén M, Ehrenberg A, et al. Emergency department triage scales and their components: a systematic review of the scientific evidence. Scand J Trauma Resusc Emerg Med 2011; 19:42.

Related topics of interest

Vascular injuries

Key points

- Approximately, 1–2% of patients with major trauma have vascular injuries, and the overall mortality from such injuries is around 20%
- Vascular trauma may be divided into compressible (CH) and noncompressible haemorrhage (NCH)
- Most vascular injuries affect the limbs (80–90%), predominantly the legs

Epidemiology

Although uncommon in civilian trauma, vascular injuries may account for up to 20% of trauma deaths. Approximately, 1–2% of patients with major trauma have vascular injuries, and the overall mortality from such injuries is about 20%. Crucially, vascular injuries are time dependent, in terms of arresting catastrophic bleeding or restoring blood supply to preserve limb function. Vascular trauma may be divided into CH and NCH. Compressible injury encompasses haemorrhage controllable by external pressure, mostly affecting the limbs. NCH includes torso and junctional injury and is not amenable to pressure control. The ultimate consequence of NCH is exsanguination and prehospital arrest, correlating with a high mortality (>80%); the long-term effects of CH impact on functional limb recovery.

Noncompressible injury

Noncompressible haemorrhage is defined as:

- Pulmonary injury
- Named torso vessel injury
- > Grade 4 solid organ injury
- Open pelvic ring fracture with a systolic blood pressure < 90 mmHg

The dominant challenge in managing NCH is applying a resuscitative-bridge to definitive surgical care. Without intervention, the natural history of NCH is rapid demise as a consequence of exsanguination. Permissive hypotensive resuscitation, maintaining adequate perfusion to the brain and heart, is key in the predefinitive care phase. Traditional resuscitative paradigms of care have now changed into damage control resuscitative techniques utilising blood products and tranexamic acid, rather than crystalloids. Adjuncts to fluid resuscitation include left lateral thoracotomy, with aortic cross clamping, resuscitative endovascular balloon occlusion of the aorta (see p. 248), abdominal tourniquets and intra-abdominal foams.

Chest and abdomen

An anterolateral thoracotomy via the fourth interspace allows access to the underlying chest; extension to a full clamshell incision provides access to the contralateral side if required. Initial actions include assessment of the pericardium for tamponade and creation of a pericardial window through an inverted T-incision avoiding the phrenic nerves. The aorta is cross-clamped avoiding caval and oesophageal injury. Different techniques can then be utilised to control bleeding in the chest. Staplers or clamps can be used to isolate areas of lung without following anatomical borders. Proximal pulmonary vessels can be controlled by clamping or twisting the lung, occluding the hilar vessels.

Abdominal tourniquets compress the aorta against the spine; intra-abdominal self-expanding foam limits exsanguination through tamponade; resuscitative endovascular balloon occlusion of the aorta involves placing a self-centering balloon into the aorta via the common femoral artery to produce aortic occlusion. The primary aim of these interventions is to maintain perfusion to the brain and heart, in addition to reducing blood loss. Circumferential binders are used in significant pelvic injuries to limit blood loss.

Definitive care involves gaining proximal and distal control and then repairing the injury. In torso injuries, ideally a single compartment is entered to gain control and affect repair. However, in straight-to-theatre situations, without cross-sectional imaging, the surgeon must be prepared to enter a second cavity if required.

The retroperitoneum

In trauma, the retroperitoneum is divided into four zones. Zone 1 is central, containing the aorta and inferior vena cava (IVC), explored through left (aorta) or right (IVC) medial visceral rotation (Mattox or Cattel-Braasch manoeuvres). Zone 2 is perirenal, usually managed conservatively in blunt trauma, but it may require repair or removal of the involved kidney. Zone 3 involves the pelvis and requires exploration if a direct vessel injury is suspected. Zone 4 includes the retrohepatic and portal areas and provides a significant management challenge: initial packing is recommended. Access requires a full midline laparotomy. Haemorrhage is usually controlled with 4-quadrant packing. In the presence of major haemorrhage, supracoeliac control of the aorta may be necessary, initially by direct pressure at the level of the crus of the diaphragm. Blunt dissection through the lesser omentum and fibres of the left diaphragmatic crus gives access to the aorta at the diaphragmatic hiatus avoiding a difficult dissection to the visceral aorta via the lesser sac. Once haemorrhage control is achieved, definitive control and repair can be undertaken.

Repairing the vessels

There are five methods of definitive repair to an artery:

- Direct repair (suturing) in low-energy incisional injuries
- Patch angioplasty, following exploration of injured vessels with suspected intimal flaps, uses a vein patch avoiding narrowing in longitudinally opened vessels
- End-to-end anastomosis for short segmental injury, where vessel ends are brought together in a tension-free fashion
- Interposition graft for segmental loss in the anatomical plane
- Bypass graft either anatomical or extra-anatomical in the presence of significant tissue injury and contamination, ideally utilising reversed long saphenous vein

In contaminated wounds, definitive repair may be deferred until contamination is controlled. Temporary vascular shunting or grafting with synthetic conduits allows this.

Endovascular control and embolisation or stenting can be an adjunct to surgery or the primary modality of treatment. Embolisation has utility in solid organ injury, often negating the need for laparotomy; stenting is utilised in junctional injuries, particularly the subclavian vessels, but both require specialist expertise and equipment.

Junctional injuries

Junctional injuries occur at the noncompressible level of the limbs (axillobrachial and proximal femoral/distal iliac arteries). Special approaches are required: axillobrachial control is obtained through a supraclavicular approach for proximal injuries and infraclavicular for distal injuries. Proximal femoral vessels require retroperitoneal control, entering the retroperitoneum through transversus abdominis, retracting the peritoneum medially to access underlying vessels prior to groin opening; midline sternotomy for Zone 1 neck injuries allows access to proximal arch and neck vessels.

Compressible haemorrhage

Most vascular injuries affect the limbs (80–90%), predominantly the legs. CH is amenable to control by external compression and is less lethal than NCH.

Direct pressure or tourniquets can be applied by nonspecialists, bystanders or the individual. Tourniquets prevent haemorrhage but put the distal limb at risk of prolonged ischemia, with little chance of limb salvage after very extended use. Novel haemostatic agents can be applied and work by either concentrating clotting factors through absorbing water or adding procoagulant to the area of bleeding.

In CH, early restoration of inline blood flow is essential. Preservation of maximal limb function requires reperfusion within 4.5 hours in the absence of major haemorrhage, or 90 minutes in the presence of significant blood loss. This can only be achieved with temporary vascular shunting, prior to repair of other injuries. Shunts range from specifically designed trauma shunts to intravenous tubing. Proximal and distal vessels are controlled, with inflow/back bleeding assessment. The shunt is placed and secured with flow evaluated by Doppler. Heparinisation is not required. Other injuries are then addressed and definitive repair performed.

At this stage, ischaemia–reperfusion injury is a significant risk. Increased intracompartmental pressures threaten the limb through decreased perfusion and neurological and muscle damage. Release of the effluent from the ischaemic limb can create significant systemic effects, leading to multiorgan failure and risk to life. Careful assessment of limb salvageability must be made prior to revascularisation to avoid causing harm, turning a limb-threatening situation into a life-threatening one. Significant vascular injury with delay to reperfusion mandates full open fasciotomies. In the future, pharmacological adjuncts may provide a means to mitigate ischaemia–reperfusion injury and improve functional recovery.

Further reading

Rasmussen TE, Tai QHS, Nigel RM (eds.). Rich's vascular trauma, 3rd edn. Amsterdam: Elsevier, 2015.

Related topics of interest

Viscoelastic assessment of coagulation in trauma

Key points

- Clotting abnormalities following major trauma are common and independently associated with increased mortality
- Viscoelastic assessment of coagulation in trauma can assist in the diagnosis of the presence and degree of trauma coagulopathy
- The viscoelastic assessment of coagulation can detect hypocoagulability, hyperfibrinolysis, hypercoagulability and platelet dysfunction and can be used to monitor and direct targeted blood component replacement therapy

Background, epidemiology and definition

In the United Kingdom, 40% of trauma deaths are as a result of haemorrhage. Coagulopathy is present at the time of admission to the emergency department in up to 25% of patients, and the presence of shock and coagulopathy are independently associated with both massive transfusion and increased mortality. Contributing factors to abnormal clotting occurring soon after injury include consumption of clotting factors, haemodilution, acidosis, hypothermia, continuing bleeding and hypoperfusion. A diagnosis of coagulopathy associated with trauma on admission to hospital carries a mortality rate amongst patients of up to 50% and is often associated with increased burdens of transfusion, greater risks of organ injury and septic complications and longer stays in critical care.

Coagulopathy has been defined within the literature using prothrombin time ratios (PTr). Two ranges have been used to define trauma-induced coagulopathy, a PTr ≥ 1.2 or a PTr ≥ 1.5 being defined as hypocoagulopathic. However, prothrombin time (and activated partial thromboplastin time) are performed on platelet-poor plasma and were developed to evaluate clotting factor deficiencies and anticoagulation therapy. These tests measure the time prior to initial thrombin generation and are known to be poor predictors of bleeding in trauma. It has been shown that neither APTT nor PT is sensitive for the diagnosis of acute trauma coagulopathy. In addition, the delay before the test results become clinically available is typically in the region of 45–60 minutes from sampling by which time the patient's condition will have potentially changed, and the results will not reflect the current condition of the patient.

Point-of-care prothrombin time devices exist but are unvalidated in the presence of active haemorrhage and major trauma. PTr remains the current standard assessment of coagulation in trauma practice but due to the limitations described, interest in near-patient functional tests of coagulation, such as thromboelastometry or thromboelastography (TEG), has grown. Viscoelastic assessment of clotting utilising rotational thromboelastometry (ROTEM) or TEG has become robust reliable tools suitable for use in the near-patient setting, although there are no universally agreed definitions of what constitutes coagulopathy using parameters derived from these methodologies. There is now extensive military experience of using viscoelastic assessment to guide the management of the critically injured, and the technique is being increasingly adopted in civilian practice.

Pathophysiology and clinical management

The aetiology of trauma-induced coagulopathy is incompletely understood. After trauma, blood clots form through a chain of actions. First, platelets form a plug on the blood vessel wall at the site of injury. This platelet plug is weak, but a cascade of clotting proteins generates fibrin, which incorporates platelets and red blood cells to produce a stronger clot. This process can become disordered in approximately a quarter of trauma patients. The reasons for this disordered coagulation are still incompletely understood. The combination of tissue damage and the presence of hypoperfusion through severe haemorrhage are known to be important factors.

Protocols for the early administration of packed red cells, plasma and platelets have been adopted to try and correct acute trauma coagulopathy. This requires an ability to predict which patients are likely to have acute trauma coagulopathy and require massive transfusion therapy and a means of determining which blood components they need. Clinical prediction algorithms are poor in predicting the presence of acute trauma coagulopathy or the requirement for massive transfusion. Consequently, a 'one-size fits all' approach with major traumatic injury can potentially expose some patients to blood products unnecessarily with all the potential risks and logistic costs, or under treat others. No independently validated, clinical tools exist for the prediction of the need for such therapy. It is recognised that a global assessment of coagulation including the initiation, dynamics, maturation of clot and clot lysis in an individual patient could aid tailored therapy.

The ROTEM and TEG are both viscoelastic assessments of clot development and offer a number of parameters that assess these aspects of coagulation, with different nomenclature (shown in parenthesis) depending on the system used:

- Time to initiate clotting (CT, R)
- Time of clot formation (CFT, K time)
- Alpha angle
- Clot amplitude (MCF, MA)
- Time to maximum clot strength (MCF-t, TMA)
- Maximum strength of clot (MA, MCF)
- Time to lysis (Ly, ML)

Early measures of the clot amplitude at 5 minutes (A05) or 10 minutes (A10) have been suggested to be a sensitive estimate of final MCF with ROTEM.

The ROTEM clot assessment may be conducted under several different conditions. The two basic tests are EXTEM (activated with tissue factor) and FIBTEM (tissue factor activation after platelet inhibition with cytochalasin D); this allows the relative contribution of platelets to clot to be assessed.

The graphical scaled representation of the EXTEM and FIBTEM allows a rapid assessment of the quality of the overall clot and which aspect of initiation, dynamics, maturation or lysis is contributing to any derangement.

European guidelines on the management of bleeding and coagulopathy following major trauma published in 2013 have suggested that repeat doses of fibrinogen concentrate or cryoprecipitate may be guided by viscoelastic monitoring (Recommendation 27).

Systematic evaluations of viscoelastic assessments of coagulation in trauma

A Cochrane Systematic Diagnostic Test Accuracy Review found no evidence on the accuracy of TEG and very little evidence on the accuracy of ROTEM in adult trauma patients with haemorrhage. The small number of studies and potential risk of bias relating to the index test undermined the value of accuracy estimates. The review was unable to offer advice on the use of global measures of haemostatic function for trauma based on the evidence it identified.

A Canadian descriptive systematic review was reported in accordance with Preferred Reporting Items for Systematic Reviews and Meta-Analyses guidelines. It suggests that TEG/ROTEM tests diagnose early trauma coagulopathy and may predict blood product transfusion and requirements and mortality in trauma.

Conclusion

Current standard laboratory-based tests that are used to define coagulopathy following trauma are inadequate, and viscoelastic assessment may provide a near-patient method, which offers a global assessment of coagulation in trauma patients allowing diagnosis, targeted therapy and monitoring of coagulopathy. There is a need to fully assess this technology and define coagulopathy with the relevant viscoelastic parameters.

Further reading

Da Luz LT, Nascimento B, Shankarakutty AK, Rizoli S, Adhikari NKJ. Effect of thromboelastography (TEG®) and rotational thromboelastometry (ROTEM®) on diagnosis of coagulopathy, transfusion guidance and mortality in trauma: descriptive systematic review. Crit Care 2014; 18:518.

Hunt H, Stanworth S, Curry N, et al. Thromboelastography (TEG) and rotational thromboelastometry (ROTEM) for trauma induced coagulopathy in adult trauma patients with bleeding (Review). Cochrane Database Syst Rev 2015: CD010438.

Spahn DR, Bouillon B, Cerny V, et al. Management of bleeding and coagulopathy following major trauma: an updated European guideline. Crit Care 2013; 17:R76.

Related topics of interest

Wrist and carpal injuries

Key points

- Fractures of the wrist and carpus are extremely common and account for one-sixth of all fractures presenting to an emergency department
- Management will be based on an assessment of each patient's individual circumstances including their age, level of normal physical activity and general health
- The potential consequences of missed hand injuries can be life changing for the patient

Fractures involving the distal radius

Distal radius fractures account for one-sixth of all fractures presenting to the emergency department. They usually occur from a fall on the outstretched hand. They are most common in children, which are usually managed conservatively, and in elderly osteoporotic females. The majority of fractures are dorsally displaced (Colles' type fractures) (**Figure 84**). In younger adult patients the fractures are more commonly high-energy injuries and often intra-articular.

Clinical features

There is usually pain, swelling and deformity, often of the dinner fork type. The patient may complain of pins and needles in the fingers due to median nerve compression. Open fractures are rare and usually occur on the ulna side of the wrist.

Imaging

Plain X-rays usually reveal the nature and direction of displacement. Intra-articular fractures, especially if the articular surface is displaced, usually need a computed tomography (CT) scan to assess the extent of the injury and to help plan treatment.

Classification

There are many classifications. Frykman's classification (1967) is the most commonly used, but in general they are all poor in predicting outcome. Melone's classification of intra-articular fractures does help in planning treatment.

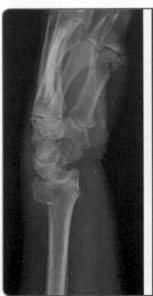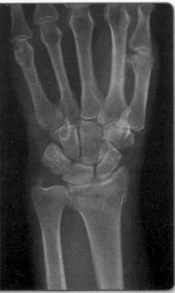

Figure 84 A Colles' fracture–dorsally displaced and angulated, shortened and radially deviated (lateral and anteroposterior views).

Extra-articular dorsally displaced fractures (Colles' fracture)

In these injuries, the distal fragment is dorsally displaced and angulated, shortened and radially deviated. As a result, if malunion occurs, there is often distortion of the radioulnar joint resulting in pain and loss of rotation, especially supination.

Initial management

In the United Kingdom, fractures in adults are manipulated in the emergency department under a Bier's block or haematoma block and a plaster back slab applied. If neurological symptoms persist, then urgent decompression should usually be performed. Manipulation usually produces a satisfactory result. Factors suggesting instability and thus unsuccessful non-operative treatment are

- Dorsal angulation > 20°
- Radial shortening > 5 mm
- Dorsal comminution
- Displaced intra-articular fractures

On-going management with plaster may be successful, but careful radiological monitoring is essential for usually three successive weeks. Plaster can usually be completed at 1 week. If the position slips postmanipulation or the reduction is inadequate, then operative intervention should be considered (remanipulation is usually unsuccessful).

Operative treatment

Options for operative management include:

- Kirschner (K) wire fixation by transfixion of the styloid and dorsoulna corner into the volar cortex or an intrafocal buttress technique. The wires are usually removed at 4–6 weeks to reduce the risk of infection. If the wires are removed too early the fracture may redisplace. The superficial radial nerve is at risk from the radial styloid wire.
- External fixation with bridging (distal pins in 2nd metacarpal) or non-bridging (distal pins in distal radius). Non-bridging possibly gives better functional and anatomical results. Fixators are usually removed at 6 weeks. If left on for longer, they may

cause more stiffness, and if removed early fracture, malunion may occur

- Internal fixation, usually with volar locking plates. There has been a very significant increase in the use of this method recently, associated with an increase in complications, especially tendon injuries

Some patients will have good functional results with significant malunion. However, in general the more accurate the anatomical result the better the functional result. Radial shortening > 2 mm, carpal malalignment and dorsal angulation > 20° from normal should be avoided. The complications of the fracture and its treatment are shown in **Table 45**.

Outcomes

The evidence as to which treatment is better is still not established. A recent study of patients randomized between K wire fixation and internal fixation showed little difference in outcome. Studies on internal fixation have suggested a quicker return to activity but no definite long-term benefit.

Volar displaced fractures (Smith's fracture)

In these fractures, which are rarer than dorsally displaced fractures, the distal fragment displaces and angulates volarly with shortening and radial deviation (**Figure 85**).

Table 45 Complications of extra-articular dorsally displaced fractures	
Fracture complications	**Treatment complications**
Pain	Pain
Stiffness	Stiffness
Malunion	Malunion (not usually as severe with fixation)
Chronic regional pain syndrome	Chronic regional pain syndrome
Median nerve compression	Median nerve compression
Extensor pollicis longus rupture (usually undisplaced fractures)	Flexor and extensor tendon rupture
	Radial and median nerve injury
	Pin track infection

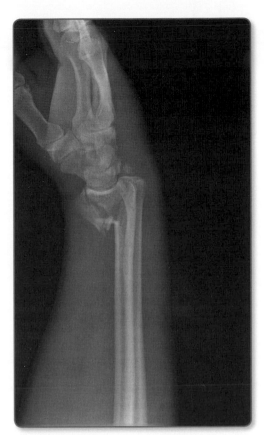

Figure 85 Distal radial fracture with volar displacement.

Initial management

Conservative treatment involves an above elbow plaster in full supination, which poorly controls the fracture. Therefore, most of these fractures are treated with volar plates.

Complications

These are the same in principle as above. Very distal fractures need placement of plates on the volar lip possibly making flexor tendon problems more common. Median nerve compression is also said to be more common.

Intra-articular fractures (Barton's fracture)

These are usually high-energy injuries in younger patients. Fractures with a simple longitudinal intra-articular split (fracture line), which reduce after manipulation, are usually treated as extra-articular fractures. All patients should have a preoperative CT scan (**Figure 86**).

Management

Most of these fractures need internal fixation using plates, although a minority of surgeons treats them with external fixation or distraction plating. Fixation may be dorsal or volar or both. Plates may need

Figure 86 Computed tomography scan of intra-articular fracture of the distal radius.

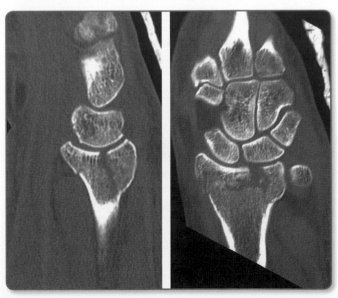

removal to improve the range of motion after fracture union.

Ulna injuries

The management of fractures of the ulnar depends on the anatomical location of the fracture:

- Injuries proximal to the distal radioulnar joint should be treated as ulna shaft injuries by internal fixation
- Injuries involving the articular surface should be reconstructed as per the radial injury
- Injuries involving the triangular fibrocartilage complex including ulnar styloid fractures only require treatment if the distal radioulnar joint is clinically unstable

Carpal injuries

Scaphoid fractures

These fractures are usually caused by a fall on an outstretched hand, although they can occur due to a forced hyperextension injury (e.g. goalkeepers in football). Scaphoid fractures are difficult to diagnose on X-ray due to the orientation and shape of the bone. They are rare in children and the elderly who tend to have radial fractures. Blood supply to bone comes in distally, and as a result, fractures may cause avascular necrosis of proximal pole.

The clinical findings include tenderness in the anatomical snuffbox, pain on longitudinal pressure along the thumb (axial compression), tenderness over the dorsum of the scaphoid and pain on wrist movement.

Management

If scaphoid fracture is suspected, then scaphoid X-rays (not wrist films) should be requested. Fractures are often not visible on plain X-rays, particularly on first presentation. If a fracture is suspected, a repeat film may be required at 10–14 days, although magnetic resonance imaging is the gold standard in diagnosis and may be required anyway if symptoms persist and plain films remain normal (bone scanning can also be used).

Conservative treatment in plaster for 6 weeks results in union in 80% of fractures. There is little evidence that plaster immobilisation for longer results in higher union rates. There is no evidence that casts including the thumb are better. Recent evidence suggests that internal fixation allows early return to activity and possible higher union rates. If partial union is visible on scanning, then union is likely to take place without further immobilisation.

Complications

Non-union is more common with proximal pole injuries and avascular necrosis. These cases need bone grafting and fixation, use of vascularized bone grafts from radius or femur is becoming increasingly common. Osteoarthritis will occur in almost all patients with non-union, and partial or total wrist fusion will usually be required.

Carpal dislocations

The commonest types of carpal dislocation are the transcaphoid perilunate or perilunate dislocation when the lunate remains in place but the distal carpus dislocates off it, and the lunate dislocation when the lunate itself is displaced (**Figure 87**).

Management

Making the diagnosis is essential and can be difficult on plain X- rays with the result that this diagnosis is sometimes missed. Median nerve symptoms may be present, and urgent reduction under general anaesthetic is required. Fractures and ligament injuries need operative repair.

Children's fractures

Almost all children's fractures involve the distal radius and sometimes ulna. Shaft fractures are usually buckle or green stick type. Epiphyseal injuries especially Salter–Harris type I and II are most common (**Figure 88**). Most displaced fractures can be treated by manipulation and plaster. If the fracture is complete and especially if both bones are involved, K-wire fixation may be needed. Teenagers may require plate fixation as in adults. Some deformity in younger children can correct with growth.

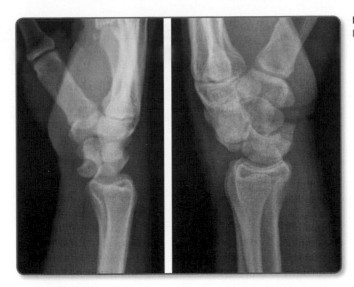

Figure 87 (a) Lunate dislocation (b) Perilunate dislocation.

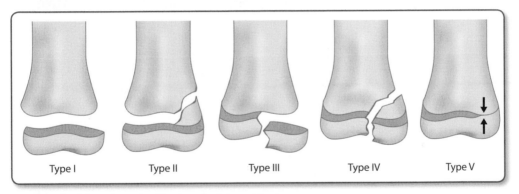

| Type I | Type II | Type III | Type IV | Type V |

Figure 88 The Salter–Harris classification of epiphyseal fractures.

Further reading

Costa ML, Achten J, Parsons NR, et al. Percutaneous fixation with Kirschner wires versus volar locking plate fixation in adults with dorsally displaced fracture of distal radius: randomised controlled trial. BMJ 2014; 349:g4807.

Leung F, Kwan K, Fang C. Distal radius fracture: current concepts and management. Focus on series, Bone Joint J 2013.

Singh HP, Dias JJ. Focus on scaphoid fractures. Focus on series, Bone Joint J 2011.

Related topics of interest

- Commonly missed injuries (p. 75)
- Hand injuries (p. 122)
- Long-bone fractures (p. 171)

Index

Note: Page numbers in **bold** or *italic* refer to tables or figures, respectively.